DISEASES
OF
THE HORSE'S FOOT
By
H. CAULTON REEKS

PREFACE

Stimulated by the reception accorded my 'Common Colics of the Horse,' both in this country and in America, and assured by my publishers that a work on diseases of the foot was needed, I have been led to give to the veterinary profession the present volume.

While keeping the size of the book within reasonable limits, no effort has been spared to render it as complete as possible. This has only been achieved by adding to my own experience a great deal of the work of others. To mention individually those who have given me permission to use their writings would be too long a matter here. In every case, however, where the quotation is of any length, the source of my information is given, either in the text or in an accompanying footnote. A few there are who will, perhaps, find themselves quoted without my having first obtained their permission to do so. They, with the others, will, I am sure, accept my hearty thanks.

The publishers have been generous in the matter of illustrations and diagrams, and although to the older practitioner some of these may appear superfluous, it is hoped they will serve to render the work an acceptable textbook for the student.

H. CAULTON REEKS.

SPALDING, *January, 1906.*

CHAPTER I
INTRODUCTION

The importance of that branch of veterinary surgery dealing with diseases of the horse's foot can hardly be overestimated. That the animal's usefulness is dependent upon his possession of four good feet is a fact that has long been recognised. Who, indeed, is there to be found entirely unacquainted with one or other of such well-known aphorisms as: 'Whoever hath charge of a horse's foot has the care of his whole body'; 'As well a horse with no head as a horse with no foot'; or the perhaps better known, and certainly more epigrammatic, 'No foot, no horse.'

Without taking these sayings literally, it will be admitted by almost everyone that they contain a vast amount of actual truth. This allowed, it at once becomes clear that a ready understanding of the diseases to which the foot is liable, the means of holding them in check, and the correct methods of treating them should figure largely in the knowledge at the command of the veterinary surgeon.

In the very great majority of instances the horse's ability to perform labour is the one thing that justifies his existence, and to that end the presence of four good, sound feet is an almost indispensable qualification. And yet how many circumstances do we see tending to militate against that one essential.

Even in colthood the foot, if neglected, may become a source of trouble. Unless periodically examined and properly trimmed, its shape is liable to serious alteration. From that in which it is best calculated to withstand the effects of the wear it will be called upon to endure in after life, it may become so changed for the worse as to seriously affect the animal's value.

In the matter of feeding, too, trouble is likely to ensue. Particularly is this the case where the colt shows points of exceptional merit. He is 'got up' for show, and the feet are likely to fall victims to the mismanagement that frequent exhibition so often carries with it. An extra allowance of peas, beans, wheat, or other equally injurious food is given. The result is a severe attack of laminitis, and an otherwise valuable and promising colt is permanently ruined.

Exposed as it is, too, to injury, the foot of a young horse, even at grass, is frequently the seat of injuries from picked up nails, stakes, or other agents which, unless detected and carefully treated, may terminate in a troublesome case of quittor and incurable lameness.

With the passing of colthood, and the coming into effect of the evils of further domestication, the troubles to which the foot is open become more numerous. Foremost among them will come those having their starting-point in errors of practice originating in the forge; for, in spite of attempts at their education, smiths, as a class, are as yet grievously unversed in even the elementary knowledge of the delicate construction of the member that is entrusted to their care.

This fact has been dilated on in books devoted to shoeing, and in the prefatory note to the last edition of Fleming's manual on this subject we find the following statement: 'The records of all humane societies show that, of prosecutions for cruelty to animals, an overwhelming majority refer to the horse; and of these, a large proportion are for working horses while suffering from lameness in one form or other.

'So frequent are such cases that observers have concluded that their prevalence must result from some specific cause, and, not unnaturally, attention has thus been directed to the various modes of management practised in relation to the horse's foot, to the manner of shoeing, and, in particular, to the way in which the foot is prepared for the shoe.'

It must be remembered, however, that although harm in the forge may frequently arise from culpable roughness or carelessness, such is not necessarily always the case, and that quite as much injury may result from careful and conscientious workmanship when it is unfortunate enough to be based upon principles wrong in themselves to commence with.

It so happens, too, that shoeing, in itself a necessary evil, may be responsible for injuries in the causation of which the smith can have played no part. Take, for example, the ill effects following upon the animal's attendant allowing him to carry his shoes for too long a time. In this case the natural growth of the horn carries the heel of the shoe further beneath the foot than is safe for a correct bearing; in fact, anterior to the point of inflection of the wall. The shoe, at the same time, is greatly thinned from excessive wear. Result, a sharp and easily-bended piece of iron situate immediately under the seat of corn. Pressure or actual cutting of the sole is bound to occur, and the animal is lamed.

Again, apart from the question of negligence or otherwise on the part of the smith or the animal's attendant, it must be remembered that the nailing on to the foot of a plate of iron is not giving to the animal an easier means of progression. The reverse is the case. In place of the sucker-like face of the natural horn is substituted a smooth, and, with wear, highly-polished surface. Slipping and sliding attempts to gain a foothold become frequent, and strains of the tendons and ligaments follow in their wake.

As, however, this treatise is not intended to deal with the art of shoeing, the reader must be referred to other works for further information. In addition to Fleming's, there may be mentioned, among others, Hunting's 'Art of Horse Shoeing,' and the very excellent volume of Messrs. Dollar and Wheatley on the same subject. Leaving the forge, we may next look to the nature of the animal's work, and the conditions under which he is kept, for active causes in the production of disorders of the foot. From the yielding softness of the pasture he is called to spend the bulk of his time upon the hard macadamized tracks of our country roads, or the still more hard and more dangerous asphalt pavings or granite sets of our towns. The former, with the bruises they will give the sole and frog from loose and scattered stones, and the latter, with the increased concussion they will entail on the limb, are active factors in the troubles with which we are about to deal. Upon these unyielding surfaces the horse is called to carry slowly or rapidly, as the case may be, not only his own weight, but, in addition, is asked to labour at the hauling of heavy loads. The effects of concussion and heavy traction combined are bound primarily to find the feet, and such diseases as side-bones, ringbones, corns, and sand-cracks commence to make their appearance.

Again, as opposed to the comparative healthiness of the surroundings when at grass, consideration must be given to the chemical changes the foot is frequently subjected to when the animal is housed.

Only too often the bedding the animal has to stand upon for several hours of the twenty-four can only be fitly described as 'filthy in the extreme.' The ammoniacal exhalations from these collected body-discharges must, and do, have a prejudicial effect upon the nature of the horn, and, though slow in its progress, mischief is bound sooner or later to occur in the shape of a weakened and discharging frog, with its concomitant of contracted heels. Lucky it is in such a case if canker does not follow on.

Observers, too, have chronicled the occurrence in horse's feet of disease resulting from the use of moss litter. Tenderness in the foot is first noticeable, which tenderness is afterwards followed by a peculiar softening of the horn of the sole and the frog. What

2

should be a dense, fairly resilient substance is transformed into a material affording a yielding sensation to the fingers not unlike that imparted by a soft indiarubber, and as easily sliced as cheese-rind.

Lastly, though the foot is extremely liable to suffer from the effects of extreme dryness or excessive humidity, especially with regard to the changes thus brought about in the nature of the horn, it is perforce exposed at all times to the varying condition of the roads upon which it must travel. The intense dryness of summer and the constant damp of winter, each in their turn take part in the deteriorating influences at work upon it.

Though this subject might be indefinitely prolonged, this brief résumé of the adverse circumstances to which the foot of the horse is exposed is sufficient to point out the extreme importance of its study to the veterinary surgeon. So long as the horse is used as a beast of burden so long will this branch of veterinary surgery offer a wide and remunerative field of labour.

CHAPTER II
REGIONAL ANATOMY

Considered from a zoological standpoint, the foot of the horse will include all those parts from the knee and hock downwards. For the purposes of this treatise, however, the word foot will be used in its more popular sense, and will refer solely to those portions of the digit contained within the hoof. When, in this chapter on regional anatomy, or elsewhere, the descriptive matter or the illustrations exceed that limit, it will be with the object of observing the relationship between the parts we are concerned with and adjoining structures.

Taking the limit we have set, and enumerating the parts within the hoof from within outwards, we find them as follows:

A. THE BONES.—The lower portion of the second phalanx or os coronæ; the third phalanx, os pedis, or coffin bone; and the navicular or shuttle bone.

B. THE LIGAMENTS.—The ligaments binding the articulation.

C. THE TENDONS.—The terminal portions of the extensor pedis and the flexor perforans.

D. THE ARTERIES.

E. THE VEINS.

F. THE NERVES.

G. THE COMPLEMENTARY APPARATUS OF THE OS PEDIS.

H. THE KERATOGENOUS MEMBRANE.

I. THE HOOF.

A. THE BONES.

THE SECOND PHALANX, OS CORONÆ, OR SMALL PASTERN BONE.— ;This belongs to the class of small bones, in that it possesses no medullary canal. It is situated obliquely in the digit, running from above downwards and from behind to before, and articulating superiorly with the first phalanx or os suffraginis, and inferiorly with the third phalanx and the navicular bone.

FIG. 1.—THE BONES OF THE PHALANX. 1, The os suffraginis; 2, the os coronæ; 3, the os pedis; 4, the navicular bone, hidden by the wing of the os pedis, is in articulation in the position indicated by the barbed line.

FIG. 2.—SECOND PHALANX OR OS CORONÆ (ANTERIOR VIEW). 1, Anterior surface; 2, superior articulatory surface; 3, inferior articulatory surface; 4, pits for ligamentous attachment.

FIG. 3.—SECOND PHALANX OR OS CORONÆ (POSTERIOR VIEW). 1, Posterior surface; 2, gliding surface for passage of flexor perforans; 3, lower articulatory surface.

Cubical in shape, it is flattened from before to behind, and may be described as possessing six surfaces: *An anterior surface*, covered with slight imprints; *a posterior surface*, provided above with a transversely elongated gliding surface for the passage of the flexor perforans; *two lateral surfaces*, each rough and perforated by foraminæ, and each bearing on its lower portion a thumb-like imprint for ligamentous attachment, and for the insertion of the bifid extremity of the perforatus tendon; *a superior surface*, bearing two shallow articular cavities, separated by an antero-posterior ridge, for the accommodation of the lower articulating surface of the first phalanx; *an inferior surface*, also articulatory, which in shape is obverse to the superior, bearing two unequal condyles, separated by an ill-defined antero-posterior groove, which surface articulates with the os pedis and the navicular bone.

Development.—The bone usually ossifies from one centre, but often there is a complementary nucleus for the upper surface.

THE THIRD PHALANX, OS PEDIS, OR COFFIN BONE.—This also belongs to the class of short bones. It forms the termination of the digit, and, with the navicular bone, is included entirely within the hoof. For our examination it offers *three surfaces, two lateral angles*, and *three edges*.

The Anterior or Laminal Surface, following closely in contour the wall of the hoof, is markedly convex from side to side, nearly straight from above to below, and closely dotted with foraminæ of varying sizes. On each side of this surface is to be seen a distinct groove, the *preplantar groove*, or *preplantar fissure*, which, commencing behind, between the basilar and retrossal processes, runs horizontally forwards from the angles or wings of the bone, and terminates anteriorly into one of the larger foraminæ. As the name 'laminal' indicates, it is this surface which in the fresh state is covered by the sensitive laminæ.

The Inferior or Plantar Surface, hollowed in the form of a low arch, presents for our inspection two regions, an anterior and a posterior, divided by a well-marked line, the *Semilunar Crest*, which extends forward in the shape of a semicircle. The anterior region, as is the laminal surface, is covered with foraminæ; in this case more minute. In the recent state it is covered by the sensitive sole. The posterior region, lying immediately behind the semilunar crest, shows on each side of a median process a large foramen, the *Plantar Foramen*. From this foramen runs the *Plantar Groove*, a channel, bounded above by the superior edge, and below by the semilunar crest of the bone, which conducts the plantar arteries into the *Semilunar Sinus*, a well-marked cavity in the interior of the bone.

The Superior or Articular Surface consists of two shallow depressions, divided by a slight median ridge. Its posterior part shows a transversely elongated facet for articulation with the navicular bone.

The Superior Edge, outlining the superior margin of the laminal surface, describes a curve, with the convexity of the curve forward. In the centre of the curve is a triangular process, the *Pyramidal Process*, which serves as the point of attachment of the extensor pedis.

The Inferior Edge, the most extensive of the three, separates the laminal from the solar surface. It is semicircular in shape, sharp, and finely dentated, and is perforated by eight to ten large foraminæ.

The Posterior Edge, very slightly concave, divides the small, transversely elongated facet of the superior surface from the posterior region of the inferior surface.

The Lateral Angles of the bone, also termed the *Wings*, are two projections directed backwards. Each is divided by a cleft into an upper, the *Basilar Process*, and a lower, the *Retrossal Process*. In old animals the posterior portion of the cleft separating the two processes gradually becomes filled in with bony deposit, thus transforming the cleft into a foramen, which gives passage to the preplantar artery. We may mention in passing that the lateral angles give attachment to the lateral fibro-cartilages, and that the lateral angles themselves in old horses become increased in size owing to ossification of portions of the adjacent lateral cartilages.

Development.—The os pedis ossifies from two centres, one of which is for the articular surface; but this epiphysis fuses with the rest of the bone before birth.

4

FIG. 4.—THIRD PHALANX OR OS PEDIS (POSTERO-LATERAL VIEW). 1, Anterior or laminal surface; 2, preplantar foramen; 3, preplantar groove; 4, basilar process of the wing; 5, retrossal process of the wing; 6, foramen caused by the ossifying together posteriorly of the basilar and retrossal processes.

FIG. 5.—THIRD PHALANX OR OS PEDIS (VIEWED FROM BELOW). 1, Plantar surface; 2, plantar foramen and plantar groove; 3, semilunar crest; 4, tendinous surface; 5, retrossal processes of the wings.

THE NAVICULAR BONE, SHUTTLE BONE, OR SMALL SESAMOID.—Placed behind the articulating point of the second and third phalanges, this small shuttle-shaped bone assists in the formation of the pedal articulation. It is elongated transversely, flattened from above to below, and narrow at its extremities. In it we see two surfaces, and two borders.

The Superior or Articular Surface of the bone, which may easily be recognised by its smoothness, is moulded upon the lower articular surface of the second phalanx, being convex in its middle, and concave on either side.

The Inferior or Tendinous Surface resembles the preceding in form, but is broader and less smooth. In the recent state it is covered with fibro-cartilage for the passage of the flexor perforans. *The Anterior Border* possesses above a small transversely elongated facet for articulation with the os pedis, and below a more extensive grooved portion, perforated by numerous foraminæ, affording attachment to the interosseous ligaments of the articulation. *The Posterior Border*, thick in the middle, but thinner towards the extremities, is roughened for ligamentous attachment. *Development.*—The bone ossifies from a single centre.

B. THE LIGAMENTS.

THE ARTICULATION OF THE FIRST WITH THE SECOND PHALANX, OR THE PASTERN JOINT.—Adhering to the limit we have set, this articulation should not receive our attention. As, however, we shall in a later page be concerned with fractures of the os coronæ, which fractures may affect the articulation above mentioned, a brief note of its formation will not be out of place.

It is an imperfect hinge-joint, permitting of extension and flexion, allowing the first phalanx to pivot on the second, and admitting of the performance of slight lateral movements. It is formed by the opposing of the inferior surface of the os suffraginis with the superior surface of the os coronæ. The articulating surface of the os coronæ is supplemented by the addition behind of a thick piece of *fibro-cartilage (the glenoid)* attached inferiorly to the posterior edge of the upper articulatory surface of the os coronæ, and superiorly by means of three fibrous slips on each side to the os suffraginis. The innermost of these three slips becomes attached to about the middle of the lateral edge of the suffraginis, and the remaining two, beneath the first, attach themselves to nearer the lower end of that bone. The posterior surface of the complementary cartilage forms a gliding surface for the passage of the perforans.

FIG. 6.—THE NAVICULAR BONE (VIEWED FROM BELOW).
1, Inferior surface (smooth for the passage of the flexor perforans); 2, anterior edge of inferior surface; 3, posterior edge of inferior surface.

FIG. 7.—THE NAVICULAR BONE (VIEWED FROM ABOVE, THE BONE TILTED POSTERIORLY TO SHOW ITS ANTERIOR BORDER).
1, Superior articulatory surface; 2, anterior border (grooved portion of); 3, anterior border (articulatory portion of).

FIG. 8.—LIGAMENTS OF THE FIRST AND SECOND INTERPHALANGEAL ARTICULATIONS (VIEWED FROM THE SIDE). (AFTER DOLLAR AND WHEATLEY.)
1, Outermost slip from the glenoidal fibro-cartilage; 2, lateral ligament of the first interphalangeal articulation; 3, prolongations of the lateral ligament of the first

5

interphalangeal articulation attached to the end of the navicular bone to form the postero-lateral ligament of the pedal joint; 4, end of the navicular bone; 5, antero-lateral ligament of the pedal joint.

The Lateral Ligaments.—These are large and thick, an outer and an inner, running obliquely from above downwards and backwards. Each is inserted superiorly into the lateral tubercle of the lower end of the first phalanx, and inferiorly to the side of the second phalanx, their most inferior fibres becoming finally fixed to the extremities of the navicular bone, where they form the postero-lateral ligaments of the pedal articulation. In front of the joint the extensor pedis plays the part of an additional ligament.

The Synovial Membrane.—This is limited in front by the tendon of the extensor pedis, on each side by the lateral ligaments of the joint, and behind by the glenoid fibro-cartilage. At this point it is prolonged upwards as a pouch behind the lower extremity of the first phalanx.

THE ARTICULATION OF THE SECOND PHALANX WITH THE THIRD, THE PEDAL, OR THE COFFIN JOINT.—This also is an imperfect hinge-joint, permitting only of flexion and extension, which movements are more restricted than in the previous articulation. Three bones enter into its formation: the second phalanx, the third phalanx, and the navicular bone. The lower articulatory surface is formed by the third phalanx and the navicular bone combined. To effect this the navicular is closely and firmly attached to the third phalanx by an interosseous ligament. The two bones, as one, are then connected to the second phalanx by four lateral ligaments, an anterior and a posterior on each side.

The Interosseous Ligament consists of extremely short fibres running from the extensively grooved portion of the anterior surface of the navicular bone to become attached to the os pedis immediately behind its articular surface.

The Antero-lateral Ligaments are attached by their superior extremities to the lateral surfaces of the second phalanx, and by their inferior extremities into the depressions on either side of the pyramidal process of the os pedis.

The Postero-lateral Ligaments.—As mentioned when describing the first interphalangeal articulation, these are in reality continuations of the lateral ligaments of that joint. Running obliquely downwards and backwards from their point of attachment to the first phalanx they curve round the lower part of the side of the second phalanx and end on the extremities and posterior surface of the navicular bone. Having reached that position, they send short attachments to the retrossal process of the os pedis and to the inner face of the lateral cartilage.

FIG. 9.—LIGAMENTS OF THE FIRST AND SECOND INTERPHALANGEAL ARTICULATIONS (VIEWED FROM BEHIND). (AFTER DOLLAR AND WHEATLEY.) 1, Suspensory ligament; 2, innermost slip from complementary cartilage of pastern joint; 3, middle slip from complementary cartilage of pastern joint; 4, outermost slip from complementary cartilage of pastern joint; 5, glenoid or complementary cartilage of pastern joint; 6, postero-lateral ligaments of the pedal joint; 7, the navicular bone; 8, interosseous ligaments of the pedal joint; 9, semilunar crest of os pedis; 10, plantar surface of os pedis.

Synovial Membrane.—This extends below the facets uniting the navicular to the pedal bone, and offers for consideration two sacs. A large one posteriorly running up behind the second phalanx to nearly adjoin the sesamoidean bursæ, and a small one, a prolongation of the synovial membrane between the antero-lateral and postero-lateral ligaments of the same side. This latter is often distended, and on account of its close proximity to the seat of operation, is liable to be accidentally opened in excision of the lateral cartilage for quittor.

C. THE TENDONS

In order to convey an intelligent understanding of the tendons it will be wise to briefly describe the course of their parent muscles from their commencement.

THE EXTENSOR PEDIS.—The extensor pedis arises from the lower extremity of the humerus in two distinct portions of unequal size, a muscular and a tendinous. These are succeeded by two tendons passing in common through a vertical groove at the lower end of the radius. Lower in the limb these tendons separate, the outer and smaller joining the tendon of the extensor suffraginis, and the inner and main tendon continuing its course downwards. With the exception of the navicular, it is attached to all the bones of the foot, and is covered internally by the capsular ligaments of the joints over which it passes, those with which we are concerned being the pastern joint and the pedal joint. Before its attachment to the os pedis it receives on each side of the middle of the first phalanx reinforcement in the shape of a strong band descending obliquely over the fetlock from the suspensory ligament. Widening out in fanlike fashion, it is inserted into the pyramidal process of the os pedis.

Action.—The action of this muscle is to extend the third phalanx on the second, the second on the first, and the first on the metacarpus. It also assists in the extension of the foot on the forearm.

FIG. 10.—THE FLEXOR TENDONS AND EXTENSOR PEDIS. (AFTER HAÜBNER.) 1, Tendon of flexor perforans; 2, its supporting check-band from the posterior ligament of the carpus; 3, tendon of the flexor perforatus; 4, ring and sheath of the flexor perforatus; 5, widening out of the flexor perforatus to form the plantar aponeurosis; 6, suspensory ligament; 7, reinforcing band from the suspensory ligament to the extensor pedis; 8, the extensor pedis.

THE FLEXOR PEDIS PERFORATUS, OR THE SUPERFICIAL FLEXOR OF THE PHALANGES.—In common with the perforans, this muscle arises from the inner condyloid ridge of the humerus. It is reinforced at the lower end of the radius by the superior carpal ligament, passes through the carpal and metacarpo-phalangeal sheaths, and, arriving behind the fetlock, forms a ring for the passage of the flexor perforans. Its termination is bifid, and it is inserted on either side to the lateral surface of the second phalanx.

FIG. 11.—THE FLEXOR PERFORANS AND FLEXOR PERFORATUS TENDONS. The metacarpo-phalangeal sheath and the ring of the perforatus laid open posteriorly, and the cut edges reflected to show the passage of the perforans. 1, Reflected cut edges of the perforatus ring and the metacarpo-phalangeal sheath; 2, the perforans tendon; 3, point of insertion of the perforans tendon into the semilunar crest of the os pedis (this widened and thickened extremity of the perforans is known as the plantar aponeurosis).

FIG. 12.—THE FLEXOR PERFORATUS AND FLEXOR PERFORANS TENDONS. The metacarpo-phalangeal sheath and the ring of the perforatus laid open posteriorly, and the cut edges reflected; the flexor perforans cut through at about the region of the sesamoids, and its inferior portion deflected. 1, Superior end of severed perforans tendon; 2, inferior end of severed perforans tendon; 3, insertion of flexor perforans into semilunar crest of os pedis; 4, the cut and reflected edges of the metacarpo-phalangeal sheath and perforatus ring; 5, the bifid insertion of the flexor perforatus into the lateral surfaces of the os corona; 6, the capsular ligament of the pedal joint; 7, the navicular bone; 8, the posterior surface and glenoid fibro-cartilage of the os coronæ.

Action.—This muscle flexes the second phalanx on the first, the first on the metacarpus, and the entire foot on the forearm. Mechanically, it acts as a stay when the animal is standing by maintaining the metacarpo-phalangeal angle.

7

FIG. 13.—MEDIAN SECTION OF FOOT. *A*, Os suffraginis; *B*, os coronæ; *C*, os pedis; *D*, navicular bone; *E*, tendon of the extensor pedis; *F*, insertion of the extensor pedis into the pyramidal process of the os pedis; *G*, the tendon of the flexor perforatus; *H*, insertion of perforatus into the os coronæ; *I*, tendon of the flexor perforans; *J*, its passing attachment to the os coronæ; *K*, its final insertion into the semilunar crest of os pedis; *a*, section of coronary cushion; *b*, section of plantar cushion; *c*, semilunar sinus of os pedis.

THE FLEXOR PEDIS PERFORANS, OR THE DEEP FLEXOR OF THE PHALANGES.—This muscle consists of three easily-divided portions: an ulnar, a humeral, and a radial, and has for points of origin the olecranon process of the ulna, the inner condyloid ridge of the humerus, and the posterior surface of the radius. These portions are continued by a common tendon which enters the carpal sheath with the tendon of the perforatus, and continues with it through the synovial sheath of the metacarpo-phalangeal region. Like the last-named tendon, it receives a supporting check-band, in this case from the posterior ligament of the carpus. Passing down between the suspensory ligament in front, and the perforatus tendon behind, it glides over the sesamoid pulley and passes through the ring formed by the perforatus. Continuing its course, it passes between the bifurcating portions of the extremity of the perforatus, glides over the smooth posterior surface of the supplementary glenoid cartilage of the articulation of the first and second phalanges, plays over the inferior surface of the navicular bone, and finally becomes inserted into the semilunar crest of the os pedis. On reaching the posterior border of the navicular bone it widens out to form the plantar aponeurosis.

In connection with the lower portion of this tendon must be noticed the Navicular Sheath. This is a synovial sheath lining the deep face of the tendon, and reflected on to the navicular bone and the interosseous ligament of the pedal joint. This will be of particular interest when we come to deal with cases of pricked foot from picked up nails. Above, it is in connection with the synovial membrane of the pedal articulation and that of the metacarpo-phalangeal sheath.

Action.—The action of the perforans is to flex the third on the second, and the second on the first phalanx. The latter it flexes in turn on the metacarpus. It also assists in the flexion of the entire foot on the forearm, and in supporting the angle of the metacarpo-phalangeal articulation when the animal is standing.

D. THE ARTERIES.

So far as the arteries supplying the foot are concerned, we shall be interested in following up the distribution of the two digitals, which are the terminal branches of the Large Metacarpal.

THE LARGE METACARPAL, OR COLLATERAL ARTERY OF THE CANNON.—This, the larger terminal branch of the posterior radial artery, needs brief mention, for the reason that we shall be afterwards concerned with it in the operation of neurectomy. Its point of origin is the inside of the inferior extremity of the radius. Descending in company with the flexor tendons, and passing behind the carpus and beneath the carpal sheath, it continues its descent, in company with the internal plantar nerve and the internal metacarpal vein, on the inner side of the flexor tendons until just above the fetlock. At this point it bifurcates into the digital arteries.

From the carpus downwards the large metacarpal artery, the internal metacarpal vein, and the internal plantar nerve are in close relation with each other. The vein holds the anterior position. The artery is between the two, and has the nerve in close contact with it behind.

THE DIGITAL ARTERIES, OR COLLATERAL ARTERIES OF THE DIGIT.— These are of large volume, and carry the blood to the keratogenous apparatus of the foot. They separate from each other at an acute angle, and pass over the side of the fetlock, one to the inside, the other to the outside, to reach the internal face of the basilar process of the os pedis, where they bifurcate to form the *Plantar* and *Preplantar* arteries. In the whole of their course the digital arteries follow the flexor tendons, and are related in front to the digital vein, and behind to the posterior branch of the plantar nerve. This is the nerve implicated in the lower operation of neurectomy, and its relation to adjoining structures will be detailed under Section F. of this chapter. During its course the digital artery gives off branches in the following positions:

1. *At the Fetlock* numerous branches to the metacarpo-phalangeal articulation, the sesamoid sheath, and the tendons.

2. *At the Upper Extremity of the First Phalanx* branches for the supply of the surrounding tissues, and for the tissues of the ergot.

3. *Towards the Middle of the Third Phalanx*, the *Perpendicular* artery of Percival. This arises at a right angle from the main vessel, and immediately divides into two series of ramifications—an ascending and a descending. The ramifications of these series freely anastomose with corresponding vessels of the opposite side.

4. *At the Superior Border of the Lateral Cartilage*, the *Artery of the Plantar Cushion*. This is directed obliquely downwards and backwards, under cover of the cartilage, and is distributed to the middle portion of the complementary apparatus of the os pedis, as well as to the villous tissue and the coronet. A branch of it is turned forwards to join with the coronary circle in forming the *circumflex artery of the coronet.*

FIG. 14.—THE ARTERIES OF THE FOOT. The digital; 2, the perpendicular—(*a*) its ascending branch, (*b*) its descending branch; 3, circumflex artery of coronary cushion; 4, the preplantar (ungual) artery—this is seen issuing from the preplantar foramen, and distributing numerous ascending (*c*) and descending (*d*) branches (the latter concur in forming the circumflex artery of the toe); 5, the circumflex artery of the toe; 6, at the point marked (*) the terminal branch of the digital—namely, the plantar ungual—is hidden behind the lateral cartilage; 7, the lateral cartilage.

5. *Under the Lateral Cartilage* two transverse branches, an anterior and a posterior, to form the *Coronary Circle*. The numerous ramifications of these branches anastomose both anteriorly and posteriorly with their corresponding branches of the artery of the opposite side. This circle closely embraces the os coronæ. Among the larger branches given off from its anterior portion are two descending, one on each side of the extensor pedis, to assist in the formation of the *Circumflex Artery of the Coronary Cushion*. The formation of this last-named artery is completed posteriorly by the before-mentioned branch from the artery of the plantar cushion.

THE PREPLANTAR (UNGUAL[A]) ARTERY.—This, the smaller of the two terminal branches of the digital, is situated inside the basilar process of the os pedis. It turns round this to gain the fissure between the basilar and retrossal processes, and becomes lodged in the preplantar fissure. Here it terminates in several divisions which bury themselves in the os pedis. Before leaving the inner aspect of the pedal wing it supplies a deep branch to the heel and the villous tissue. Gaining the outer aspect of the wing, it distributes a further backward branch, which passes behind the circumflex artery of the pedal bone, and, during its passage in the preplantar fissure, gives off ascending and descending branches, which ramify in the laminal tissue.

THE PLANTAR (UNGUAL[A]) ARTERY.—This, the larger of the two terminals of the digital, may be looked upon as a continuation of the main vessel. Running along the plantar groove, it gains the plantar foramen. Here it enters the interior of the bone (the semilunar sinus) and anastomoses with the corresponding artery of the opposite side. The circle of vessels so formed is called the *Plantar Arch* or the *Semilunar Anastomosis*.

[Footnote A: The epithet 'ungual' is added by Chauveau to distinguish these arteries from the properly so-called plantar arteries—the terminal divisions of the posterior tibial artery.]

From the semilunar anastomosis radiate two main groups of arterial branches, an ascending group and a descending one. The *ascending* branches penetrate the substance of the os pedis, and emerge by the numerous foraminæ on its laminal surface.

The *descending* branches, larger in size, also penetrate the substance of the pedal bone, and emerge in turn from the foraminæ cribbling its outer surface—in this case the set of larger foraminæ opening on its inferior edge. Having gained exit from the bone, their frequent anastomosis, right and left, with their fellows forms a large vessel following the contour of the inferior edge of the os pedis. This constitutes the *Circumflex Artery of the Toe.*

E. THE VEINS.

These commence at the foot with a series of plexuses, which may be described as forming (1) AN INTERNAL OR INTRA-OSSEOUS VENOUS SYSTEM, and (2) AN EXTERNAL OR EXTRA-OSSEOUS VENOUS SYSTEM.

1. THE INTRA-OSSEOUS VENOUS SYSTEM.—This is a venous system within the structure of, and occupying the semilunar sinus of the os pedis. It follows in every respect the arrangement of the arteries as before described in the same region. Efferent vessels emerge from the plantar foraminæ, follow the plantar fissures, and ascend within the basilar processes of the os pedis. Here they lie under shelter of the lateral cartilages, and assist in the formation of the deep layer of the coronary plexus of the extra-osseous system.

2. THE EXTRA-OSSEOUS VENOUS SYSTEM.—This may be regarded as a close-meshed network enveloping the whole of the foot. Although a continuous system, it is best described by recognising in it three distinct parts:

(a) The Solar Plexus.
(b) The Podophyllous Plexus.
(c) The Coronary Plexus.

(a) The Solar Plexus.—The veins of this plexus discharge themselves in two directions: (1) By *a central canal* or canals running along the bottom of the lateral lacunæ of the plantar cushion to gain the deep layer of the coronary plexus. (2) By *the Circumflex or Peripheral Vein of the Toe,* a canal formed by ramifications from the solar and the podophyllous plexuses, and following the direction of the artery of the same name. The circumflex vein terminates by forwarding branches to concur in the formation of the superficial coronary plexus.

(b) The Podophyllous or Laminal Plexus.—The podophyllous veins anastomose below with the circumflex vein of the solar plexus, and above with the veins of the coronary plexus.

(c) The Coronary Plexus.—This proceeds from the podophyllous, the intra-osseous, and the solar networks, and consists of a *central* and *two lateral parts.*

The *central* portion lies between the lateral cartilages and immediately under the coronary cushion. The *lateral portions* are ramifications on both surfaces of the lateral cartilages. The ramifications on the lateral cartilages may be again distinguished as *superficial* and *deep.* The superficial layer is distributed over the external face of the cartilage, forming thereon a dense network, and finally converges towards the superior limit of the plexus to form ten or twelve principal branches, which again unite to form two large vessels. These vessels, by their final fusion at the lower end of the first phalanx, constitute the digital vein. The deep layer is formed, as before described, by ascending branches from the posterior parts of the podophyllous and solar plexuses, and by branches from the intra-osseous system of the pedal bone. The veins of this deep layer finally drain into the two vessels proceeding from the superficial layer, which go to the formation of the digital vein.

THE DIGITAL VEINS—These arise from the network formed on the surfaces of the lateral cartilages, and ascend in front of the digital arteries to unite above the fetlock, where they form an arch between the deep flexor and the suspensory ligament. From this arch (named the *Sesamoidean)* proceed the Metacarpal Veins.

THE METACARPAL VEINS.—Three in number, they are distinguished as an *Internal* and an *External Metacarpal,* and a *Deep* or *Interosseous Metacarpal.* As we shall be concerned with these in the higher operation of neurectomy, we may give them brief mention.

THE INTERNAL METACARPAL VEIN, the largest of the three, has relations with the internal metacarpal artery and the internal plantar nerve. These relations were shortly discussed under the section devoted to the arteries, to which the reader may refer.

THE EXTERNAL METACARPAL VEIN.—This ascends on the external side of the flexor tendons in company with the external plantar nerve.

The Interosseous Vein.—This is an irregular vessel running up between the suspensory ligament and the posterior face of the large metacarpal bone.

F. THE NERVES.

THE PLANTAR NERVES.—These are two in number, and are distinguished as Internal and External.

THE INTERNAL PLANTAR NERVE lies behind and in close contact with the great metacarpal artery during that vessel's course down the region of the cannon. A point of interest is that it gives off at about the middle of the cannon a branch which bends obliquely downwards and behind the flexor tendons to join its fellow of the opposite side—namely, the external plantar. This it joins an inch or more above the bottom of the splint bone. Measured in a straight line, this is about 2-1/2 inches below its point of origin. Near the fetlock, at the level of the sesamoids, the internal plantar nerve ends in several digital branches.

THE EXTERNAL PLANTAR NERVE.—This holds a position to the outside of the metacarpal region, analogous to that of the internal plantar nerve on the inside of the limb, running down on the external edge of the flexor tendons. Unlike the internal nerve, it is accompanied by a single vessel only, the external metacarpal vein, behind which it lies. At the level of the sesamoid bones it divides, as does the *internal* nerve, into three main branches—the digital nerves.

FIG. 15.—THE VEINS AND NERVES OF THE FOOT. 1, The digital vein; 2, its main tributaries, draining the podophyllous plexus, and concurring to form the digital; 3. the digital artery (the main trunk only of this is shown, in order to show its relationship with the vein and nerve); 4, the plantar nerve, with its three branches—(*a*) the anterior digital, (*b*) the middle digital, (*c*) the posterior digital; 5, the podophyllous plexus; 6, superficial portion of the coronary plexus; 7, the peripheral or circumflex vein of the toe.

THE DIGITAL NERVES.—These are distinguished as Anterior, Middle, and Posterior.

The Anterior Branch descends in front of the vein, distributing cutaneous branches to the front of the digit, and terminating in the coronary cushion.

The Middle Branch descends between the artery and the vein, and freely anastomoses with the two other branches. It terminates in the coronary cushion and the sensitive laminæ.

The Posterior Branch.—This is the largest of the three, and may be regarded as the direct continuation of the plantar. At the fetlock it is placed immediately above the digital artery, but afterwards takes up a position directly behind that vessel. Together with the digital artery it descends to near the basilar process of the os pedis. Here it passes with the plantar artery into the interior of the os pedis, and continues its main branch, with the preplantar artery, in the fissure of the same name, to finally furnish supply to the os pedis and the sensitive laminæ. It is this nerve which is divided in the low operation of neurectomy.

Beyond the fact of this branch descending, in the region of the pastern, 1 inch behind the digital artery, a further point of interest presents itself to the surgeon, and one to which attention must be paid. This is the presence in close proximity to the nerve of the Ligament of the Pad (Percival), or the Ligament of the Ergot (McFadyean). This is a subcutaneous glistening cord originating in the ergot of the fetlock, passing in an oblique direction downwards and forwards, and crossing over on its way both the digital artery and the posterior branch of the digital nerve.

In the foregoing description of the anatomy, we have taken the fore-limb as our guide. In the hind-limb, where they reach the foot, the counterparts of the tendons, arteries, veins, and nerves differ in no great essential from their fellows in the fore. They will therefore need no special mention.

G. THE COMPLEMENTARY APPARATUS OF THE OS PEDIS.

This consists of two lateral pieces, the LATERAL CARTILAGES or *Fibro-cartilages* of the pedal bone, united behind and below by the *Plantar Cushion*.

1. THE LATERAL CARTILAGES.—Each is a flattened plate of cartilage, possessing two faces and four borders separated by four angles.

11

The external face is convex, covered by a plexus of veins, and slightly overhangs the pedal bone. The internal face is concave, and covers in front the pedal articulation and the synovial sac, already mentioned as protruding between the antero- and postero-lateral ligaments of that joint. We have already remarked that this is a point of interest to be remembered in connection with the operation for quittor. Below and behind, the internal face of the cartilage is united to the plantar cushion.

FIG. 16.—EXTERNAL FACE OF THE OUTER LATERAL CARTILAGE. 1, External face of cartilage—(*a*) its upper border, (*b*) its posterior border, (*c*) its anterior border, (*d*) its inferior border; 2, the os pedis; 3, wing of os pedis.

The upper border, sometimes convex, sometimes straight, is thin and bevelled, and may easily be felt in the living animal. It is this border that the digital vessels cross to gain the foot, and the border is often broke by a deep notch to accommodate them. The inferior border is attached in front to the basilar and retrossal processes, behind which it blends with the plantar cushion. The posterior border is oblique from before to behind, and above to below, and joins the preceding two. The anterior border is oblique in the same direction, and is intimately attached to the antero-lateral ligament of the pedal articulation. The cartilages of the fore-feet are thicker and more extensive than those of the hind.

2. THE PLANTAR CUSHION on FIBRO-FATTY FROG.—Composed of a fibrous meshwork, in the interstices of which are lodged fine elastic and connective fibres and fat cells, this wedge-shaped body occupies the space between the two lateral cartilages, the extremity of the perforans tendon, and the horny frog. It offers for consideration an antero-superior and an infero-posterior face, a base, an apex, and two borders.

The antero-superior face is in contact with the terminal expansion of the perforans tendon. The infero-posterior face is covered by the keratogenous membrane, and follows closely the shape of the horny frog, on whose inner surface it is moulded. It presents, therefore, at its centre a single conical prolongation, the*Pyramidal Body*, which is continued behind, as is the horny frog, in the shape of two lateral ridges divided by a median cleft. The *base* of the cushion lies behind, and consists of two lateral masses, *the Bulbs of the Plantar Cushion*. In front these are continuous with the ridges of the pyramidal body, while behind they become confounded with the lateral cartilages and the coronary cushion. The *apex* is fixed into the plantar surface of the os pedis, in front of its semilunar ridge. The *borders*, right and left, are wider behind than before, and are in relation with the inner faces of the lateral cartilages.

H. THE KERATOGENOUS MEMBRANE.

THE KERATOGENOUS, OR HORN-PRODUCING MEMBRANE, is in reality an extension of the dermis of the digit. It covers the extremity of the digit as a sock covers the foot, spreading over the insertion of the extensor pedis, the lower half of the external face of the lateral cartilages, the bulbs of the plantar cushion, the pyramidal body, the anterior portion of the plantar surface of the os pedis, and over the anterior face of the same bone. In turn, as the human foot with its sock is covered by the boot, this is encased by the hoof, the formation of which we shall study later.

To expose the membrane for study the hoof must be removed. This may be done in two ways. By roasting in a fire, and afterwards dragging off the horny structures with a pair of pincers, a knife having first been passed round the superior edge of the horny box. Or by maceration in water for several days, when the hoof will become loosened by the process of decomposition, and may be easily removed by the hands. The latter method is less likely to injure the sensitive structures, and will expose them with a fresh appearance for observation.

For purposes of description the keratogenous membrane is divided into three regions:

1. The Coronary Cushion.
2. The Velvety Tissue.
3. The Podophyllous Tissue, or the Sensitive Laminæ.

1. THE CORONARY CUSHION. In the foot stripped of the hoof the coronary cushion is seen as a rounded structure overhanging the sensitive laminæ after the manner of a cornice. It extends from the inner to the outer bulbs of the plantar cushion, and is bounded above by the perioplic ring, and below by the laminæ.

When *in situ* it is accommodated by the *Cutigeral Groove*, a cavity produced by the bevelling out of the superior portion of the inner face of the wall of the hoof. Its superior surface is covered by numerous elongated papillæ, set so closely as to give the appearance of the 'pile' of velvet. This is observed to the best advantage with the foot immersed in water.

The Superior Border of the cushion is bounded by the *Perioplic Ring*, the cells of which have as their function the secreting of the *Periople*, a layer of thin horn to be noted afterwards as covering the external face of the wall. From the perioplic ring the cushion is separated by a narrow and shallow, though well-marked, groove.

The inferior border is bounded by the sensitive laminæ.

FIG. 17.—THE KERATOGENOUS MEMBRANE (VIEWED FROM THE SIDE). (THE HOOF REMOVED BY MACERATION.) 1. The sensitive laminæ, or podophyllous tissue; 2, the coronary cushion; 3, the perioplic ring; 4, portion of plantar cushion; 5, groove separating perioplic ring from coronary cushion; 6. the sensitive sole.

The upper portions of the laminæ, those in contact with the cushion, are pale in contrast with the portions immediately below, and thus there is given the appearance of a white zone adjoining the inferior border of the cushion.

Widest at its centre, the cushion narrows towards its extremities, which, arriving at the bulbs of the plantar cushion, bend downwards into the lateral lacunæ of the pyramidal body, where they merge into the velvety tissue of the sole and frog.

The papillæ of the coronary cushion secrete the horn tubules forming the wall, and the papillæ of the perioplic ring secrete the varnish-like veneer of thin horn covering the outside surface of the hoof.

FIG. 18.—THE KERATOGENOUS MEMBRANE (VIEWED FROM BELOW). (THE HOOF REMOVED BY MACERATION.) 1, The sensitive sole; 2, the sensitive frog[A]—(a) its median lacuna, (6) its lateral lacuna; 3. V-shaped depression accommodating the toe-stay; 4, the sensitive laminæ which interleave with the horny laminæ of the bar.

[Footnote A: The sensitive frog thinly invests the plantar cushion or fibre-fatty frog, the outline of which is here indicated.]

2. THE VELVETY TISSUE.—This is the portion of the keratogenous membrane covering the plantar surface of the os pedis and the plantar cushion. To the irregularities of the latter body—its bulbs, pyramidal body, and its lacunæ—it is closely adapted. Its surface may, therefore, be divided into *(a) The Sensitive Frog*, and *(b) The Sensitive Sole*.

(a) The Sensitive Frog is that part of the velvety tissue moulded on the lower surface of the plantar cushion. The shape of the plantar cushion has already been described as identical with that of the horny frog. It only remains to state that, like the coronary cushion, the surface of the sensitive frog is closely studded with papillæ. The cells clothing the papillæ are instrumental in forming the horny frog.

(b) The Sensitive Sole.—As its name indicates, this is the portion of the keratogenous membrane that covers the plantar surface of the os pedis. It also is clothed with papillæ, which again give rise to the formation of that part of the horny box to which they are adapted—namely, the sole.

3. THE PODOPHYLLOUS TISSUE, OR SENSITIVE LAMINÆ.—This portion of the keratogenous membrane is spread over the anterior face and sides of the os pedis,

13

limited above by the coronary cushion, and below by the inferior edge of the bone. It presents the appearance of fine longitudinal streaks, which, when closely examined with a needle, are found to consist of numerous fine leaves. These extend downwards from the lower border of the coronary cushion to the inferior margin of the os pedis. At this point each terminates in several large villous prolongations, which extend into the horny tubes at the circumference of the sole. At the point of the toe this membrane sometimes shows a V-shaped depression, into which fits a inverted V-shaped prominence on the inner surface of the wall at this point.

The sensitive laminæ increase in width from above to below. Their free margin is finely denticulated, while their sides are traversed from top to bottom by several folds (about sixty), which, examined microscopically, are seen to consist of secondary leaves, or *laminellæ*.

Examined on the foot, deprived of its horny covering, the sensitive laminæ are, the majority of them, in close contact with each other. In the normal state this is not so. The interstices between the leaves are then occupied by the horny leaves, to be afterwards described as existing on the inner surface of the wall.

Reaching and rounding the heels, the sensitive laminæ extend forward for a short distance, where they interleave with the horny laminæ of the bars.

Much discussion has centred round the point as to whether or no the cells of the sensitive laminæ take any share in the formation of the horn of the wall. This will be alluded to in a future chapter.

I. THE HOOF.

Removed from the foot by maceration a well-shaped hoof is cylindro-conical in form, and appears to the ordinary observer to consist of a box or case cast in one single piece of horn. Prolonged maceration, however, will show that the apparently single piece is divisible into three. These are known as (1) THE WALL, (2) THE SOLE, and (3) THE FROG. In addition to these, we have also an appendage or circular continuation of the frog named (4) THE PERIOPLE, or CORONARY FROG BAND. These various divisions we will study separately.

1. THE WALL is that portion of the hoof seen in front and laterally when the horse's foot is on the ground. Posteriorly, instead of being continued round the heels to complete the circle, its extremities become suddenly inflected downwards, forwards, and inwards. These inflections can only be seen with the foot lifted from the floor, and form the so-called *Bars*. It will be noticed, too, with the foot lifted, that the wall projects beyond the level of the other structures of the plantar surface, taking upon itself the bearing of the greatest part of the animal's weight.

The horn of the wall, viewed immediately from the front, is known as the *Toe*, which again is distinguished as *Outside Toe* or *Inside Toe*, according as the horn to its inner or outer aspect is indicated. The remainder of the external face of the wall, that running back to the heels, is designated the *Quarters*.

In the middle region of the toe, the wall following the angle of the bones is greatly oblique. This obliquity decreases as the quarters are reached, until on reaching the heels the wall is nearly upright.

FIG. 19.—THE WALL OF THE HOOF. 1, The toe; 2, inner toe; 3, outside toe; 4, the quarter; 5, entigeral groove; 6, horny laminæ.

For observation the wall offers two faces, two borders, and two extremities.

The External Face is convex from side to side, but straight from the upper to the lower border. Examined closely, it is seen to be made up of closely-arranged parallel fibres running in a straight line from the upper to the lower border, and giving the surface of the foot a finely striated appearance. In addition to these lines, which are really the horn tubules, the external face is marked by a series of rings which run horizontally from heel to heel. These are due to varying influences of food, climate, and slight or severe disease. This will be noted again in a later page. In a young and healthy horse the whole of the external face of the wall is smooth and shining. This appearance is due to a thin layer of horn, secreted independently of the wall proper, termed the periople.

FIG. 20.—INTERNAL FEATURES OF THE WALL, FROG, AND SOLE (MESIAN SECTION OF HOOF). 1, Horny laminæ covering internal face of wall; 2, superior border of wall; 3, junction of wall with horny sole; 4, the cutigeral groove; 5, the horny sole; 6, the horny frog (that portion of it known as the 'frog-stay'); 7, inverted V-shaped ridge on wall and sole (known as the 'toe-stay'); 8, anterior face of wall; 9, inferior border of wall.

The *Internal Face* of the wall, that adapted to the sensitive laminæ, is closely covered over its entire surface with white parallel leaves *(Keraphyllæ,* or horn leaves, to distinguish them from the *Podophyllæ,* or sensitive leaves). These keraphyllæ dovetail intimately with the sensitive laminæ, covering the os pedis. Running along the superior portion of the inner face is the *Cutigeral Groove.* This cavity has been mentioned before as accommodating the coronary cushion, whose shape and general contour it closely follows, being widest and deepest in front, and gradually decreasing as it proceeds backwards. It is hollowed out at the expense of the wall, and shows on its surface numberless minute openings which receive the papillæ of the coronary cushion.

At the bottom of the internal face, at the point where the toe joins the sole, will be noted the before-mentioned inverted V-shaped prominence. Its position will be clearly understood when we say that it gives the appearance of having been forced there by the pressure of the toe-clip of the shoe. This will be noted again when dealing with the sole.

The *Inferior Border* of the wall offers little to note. It is that portion in contact with the ground, and subject to wear. A point of interest is its union with the sole. This will be noticed in a foot which has just been pared as a narrow white or faint yellow line on the inner or concave face of the wall at its lower portion. It marks the point where the horny leaves of the wall terminate and become locked with corresponding leaves of the circumference of the sole.

The *Superior Border* follows closely the line marked by the perioplic ring and the groove separating the latter from the coronary cushion.

The *Extremities* of the wall are formed by the abruptly reflected portions of the wall at the heels. Termed by some the 'Inflexural Nodes,' they are better known to us as the '*Points of the Heels.*'

2. THE SOLE.—The sole is a thick plate of horn which, in conjunction with the bars and the frog, forms the floor of the foot. In shape it is irregularly crescentic, its posterior portion, that between the horns of the crescent, being deeply indented in a V-shaped manner to receive the frog. Its upper surface is convex, its lower concave. It may be recognised as possessing two faces and two borders.

The *Superior or Internal Face* is adapted to the sole of the os pedis. Its highest point, therefore, is at the point of its V-shaped indentation. From this point it slopes in every direction downwards and outwards until near the circumference. Here it curves up to form a kind of a groove in which is lodged the inferior edge of the os pedis. In the centre of its anterior portion—that is to say, at the toe—will be seen a small inverted V-shaped ridge, which is a direct continuation of the same shaped prominence before mentioned on the internal face of the wall. This Fleming has termed the toe-stay, from a notion that it serves to maintain the position of the os pedis. The whole of the superior face of the sole is covered with numerous fine punctures which receive the papillæ of the sensitive sole.

The *Inferior Face* is more or less concave according to circumstances, its deepest part being at the point of the frog. Sloping from this point to its circumference, it becomes suddenly flat just before joining the wall. Its horn in appearance is flaky.

15

FIG. 21.—INFERIOR ASPECT OF HOOF. *a* The inferior face of horny sole; *b*, inferior border of the wall; *c*, body or cushion of the frog; *d*, median lacuna of the frog; *e*, lateral lacuna of the frog; *f*, the bar; *g*, the quarter; *h*, the point of the frog; *i* the heel.

The *External Border* or Circumference is intimately dovetailed with the horny laminæ of the wall. At its circumference the sole, if unpared, is ordinarily as thick as the wall. This thickness is maintained for a short distance towards its centre, after which it becomes gradually more thin.

The *Internal Border* has the shape of an elongated V with the apex pointing forwards. It is much thinner than the external border, and, like it, is dovetailed into the horny laminæ of the inflections of the wall—namely, the bars. In front of the termination of the bars it is dovetailed into the sides and point of the frog. Where unworn by contact with the ground, the horn of the sole is shed by a process of exfoliation.

3. THE FROG.—Triangular or pyramidal in shape, the frog bears a close resemblance to the form of the plantar cushion, upon the lower surface of which body it is moulded. It offers for consideration two faces, two sides, a base, and a point or summit.

FIG. 22.—HOOF WITH THE SENSITIVE STRUCTURES REMOVED. 1, Superior face of horny frog; 2, the frog-stay; 3, the lateral ridges of the frog's superior surface; 4, the horny laminæ at the inflections of the wall.

The *Superior Face* is an exact cast of the lower surface of the plantar cushion. It shows in the centre, therefore, a triangular depression, with the base of the triangle directed backwards. Posteriorly, the depression is continued as two lateral channels divided by a median ridge. The median ridge widens out as it passes backwards, forming the larger part of the posterior portion of the frog. This median ridge fits into the cleft of the plantar cushion. It serves to prevent displacement of the sensitive from the horny frog, and has been rather aptly termed the '*Frog-stay*.'

The *Inferior Surface* is an exact reverse of the superior. The triangular depression of the superior surface is represented in the inferior surface by a triangular projection, and the ridge-like frog-stay of the upper surface is represented below by a median cleft, the *Median Lacuna* of the frog. The triangular projection in front of the median lacuna is the body or cushion of the frog. It is continued backwards as two ridge-like branches, which, at the points of the heels, form acute angles with the bars. On the outer side of each lateral ridge is a fissure. These are known as the Lateral Lacunæ.

The *Sides* of the frog are flat and slightly oblique. They are closely united to the bars and to the triangular indentation in the posterior border of the sole.

The *Base* of the frog is formed by the extremities of its branches, which, becoming wider and more convex as they pass backwards, form two rounded, flexible, and elastic masses separated from each other by the median lacuna. These constitute the 'glomes' of the frog. They are continuous with the periople.

The *Point of the Frog* is situated, wedge-like, within the triangular notch in the posterior border of the sole.

4. THE PERIOPLE, OR CORONARY FROG BAND.—This is a continuation of the substance of the frog around the extreme upper surface of the hoof. It is widest at the heels over the bulbs or glomes of the frog, and gradually narrows as it reaches the front of the hoof. It is, in reality, a thin pellicle of semi-transparent horn secreted by the cells of the perioplic ring. When left untouched by the farrier's rasp it serves the purpose, by acting as a natural varnish, of protecting the horn of the wall from the effects of undue heat or moisture.

CHAPTER III

GENERAL PHYSIOLOGICAL AND ANATOMICAL OBSERVATIONS

The matter embraced by the heading of this chapter will offer for discussion many subjects of great interest to the veterinary surgeon. Around some of them debate has for many years waxed more than keen. Of the points in dispute, some of them may be regarded as satisfactorily settled, while others offer still further room for investigation.

In this volume we can only hope to deal with them in brief, and must select such as appear to have the greatest bearing on the veterinarian's everyday practice.

Always prolific of heated discussion has been one question: 'Are the horny laminæ secreted by the sensitive?' To answer this satisfactorily, it will be best to give a short account of the mode of production of the hoof in general.

A. DEVELOPMENT OF THE HOOF.

Starting with the statement that it is epidermal in origin, we will first consider the structure of the skin, and follow that with a brief description of the structure and mode of growth of the human nail, a short study of which will greatly assist us when we come to investigate the manner of growth of the horse's hoof.

THE SKIN is composed of two portions, the EPIDERMIS and the CORIUM.

THE EPIDERMIS is a stratified epithelium. The superficial layers of the cells composing it are hard and horny, while the deeper layers are soft and protoplasmic. These latter form the so-called *Rete Mucosum* of Malpighi.

FIG. 23.—VERTICAL SECTION OF EPIDERMIS (HUMAN). (AFTER RANVIER) *A*, The horny layer of the epidermis; *B*, the rete mucosum; *a*, the columnar pigment-containing cells of the rete; *b*, the polyhedral cells; *c*, the stratum granulosum; *d*, the stratum lucidum; *e*, swollen horny cells; *f* the stratum squamosum.

Commencing from below and proceeding upwards, we find that the lowermost cells of the rete mucosum, those that are set immediately on the corium, are columnar in shape. In animals that have a coloured skin these cells contain pigment granules. Directly superposed to these we find cells which in shape are polyhedral. Above them, and forming the most superficial layer of the rete mucosum, is a series of flattened, granular-looking cells known as the *stratum granulosum*.

Immediately above the stratum granulosum the horny portion of the epidermis commences. In the human skin this is formed of three distinct layers. Undermost a layer of clear compressed cells, the *stratum lucidum*. Next above it a layer of swollen cells, the nuclei of which are indistinguishable. Finally, a surface layer of thin, horny scales, the *stratum squamosum*, which become detached and thrown off in the form of scurf or dandruff. In the skin of the horse, except where it is thickest, these layers are not clearly defined.

It is the Malpighian layer of the epidermis that is most active in cell division. As they are formed the new cells push upwards those already there, and the latter in their progress to the surface undergo a chemical change in which their protoplasm is converted into horny material. This change, as we have already indicated, takes place above the stratum granulosum.

In addition to its constant formation of cells to replace those cast off from the surface, the active proliferation of the elements of the Malpighian layer is responsible for the development of the various appendages of the skin, the hairs with their sebaceous glands, the sweat glands, horny growths and the hoof, and, in the human subject, the nail. These occur as thickenings and down-growths of the epithelium into the corium.

The epidermis is devoid of bloodvessels, but is provided with fine nerve fibrils which ramify between the cells of the rete mucosum.

THE CORIUM is composed of dense connective tissue, the superficial layer of which bears minute papillæ. These project into the epidermis, which is moulded on them. For the most part the papillæ contain looped capillary vessels, rendering the superficial layer of the corium extremely vascular. Why this must be a moment's reflection will show. The epidermis, as we have already said, is devoid of bloodvessels. It therefore depends entirely for its nourishment upon the indirect supply it receives from the vessels of the corium. The need for extreme vascularity of the corium is further explained when we call to mind the constant proliferation and casting off of the cells of the epidermis, the growth of the hairs, the production of the horn of the hoof, and the work performed by the numerous sweat and other glands.

Others of the papillæ contain nerves, ending here in tactile corpuscles, or continuing, as we have mentioned before, to ramify as fine fibrils in the rete mucosum of the epidermis.

THE HAIRS are growths of the epidermis extending downwards into the deeper part of the corium. Each is developed in a small pit, the *Hair Follicle*, from the bottom of which it grows, the part lying within the follicle being known as the *Root*. It is important to note their structure, as it will be seen later that they bear an extremely close relation to the horn of the hoof.

Under a high power of the microscope, and in optical section, the central portion of a hair is tube-like. In some cases the cavity of the tube is occupied by a dark looking substance formed of angular cells, and known as the *Medulla*. The walls of the tube, or the main substance of the hair, is made up of a pigmented,*horny, fibrous material.* This fibrous structure is covered by a delicate layer of finely imbricated scales, and is termed the *Hair Cuticle.*

The root of the hair, that portion within the follicle, has exactly the same formation save at its extreme end. Here it becomes enlarged into a knob-like formation composed of soft, growing cells, which knob-like formation fits over a vascular papilla projecting up in the bottom of the follicle.

We have already stated that the hairs are down-growths of the epidermis. It follows, therefore, that the hair follicles, really depressions or cul-de-sacs of the skin itself, are lined by epithelial cells and connective tissue. So closely does the epidermal portion of the follicle invest the hair root that it is often dragged out with it, and is known as the *Root Sheath*. This is made up of an outer layer of columnar cells (*the outer root sheath*) corresponding to the Malpighian layer of the epidermis, and of an inner horny layer, next to the hair, corresponding to the more superficial layer of the epidermis, and known as the *inner root sheath.*

The hair grows from the bottom of the follicle by a multiplication of the cells covering the papilla upon which its root is moulded. When a hair is cast off a new one is produced from the cells covering the papilla, or, in case of the death or degeneration of the original papilla, the new hair is produced from a second papilla formed in place of the first at the bottom of the follicle.

FIG. 24.—SECTION OF SKIN WITH HAIR FOLLICLE AND HAIR. *a*, The hair follicle; *b*, the hair root;*c*, the medulla; *d*, the hair cuticle; *e*, the outer root sheath; *f*, the inner root sheath; *g*, the papilla from which the hair is growing; *h*, a sebaceous gland; *i*, a sudoriferous gland.

THE SEBACEOUS GLANDS are small saccular glands with their ducts opening into the mouths of the hair follicles. They furnish a natural lubricant to the hairs and the skin.

THE SUDORIFEROUS OR SWEAT GLANDS are composed of coiled tubes which lie in the deeper portion of the skin, and send up a corkscrew-like duct to open on the surface of the epidermis. They are numerous over the whole of the body.

FIG. 25.—LONGITUDINAL SECTION THROUGH NAIL AND NAIL-BED OF A HUMAN FOETAL FINGER.[A] *a*, The nail; *b*, the rete mucosum; *c*, the longitudinal ridges of the corium.

THE HUMAN NAILS are thickenings of the lowermost layer of the horny portion of the epidermis, the stratum lucidum. They are developed over a modified portion of the corium known as the nail-bed. The horny substance of the nail is composed of clear horny cells, and rests immediately upon a Malpighian layer similar to that found in the epidermis generally. Instead of the papillæ present elsewhere in the skin, the corium of the nail-bed is marked by longitudinal ridges, a similar, though less distinct, arrangement to that found in the laminæ of the horse's foot.

Having thus paved the way, we are now in a better position to discuss our original question (Are the horny laminæ secreted by the sensitive?), and better able to appreciate the work that has been done towards the elucidation of the problem.

A most valuable contribution to this study is an article published in 1896 by Professor Mettam.[A] Here the question is dealt with in a manner that must effectually silence all other views save such as are based upon similar methods of investigation—namely, histological examination of sections of equine hoofs in various stages of foetal development.

Professor Mettam commences by drawing attention to the error that has been made in this connection by studying the soft structures of the foot separated by ordinary putrefactive changes from the horny covering. "In this way," the writer points out, "a wholly erroneous idea has crept in as to the relation of the one to the other, and the two parts have been treated as two anatomical items, when, indeed, they are portions of one and the same thing. As an illustration, and one very much to the point at issue, the soft structures of the foot are to the horny covering what the corium of the skin and the rete Malpighii are to the superficial portions of the epidermis. Indeed, the point where solution of continuity occurs in macerating is along the line of the soft protoplasmic cells of the rete."

In the foregoing description of the skin we have seen that the corium is not a *plane* surface, but that it is studded by numerous papillary projections, and that these projections, with the depressions between them, are covered by the cells of the epidermis.

The corium of the horse's foot, however, although possessed of papillæ in certain positions (as, for example, the papillæ of the coronary cushion, and those of the sensitive frog and sole), has also most pronounced ridges (laminæ) which run down the whole depth of the os pedis. Each lamina again carries ridges (laminellæ) on its lateral aspects, giving a section of a lamina the appearance of being studded with papillæ. We have already pointed out the ridge-like formation of the human nail-bed, and noted that, with the exception that the secondary ridges are not so pronounced, it is an exact prototype of the laminal formation of the corium of the horse's foot.

The distribution of the laminæ over the foot we have discussed in the chapter devoted to the grosser anatomy. In a macerated foot the sensitive laminæ of the corium interdigitate with the horny laminæ of the hoof; that is to say, there is no union between the two, for the simple reason that it has been destroyed; they simply interlock like the *unglued* junction of a finely dovetailed piece of joinery. But no further, however, than the irregularities of the underneath surface of the epidermis of the skin can be said to interlock with the papillæ of the corium does interlocking of the horny and sensitive laminæ occur. It is only apparent. The horny laminæ are simply beautifully regular epidermal ingrowths cutting up the corium into minute leaf-like projections.

In a macerated specimen, then, the exposed sensitive structures of the foot exhibit the corium as (1) the *Coronary Cushion*, fitting into the cutigeral groove; (2) the *Sensitive Laminæ*, clothing the outer surface of the terminal phalanx, and extending to the bars; (3) the *Plantar Cushion*, or sensitive frog; and (4) the *Sensitive Sole*.

The main portion of the wall is developed from the numerous papillæ covering the corium of the coronary cushion. We have in this way numberless down-growing tubes of horn. Professor Mettam describes their formation in a singularly happy fashion: "Let the human fingers represent the coronary papillæ, the tips of the fingers the summits of the

19

papillæ, and the folds of skin passing from finger to finger in the metacarpo-phalangeal region the depressions between the papillæ. Imagine that all have a continuous covering of a proliferating epithelium. Then we shall have a more or less continuous column of cells growing from the tip of the finger or papilla (a hollow tube of cells gradually moving from off the surface of the finger or papilla like a cast), and similar casts are passing from off all the fingers or papillæ."

From this description it will be noticed that each down-growing tube of horn bears a striking resemblance to the growth of a hair, described on p. 47. In fact, the horn tube may be regarded as what it really is, a modified hair.

We next continue Professor Mettam's illustration, and note how the modified hairs or horn tubes become as it were matted together to form the hoof wall. The cells lining the depressions are also proliferating, and their progeny serve to cement together the hollow casts of the papillæ, thus giving the *inter*-tubular substance. We have thus produced hollow tubes, united together by cells, all arising from the rete Malpighii of the coronary corium. Section of the lower part of the horn tubes shows them to contain a cellular debris.

Thus, in all, in the horn of the wall we find a tubular, an intertubular, and intratubular substance. In fact, hairs matted together by intertubular material, and only differing from ordinary hairs in their development in that they arise, not from papillæ sunk in the corium, but from papillæ projecting from its surface.

Although this disposes of the wall proper, there still confronts us the question of the development of the horny laminæ. To accurately determine this point it is absolutely essential to examine, histologically, the feet from embryos.

In the foot of any young ungulate in the early stages of intra-uterine life horizontal sections will show a covering of epidermis of varying thickness.[A] This may be only two or three cells thick, or may consist of several layers. Lowermost we find the cells of the rete Malpighii. As some criterion of the activity with which these are acting, it may be noted that with the ordinary stains their nuclei take the dye intensely. The cells of this layer rest upon a basement membrane separating the epidermis from the corium. At this stage *the corium has a perfectly plane surface.*

[Footnote A: Equine foetus, seventy-seven days old.]

FIG. 26.—SECTION OF FOOT OF EQUINE FOETUS, SEVENTY-SEVEN DAYS OLD. The rete Malpighii rests on a plane corium; the rent in the section is along the line of the cells of the rete (Mettam).

FIG. 27.—SECTION FROM FOOT OF SHEEP EMBRYO. It shows a pronounced epithelial ingrowth into the corium (Mettam).

The next stage will demonstrate the first step in the formation of the sensitive laminæ.[A] The plain surface of the corium has now become broken up, and what is noticed is that the broken-up appearance is due to the epithelial cells irrupting and advancing *en échelon* into its connective tissue. Each point of the ingrowing lines of the *échelon* has usually one cell further advanced into the corium than its neighbours, and may be termed the *apical cell.* The fine basement membrane separating epithelium from corium is still clearly evident. This epidermal irruption of the corium takes place at definite points right round the foot. It is extremely probable, however, that it commences first at the toe and spreads laterally.

[Footnote A: Sheep embryo, exact age unknown.]

As yet, these cellular ingrowths (which are destined to be the *horny* laminæ, and cut up the corium into *sensitive* laminæ) are free from irregularities or secondary laminæ. Before these are to be observed other changes in connection with the ingrowths are to be noticed.

FIG. 28.—SECTION FROM CALF EMBRYO. The epithelial ingrowths hang down from the epidermis into the corium like the teeth of a comb (Mettam).

The first is merely that of elongation of the epithelial processes into the connective tissue, until the rete Malpighii gives one the impression that it has hanging to its underneath surface and into the corium a number of thorn-like processes. These extend all round the front of the foot, and even in great part behind. Accompanying this elongation of the processes is a condensation of the epithelial cells immediately above the rete Malpighii, with a partial or total loss of their nuclei. This is the first appearance of true horn, and its commencement is almost coincident with the first stages of ossification of the os pedis.

FIG. 29.—SECTION OF AN EPITHELIAL INGROWTH FROM AN EQUINE FOETUS. It shows commencing secondary laminar ridges. In the centre are epithelial cells which are undergoing change into horny elements to form the horn core, or 'horny laminæ' (Mettam).

With the appearance of horn comes difficulty of sectioning. The last specimen that Professor Mettam was able to satisfactorily cut upon the microtome was from a foetus between three and four months old. In this the secondary laminar ridges were clearly indicated, and the active layer of the rete Malpighii could be traced without a break from one ingrowing epithelial process to the next, and around this, following all the irregularities of its outline, and covering the branches of the nascent laminæ. The laminæ mostly show this branching as if a number of different growing points had arisen, each to take on a function similar to the epithelial process as it at first appeared.

In the centre of the processes a few nuclei may be observed, but they are scarce, and stain only faintly; they have arisen from the cells of the rete Malpighii which have grown into the corium. In fact, the active cells are passing their daughters into the middle of the process, and these pass through similar stages as those derived from the ensheathing epidermis. In other words, the daughter cells of the constituents of the rete Malpighii which have grown into the corium pass through a degeneration precisely similar to that undergone by cells shed at desquamation, or those which eventually give rise by their agglutination to a hair.

This is the real origin of the horny laminæ, and the thickness of these is increased merely by an increase in the area covered by the cells of the rete Malpighii—*i.e.*, by the development of secondary laminar ridges. If a section from a foal at term be examined, the processes will be found far advanced into the corium, and, occupying the axis of each process, will be seen a horny plate, continuous with the horn of the wall. No line of demarcation can be observed between the horn so formed and the intertubular material of the wall. They merge into and blend with each other, with no indication of their different origins. The cells that have invaded the corium have thus *not lost their horn-forming function*. There has merely been an increase in the area for horn-producing cells. The horny processes are continuous with the hoof proper at the point where the epithelial ingrowth first commenced to invade the corium, and fuses here with the horn derived from the cells of the rete Malpighii which have *not* grown inwards, and which are found between the processes in the intact foot. From this it is clear that some considerable portion of the horn of the wall is derived from the cells of the rete Malpighii covering the corium of the foot. It becomes even more clear when we remember the prompt appearance of horn in cases where a portion, or the whole, of the wall has been removed by operation or by accident (see reported cases in Chapter VII.).

The activity of the cells of the rete Malpighii of the corium covering the remainder of the foot will be quite as necessary as the activity of the cells of the coronary papillæ which form the horn tubes themselves. 'For,' in Professor Mettam's own words, 'I am inclined to believe that much of the "white line" which is found uniting the wall of the hoof to the sole has been derived from the horn formed from the rete of the foot corium. This origin will explain the absence of pigment from this thin uniting "line," as it does from the horn lining the interior of the wall. The cells of the rete are free of colouring matter.'

FIG. 30.—SECTION THROUGH HOOF AND SOFT TISSUES OF A FOAL AT TERM. The horn of the wall is shown, and the horn-core ('horny laminæ') of the epithelial ingrowth. The latter has advanced far into the corium, and is now provided with abundant secondary laminar ridges (Mettam).

From the matter here given us it is easy to understand how, in a macerated foot, the appearance is given of interlocking of the sensitive and horny laminæ. We see that the horny laminæ are ingrowths of the rete Malpighii, ploughing into and excavating the corium into the shape of leaves—the sensitive laminæ. Putrefactive changes simply break into two separate portions what originally was one whole, by destroying the cells along its weakest part. This part is the line of soft protoplasmic cells of the rete Malpighii. Thus the more resistant parts (the horn on the one hand, and the corium covering the foot on the other) are easily torn asunder.

As a result of the evidence we have quoted, we are able to answer our original question in the affirmative. Seeing that the horny and the sensitive laminæ are both portions of the same thing—namely, a modified skin, in which the epidermis is represented by the horny laminæ, and the corium by the sensitive—it is clear to see that the cells covering the inspreading horny laminæ are dependent for their growth and reproduction upon the cells with which they are in immediate contact—namely, those of the sensitive laminæ—and that therefore the sensitive laminæ are responsible for the growth of the horny.

B. CHEMICAL PROPERTIES AND HISTOLOGY OF HORN.

Horn is a solid, tenacious, fibrous material, and its density in the hoof varies in different situations. It is softened by alkalies, such as caustic potash or soda and ammonia, the parts first attacked being the commissures, then the frog, and afterwards the sole and wall. Strong acids, such as sulphuric acid and nitric acid, also dissolve it.

The chemical composition of the hoof shows it to be a modification of albumin, its analysis yielding water, a large percentage of animal matter, and materials soluble and insoluble in water. The proportions of these, as existing in the various parts of the hoof, have been given by Professor Clement as follows:

	Wall.	Sole	Frog.
Water	16.12	36.0	42.0
Fatty matter	0.95	0.25	0.50
Matters soluble in water	1.04	1.50	1.50
Insoluble salts	0.26	0.25	0.22
Animal matter	81.63	62.0	55.78

Horn appears to be identical with epidermis, hair, wool, feathers, and whalebone, in yielding 'keratin,' a substance intermediate between albumin and gelatine, and containing from 60 to 80 per cent. of sulphur.

That horn is combustible everyone who has watched the fitting of a hot shoe knows. That it is a bad conductor of heat, the absence of bad after-effects on the foot testifies.

FIG. 31.—PERPENDICULAR SECTION OF HORN OF WALL.

In a previous page we have described the manner of growth of the horn tubules, and noted the direction they took in the wall; also, we have noticed the existence between them of an intertubular horn or cement.

Those who wish to give this subject further study will find an excellent series of articles by Fleming in the *Veterinarian* for 1871. We shall content ourselves here with introducing one or two diagrams and photo-micrographs, and dealing with the histology very briefly.

Under the microscope the longitudinal striation of the wall is found to be due to the direction taken by the horn tubules.

Fig. 31 is a magnified perpendicular section of the wall. In it the parallel dark striæ are the horn tubules in longitudinal section. The lighter striæ represent the intertubular material.

Fig. 32 gives us the wall in horizontal section. To the left of this picture we find the horn tubules cut across, and standing out as so many concentrically ringed circles. In the centre of the figure are seen the horny laminæ, with their laminellæ, and the sensitive laminæ. The right portion of the figure pictures the corium.

FIG. 32.—HORIZONTAL SECTION OF HORN OF WALL.

Fig. 33 is, again, a horizontal section, cut this time at the junction of the wall with the sole. To the left are seen, again, the horn tubules of the wall, and to the centre the horny laminæ. In this position, however, the structures interdigitating with the horny laminæ are not sensitive, but are themselves horny. As the diagram shows, they contain regularly arranged horn tubules cut across obliquely. It is this horn which forms the 'white line.' To the extreme right of the figure are seen the horn tubules of the sole.

There remains now but to notice the arrangement of the horn tubules in the frog. The peculiar, indiarubber-like toughness of this organ is well known. Histological examination gives a reason for this.

FIG. 33.—HORIZONTAL SECTION OF HORN THROUGH THE JUNCTION OF THE WALL WITH THE SOLE. *a*, Horn tubule of the wall; *b*, horn tubule of the sole; *c, d*, horny laminæ.

FIG. 34.—SECTION OF FROG THROUGH CORIUM AND HORN. The long finger-like projections of corium into epidermis are sections of the long papillæ from which the horn-tubes of the sole grow. In the stainable portion of the epidermis are to be clearly seen light and dark streaks pointing out the alternate strata-like arrangement of cells mentioned in the text (Mettam).

The horn tubules of the frog are sinuous in their course. This is accounted for by the fact that in the horn of the frog there is a large amount of intertubular material, this having the effect of frequently turning the horn tubules from the straight. In addition to this, the intertubular material has a peculiar arrangement of the cells composing it. These are laid down in alternating striæ (1) of cells with their long axes longitudinal, and (2) of cells with their long axes horizontal. This is seen in Fig. 34, between the long papillæ of the corium, where the lines of longitudinally arranged cells in horizontal section stand out darker than the adjoining strata in which their arrangement is horizontal. The tortuous direction of the horn tubules, and the almost interlocking nature of the alternating strata of the intertubular material, together combine to give the frog its characteristic toughness and resiliency.

C. EXPANSION AND CONTRACTION OF THE HOOF.

Among other questions productive of heated argument come those relating to expansion of the horse's hoof. In the past many observers have strenuously insisted on the fact that expansion and contraction regularly occur during progression. Opposed to them have been others equally firm in the belief that neither took place. Quite within recent times this question also has been settled once and for all by the experiments of A. Lungwitz, of Dresden. His conclusions were published in an article entitled 'Changes in Form of the Hoof under the Action of the Body-weight.'[A]

[Footnote A: *Journal of Comparative Pathology and Therapeutics*, vol. iv., p. 191. The whole of the matter in this article, from which we have borrowed Figs. 35 and 36, is too long for reproduction here. It forms, however, most instructive reading, and its careful perusal will well repay everyone interested in this most important question (H.C.R.).]

In connection with this it is interesting to note how, all unconsciously, two separate observers were simultaneously arriving by almost identical means at an equally satisfactory answer to the question. Prior to the publication of Lungwitz's article on the subject, Colonel F. Smith, A.V.D., had arrived at similar conclusions by working on the same methods.

Fig. 35. I. Electric Bell with Dry Element. a, Under part, with box, for the dry element; 6, roller for winding up the conducting-wires; c, dry element, with screw-clamp for attachment of the conducting-wires; c', conducting-wire leading to the screw-clamp, with contact-spring in c', Fig. 2, or to the wall in Fig. 3; d, upper part, with bell; d', conducting-wire to the shoe d' in Figs. 2 and 3; e, strap for slinging the apparatus around the body of the assistant or rider; f, connecting-wire between bell and dry element.

Fig. 35. II. Hoof Shod with Shoe provided with Toe-piece and Calkins; Wall of the Hoof covered with Tinfoil. a, Heel angle, with b, the contact-screws; c, screw-clamp, with contact-spring (isolated from the shoe); c' conducting-wire from the same; d, screw-clamp, with conducting-wire (d') screwed into the edge of the shoe; e, nails isolated by cutting a small window in the tinfoil.

Fig. 35. III. Hoof Shod with Plain Shoe; Horny Wall covered with Tinfoil. a, Toe and heel angle, with b, the contact-screws; c, conducting-wire passing from the tinfoil on the wall; d, conducting-wire passing from the shoe; c', d', ends of the conducting-wires, which must be imagined connected with the ends c', d', passing from the apparatus.

It is unnecessary for our purpose here to minutely describe the exact *modus operandi* of these two experimenters. Briefly, the method of inquiry adopted in each case was the 'push and contact principle' of the ordinary electric bell, and the close attention which was paid to detail will be sufficiently gathered from Figs. 35 and 36.

Fig. 36. I. LEFT FORE-FOOT SHOD AND MOUNTED TO RECOGNISE THE SINKING OF THE SOLE. *a*, Iron plate covering the inner half of the horny sole; *b*, openings in the same, with screw-holes for the reception of the contact-screw *c* (the part of the sole under the plate is covered with tinfoil, which at *d* passes out under the outer branch of the shoe, and becomes connected with the tinfoil of the wall; in order to give the freshly applied tinfoil a better hold, copying-tacks are at *e* passed through it into the horn, and one is similarly used to protect the tinfoil at the place where the contact-screw touches the latter); *f*, holes with screw thread for the fastening of the angle required to measure the movement of the wall, and also for the fastening of the conducting-wire; *g; h*, conducting-wire passing from the tinfoil; *i*, isolated nails.

Fig. 36. II. BAR-SHOE WITH OPENINGS. *a*, Near the inner margin and in the longitudinal bar; *b*, for the reception of the contact-screw *c; d*, openings for fastening the angle and the conducting-wires.

After numerous experiments with the depicted contact-screws, moved to the various positions indicated in the drawings, the following conclusions were arrived at:

1. BEHAVIOUR OF THE CORONARY EDGE.—During uniform weighting of all four hoofs the coronary edge shows a tendency to contraction in the anterior and lateral regions of the hoof, and a tendency to expansion posteriorly. With heavy weighting of the hoof, which is shown by a backward inclination of the fetlock, contraction in the anterior and lateral regions is slight, but the expansion behind, in the region of the heels, is distinct, commencing gradually in front, becoming stronger, and diminishing again posteriorly. The coronary edge of the heels becomes slightly bulged outwards. The bulbs of the heels swell up and incline a little backwards and downwards.

When the fetlock is raised the expansion of the coronary edge of the heels disappears from behind forwards, passing forwards like a fluid wave. In the lateral and anterior regions of the coronary edge the contraction disappears; and when the weight is thrown off the foot it passes into a gentle expansion of the coronary edge of the toe. During the opposite movement of the fetlock, that of sinking backwards, this change of form is executed in the converse manner.

In short, the coronary edge resembles a closed elastic ring, which yields to pressure, even the most gentle, of the body-weight, in such a way that a bulging out of any one part is manifested by an inward movement of another part.

In Fig. 37, *b*, the dotted line represents the changes of form in comparatively well-formed and sound hoofs at the moment of strongest over-extension[A] of the fetlock-joint.

[Footnote A: The term 'over-extension,' as employed by Lungwitz, is intended to indicate that position assumed by the fetlock-joint when the opposite foot is raised from the ground.]

2. BEHAVIOUR OF THE SOLAR EDGE.—Under the action of the body-weight this is somewhat different from that of the coronary edge. Anteriorly, and at the sides, as far as the wall forms an acute angle with the ground, the tendency to expansion exists, but the change of form first becomes measurable in the region where the lateral cartilages begin. Quite posteriorly the expansion again diminishes.

Fig. 37, *a*, by the dotted line represents the expansion at the moment of over-extension of the fetlock-joint. This expansion is itself rather less than at the coronary edge, and it shows itself distinctly *only when the weighted hoof is exposed to a counter-pressure on the sole and frog*, no matter whether the counter-pressure is produced naturally or artificially. Thus anything tending to the removal of the pressure from below, such as a decayed condition of the frog or excessive paring in the forge, will diminish the extent of expansion of the solar edge.

Contraction of the solar edge of the heels occurs at the moment of greatest over-extension of the fetlock-joint—that is, in a foot with pressure from below absent. On the face of it, this appears impossible. Lungwitz, however, has perfectly demonstrated it; and, when dealing with the functions of the lateral cartilages in a later paragraph, we shall show reason for why it is but a simple and natural result of the foot dynamics.

3. BEHAVIOUR OF THE SOLE.—The horny sole becomes flattened under the action of the body-weight. This is most distinct at the solar branches, and gradually shades

off anteriorly and towards the circumference. As might be supposed, width of hoof and thickness of the solar horn exert an influence on the extent of this movement. The sinking of the horny sole is most marked in flat hoofs.

D. THE FUNCTIONS OF THE LATERAL CARTILAGES.[A]

[Footnote A: Extracted from a paper by J.A. Gilruth, M.R.C.V.S., in the *Veterinary Record*, vol. v., p. 358.]

We have just referred to contraction of the heels as taking the place of a normal expansion in those cases where ground frog-pressure was absent. We shall readily understand this when we bear in mind the anatomy of the parts concerned, especially that of the plantar cushion. This wedge-shaped structure we have already described as occupying the irregular space between the two lateral cartilages, the extremity of the perforans tendon, and the horny frog.

Now, when weight or pressure is exerted from above on to this organ, and the *frog is in contact with the ground below*, it is clear from the position the cushion occupies that, whatever change of form pressure from above will cause it to take, it must certainly be limited in various directions.

FIG. 37. *a*, The dotted lines in this diagram represent the expansion of the solar edge of the hoof at the moment of over-extension of the fetlock-joint; *b*, the dotted line represents the change in form of the coronary edge under similar circumstances.

Because of the shape of the cushion its change of form cannot be forwards (simultaneous pressure from above and below on to this wedge with its apex forwards must tend to give it a backward change of form). Because of the pastern being horizontal, and aiding in the downward pressure, its change of form cannot be upwards. And because of the ground it cannot be downwards. It follows, therefore, that the movement must be backwards and outwards, being especially directed outwards because of its shape and the median lacuna in its posterior half—this latter, the lacuna, accommodating as it does the frog-stay, preventing the tendency to backward movement becoming excessive, and directing the change of form to the sides. Where the greatest pressure is transmitted, then, is to the inner aspects of the flexible lateral cartilages. The coronary cushion being continuous with the plantar, the backward and outward movements of the latter will tend to pull upon and tighten the former, especially *in front*. This will account for the contraction noted by Lungwitz in the *anterior half* of the coronary edge of the hoof.

Remove the body-weight, and naturally the elastic nature of the lateral cartilages and the coronary and plantar cushions, with, in a less degree, that of the hoof, cause things to assume their normal position.

Repeat the weighting of the hoof, in this second case *without frog-pressure*, and we shall see at once that we have done away with one of the greatest factors in determining the outward and backward movements of the plantar cushion—namely, the pressure from below on its wedge-shaped mass. The movement of the plantar cushion will now be *downwards* as well as backwards; and, seeing that it is attached to the inner aspect of each lateral cartilage, we shall expect these latter, by the downward movement of the plantar cushion, to be drawn *inwards*. This Lungwitz has shown to occur.

The chief function of the lateral cartilages, therefore, is to *receive the concussion engendered by locomotion*, which concussion is directed backwards and outwards by the pad-like plantar cushion.

In addition to this, the lateral cartilages, together with the plantar and coronary cushions, *play the part of a valve to the whole of the veins of the foot*.

It is in this way: We have only to refer to the chapter on anatomy to see that the whole of the foot is covered with a tissue of extreme vascularity. Thus we find papillæ—the over the coronary cushion; enlarged and modified papillæ sensitive laminæ—covering the anterior face of the os pedis; and numberless papillæ again covering the sole. There can be no doubt that the quantity of fluid brought by the bloodvessels of these papillæ to the foot acts largely as a means of hydraulic protection to the soft structures.[A] In like manner as that delicate organ, the brain, is best protected by being floated upon the cerebro-spinal fluid and bloodvessels (which fluids transmit waves of concussion or pressure *through* the organ without injury to the delicate cells forming it), so, in like manner, does the extreme vascularity of the foot protect the cells of its softer structures from the effects of pressure and concussion.

[Footnote A: The *Veterinary Record*, vol. iii., p. 518.]

That this law of hydraulics may operate in the horse's foot to the best

advantage, the veins must be provided with valves, and valves of no mean strength. These we know to be absent. It is here that the lateral cartilages and the elastic substances of the coronary and plantar cushions step in to supply the deficiency.

At the time when weight is placed upon the foot (with, of course, a tendency to drive the blood upwards in the limb), and, therefore, the time when a valvular apparatus is needed to retain the fluid in the foot, we find the wanting conditions supplied by the pressure outwards of the plantar cushion compressing the large plexuses of veins on each side of the lateral cartilages, to which plexuses, it will be remembered, the bulk of the venous blood from the foot was directed. A more perfect valvular apparatus, automatic and powerful, it would be difficult to imagine.

E. GROWTH OF THE HOOF.

We will conclude this chapter with a few brief remarks on the growth of the hoof. That the rate of growth is slow is a well-known fact to every veterinarian, and it will serve for all practical purposes when we state that, roughly, the growth of the wall is about 1/4 inch per month. This rate is regular all round the coronet, from which it follows that the time taken for horn to grow from the coronary edge to the inferior margin will vary according as the toe, the quarters, or the heels are under consideration.

As might naturally be expected, the rate of growth will depend on various influences. Any stimulus to the secreting structures of the coronet, such as a blister, the application of the hot iron, or any other irritant, results in an increased growth. Growth is favoured by moisture and by the animal going unshod, as witness the effects of turning out to grass. Exercise, a state of good health, stimulating diets—in fact, anything tending to an increased circulation of healthy blood—all lead to increased production of horn. With the effects of bodily disease and of ill-formed legs and feet on the wear of the hoof, and the growth of horn, we shall be concerned in a future chapter.

CHAPTER IV
METHOD OF EXAMINING THE FOOT

As a general rule, it may be taken that most diseases of the foot are comparatively easy of diagnosis. When, however, the condition is one which commences simply with an initial lameness, the greatest care will have to be exercised by the practitioner.

What remarks follow here should rightly be confined to a treatise on lameness. This much, however, we may state: As compared with lameness arising from abnormal conditions in other parts of the limb, that emanating from abnormalities of the foot is easy of detection. With a case of lameness before him, concerning which he is in doubt, the practitioner remembers that a very large percentage may safely be referred to the foot, and, if wise, subjects the foot to a rigorous examination.

Much may be gathered by first putting the animal through his paces. When at a trot, notice the peculiarity of the 'drop,' whether any alteration in going on hard or soft ground, and watch for any special characteristic in gait. At the same time inquiry should be made as to the history of the case; its duration; whether pain, as evidenced by lameness, is constant or periodic; the effect of exercise on the lameness; and the length of time elapsed since the last shoeing.

This failing to reveal adequate cause for the lameness in any higher part of the limb, one is led, by a process of negative deduction, to suspect the foot. If 'pointing' is a symptom, its manner is noticed. The foot is compared with the other for any deviation from the normal. In some cases the two fore or the two hind feet may differ in size. Though this may not necessarily indicate disease, it may, nevertheless, be taken into account if the lameness is not easily referable to any other member. Measurement with calipers will then be of help, and a pronounced increase in size, especially if marked in one position only, given due consideration. The hand is used upon each foot alternately to look for change of temperature, to detect the presence of growths small enough to escape the eye, and to discover evidence of painful spots along the coronet.

At this stage the method of percussion recommends itself, and in many cases no more useful diagnostic agent is to be found than the ordinary hammer. As a preliminary, the foot of the sound limb should be always tapped first. This precaution will serve to bring to light what is frequently met with—the aversion nervous animals sometimes exhibit to this manner of manipulation of the hoof. Unless this is done, the ordinary objection to interference is apt to be read as evidence of pain. No aversion to the method being shown, the suspected foot is gently tapped in various places round the wall, a keen look-out being kept for any manifestation of tenderness. This may vary from a slight resentment to each tap, indicated by a sudden lifting and setting down again of the foot, to a complete removal of the foot from the ground, and a characteristic pawing of the air that points out clearly enough the seat of pain.

Evidence of pain once given, the tapping is persisted in until, in some cases, the exact position of the tender spot is definitely located.

Failing evidence obtained from percussion, attention should next be given to the shoeing. We may add here that, even when difficulties have to be encountered in doing it, it is always a wise plan to have the shoe removed.

The nails should be removed one by one, the course they have taken, their point of emergence on the wall, and the condition of their broken ends all being carefully noted as they are withdrawn.

The removed shoe should next be examined as to the coarseness or fineness of its punching and the 'pitch' of its nail-holes, and close attention given to the shape of its bearing surface.

From that we may pass to a consideration of the underneath surface of the foot. The drawing-knife should be run lightly over the whole of its surface, the first thing to be noticed being the point of entrance of the nails as compared with the coarseness or fineness of the punching, and the staining or otherwise of the horn immediately around. We may thus be guided towards mischief arising from tight nailing apart from actual prick of the foot.

This done, more than usual care should be taken in following up any other small prick or dark spot that may show itself upon the white surface of the cleaned sole. In any case, a suspicious-looking speck should be followed up with the searcher until it is either cut out or is traced to the sensitive structures.

While this is done, we should also have noticed the condition of the horn at the seat of corn; should have noticed the shape of the heels, contracted or otherwise; and the appearance of the frog, clean or discharging.

A point to be remembered in making this exploratory paring of the foot is the peculiar consistency of the horn of the frog, and its tendency to hide the existence of punctures. In like manner, as a pin pierces a piece of indiarubber, and leaves no clearly visible trace of the hole it has made, so does a nail or other sharp object penetrate the frog, leaving but little to show for the mischief that has been done.

28

After all, even though we may have fully decided the foot is at fault, our case of lameness may remain obscure so far as a cause is concerned. Nothing remains, then, but to acknowledge the inability to discover it, to advocate poulticing, or some other expectant palliative measure, and to bring the case up for further examination at no distant date. Where, though we may have suspected the foot, we have not been able to definitely assure ourselves that there the mischief is to be found, a further method of examination presents itself—namely, subcutaneous injections of cocaine along the course of the plantar nerves.

The salt of cocaine used is the hydrochlorate, 2-1/2 grains for a pony, 4 grains for a medium-sized animal, and 6 grains for a large horse. A solution of this is made in boiled water (about 3 drams), and injected at the seat of the lower operation of neurectomy.

It is advisable to first render aseptic the seat of operation, and no sterilize both the needle and the syringe by boiling. A suitable point to choose for the injection is exactly over the upper border of the lateral faces of the two sesamoids, the needle being introduced behind the cord formed by the nerve and accompanying vessels, and parallel with it.

It is possible that the vein or the artery may be wounded, but such accident is of little importance. All that is necessary in that case is to partly withdraw the needle and again insert it. It is advisable to use a twitch.

When the needle is in position, the injection should be made slowly, and at the same time the point of the needle should be made to describe a semicircular sweep, so as to spread the solution over as wide an area as is possible.

Anæsthesia ensues in from six to twenty minutes, and if the cause of the lameness is below the point of injection the animal moves sound.

Regarding this method of diagnosis, Professor Udriski of Bucharest, after a series of trials, sums up as follows:

1. For the diagnosis of lameness cocaine injections are of very considerable value.

2. These injections should be made along the course of the nerves.

3. Solutions heated to 40° or 50° C. produced quicker, deeper, and longer anæsthesia than equally strong cold solutions.

4. In the sale of horses cocaine injections conceal fraud.

Cocaine being an irritant, it must be remembered that after the anæsthesia the lameness is somewhat more marked than before.

To the cocaine other practitioners add morphia in the following proportions:

Cocaine hydrochlorate	2-1/2 grains.
Morphia	1-1/2 "
Aqua destil	1-1/2 drams.

As a diagnostic this mixture of the two is said to be far superior to either cocaine or morphia alone.

In connection with this subject, Professor Hobday has published, among others, the following cases illustrating the practical value of this method of diagnosis:[A]

[Footnote A: The *Journal of Comparative Pathology and Therapeutics* vol. viii., pp. 27, 43.]

CASE I.—Cab gelding. Seat of lameness somewhat obscure; navicular disease suspected. Injected 2 grains of cocaine in aqueous solution on either side of the limb, immediately over the metacarpal nerves.

Five Minutes.—Lameness perceptibly diminished.

Ten Minutes.—Lameness scarcely perceptible.

CASE II.—Mare. Obscure lameness; foot suspected. Injected 30 minims of a 5 per cent. solution on either side of the leg just above the fetlock.

Ten Minutes.—No lameness, thus proving that the seat of lameness was below the point of injection.

CASE III.—Cab gelding, aged, free clinique; Messrs. Elme's and Moffat's case. Obscure lameness; foot suspected of navicular disease; very lame. Injected 30 minims of a 5 per cent. solution of cocaine on either side of the leg over the metacarpal nerves.

Six Minutes.—Lameness perceptibly less; there was no response whatever on the inside of the leg to the prick of a pin. On the outside, which had not been injected so thoroughly, there was sensation, although not so much as in a healthy foot.

Ten Minutes.—Lameness had almost disappeared; so much so, that the opinion as to navicular disease was confirmed, and neurectomy was performed. Immediately after this operation there was no lameness whatever.

The same author also reports numerous cases among horses and cattle, dogs and cats, pointing out the toxic properties of the drug. The symptoms following an overdose are interesting enough to relate here, and I select the following case of Professor Hobday's as being fairly typical:[A]

[Footnote A: *Loc. cit.*]

CASE IV.—Cart gelding. Free clinique; navicular disease. Injected subcutaneously over the metacarpal nerves on each side 6 grains of cocaine in aqueous solution. During the operation the animal manifested no signs of pain whatever, not even when the nerve was cut. This animal received altogether 12 grains of cocaine (3 grains were given on either side first, then fifteen minutes afterwards the same dose repeated). The effect was manifested on the system in ten minutes after the second injection by clonic spasms of the muscles of the limbs (the legs being involuntarily jerked backwards and forwards at intervals of about twenty seconds), which materially interfered with the performance of the operation. The animal was also continually moving the jaws, and was very sensitive to sounds, moving the ears backwards and forwards. This hyperæsthesia, as evinced by the movement of the ears, lasted for some considerable time after the animal had been allowed to get up.

Cocaine hydrochlorate solutions, if intended to be kept for any length of time, should have added to them when freshly made 1/200 part of boric acid in order to preserve them. Even then they are liable to spoil, and should, for subcutaneous injection, be made up just before needed for use.

CHAPTER V
GENERAL REMARKS ON OPERATIONS ON THE FOOT
A. METHODS OF RESTRAINT.

Many of the simple operations on the foot, such as the probing of a sinus, the paring out of corns, or the searching of pricks, may most suitably be performed with the animal's leg held by the operator as a smith holds it for shoeing. According to the temperament of the animal, even the operation for the removal of a portion of the sole, or the injection of sinuses with caustics, may be carried out with the animal simply twitched.

When the operation is still a simple one, casting inconvenient or impossible, and the animal restive, the twitch must be supplemented by some other method. The most simple and one of the most effective is the blind, cap, or bluff (Fig. 38). With it the most vicious animal or the most nervous is in many instances either cowed into submission or soothed into quietness.

At the same time, more forcible means than the operator's own strength must be taken to hold the animal's foot from the ground. If the foot is a fore-foot, and the point desired to be operated on is to the outside, the pastern should be firmly lashed to the forearm by means of a thin, short cord, or a leather strap and buckle. Much may then be done in the way of paring and probing that would otherwise be impossible.

Fig. 38—The BLIND.

Fig. 39—THE SIDE-LINE.

If the foot is a hind one, one of the many methods of using what is termed by Liautard, in his 'Manual of Operative Veterinary Surgery,' the plate-longe, must be adopted. This, in its most useful form, is a length of closely-woven cotton webbing, from about 2 to 2-1/2 inches wide, and from 5 to 6 yards long, provided with a small loop formed on one of its ends, and perhaps better known to English readers as a 'side-line.' If webbing be not available, a length of soft cotton rope, or a rope plaited and sold for the purpose, as Fig. 39, will serve equally well. One of the most convenient methods of using the side-line for securing the hind-foot is depicted in Figs. 40 and 41.

FIG. 40.—THE SIDE-LINE ADJUSTED PREPARATORY TO SECURING THE NEAR HIND-FOOT.

FIG. 41.—THE NEAR HIND-FOOT SECURED WITH THE SIDE-LINE.

Here the side-line has formed upon it a loop sufficiently large to form a collar. This is placed round the animal's neck, the free end of the line run round the pastern of the desired foot, and the foot drawn forward, as in Fig. 40.

The loose end of the line is then twisted once or twice round the tight portion, and finally given to an assistant to hold (see Fig. 41). The foot is thus held from the ground, and violent kicking movements prevented.

Where the operation is a major one, restraint of a distinctly more forcible nature becomes imperative. Many of the more serious operations can most advantageously be performed with the patient secured in some form or other of stock or trevis, and the foot suitably fixed. It is not the good fortune of every veterinary surgeon, however, to be the lucky possessor of one of these useful aids to successful operating. Perforce, he must fall back on casting with the hobbles (Fig. 42).

FIG. 42.—CASTING HOBBLES.

With the use of these we will assume our readers to be conversant, and will imagine the animal to be already cast. It remains, then, but to detail the most suitable means for firmly fixing the foot to be operated on.

Here the side-line is again brought into use. Care should previously have been taken when casting to throw the animal so that the portion of the foot to be operated on, whether inside or outside, falls uppermost, and that the buckle of the hobble on that particular foot is placed so that it also is within easy reach when the animal is down.

In the case we are illustrating the point of operation was the outside of the near hind coronet. We will, therefore, describe the mode of fixing the near hind-foot upon the cannon of the near fore-limb.

FIG. 43.—PHOTOGRAPH ILLUSTRATING METHOD OF ADJUSTING THE SIDE-LINE PREPARATORY TO FIXING THE HIND-LEG UPON THE FORE.

The side-line is first adjusted as follows: It is fixed upon the cannon of the near hind-leg (A) by means of its small loop. From there it is passed under the forearm of the same limb, over the forearm, under the rope running from A to B; from there over and under the thigh, to be finally brought in front of the thigh, and below the portion of rope running from arm to thigh. The loose end of the side-line is then given to an assistant standing behind the animal's back, the buckle of the hobble restraining the foot unloosed, and strong but steady traction brought to bear from behind upon the line. The operator should now stand in front of the fore-limbs, and, by placing a hand on the rope passing round the arm, prevent the line from slipping below the knee.

By this means the hind-limb is pulled forward until the foot projects beyond the cannon of the front-limb. When that position is reached, the operator grasps the hock firmly with one hand, and, directing the side-line to be slackened, gently slides downward the coils of rope round the arm and thigh until they encircle the cannons of both limbs. The cannon of the hind-limb is firmly lashed to the cannon of the fore, and the foot firmly and securely fixed in the best position for operating (see Fig. 44).

FIG. 44.—PHOTOGRAPH SHOWING THE NEAR HIND-FOOT SECURED UPON THE CANNON OF THE NEAR FORE-LIMB.

Similarly, with the horse still on his off side, the off hind-limb may be fixed to the near fore, and the near fore and the off fore to the near hind.

With the animal on his near side, we may fix the near hind and the off hind to the off fore, and the off fore and near fore to the near hind.

The points to be remembered in fixing the limbs thus are: (1) The side-line should always commence upon the cannon of the limb to be operated on; (2) it should next pass under and over (or over and under, it is immaterial which) first the arm and then the thigh, or the thigh and the arm, as the case may be; (3) in every case, whether rounding the thigh and the arm from above or below, the piece of rope completing the round should always finish below that portion preceding it, so that traction upon it from behind the animal's back should tend to keep all portions of it from slipping below the knee and the hock.

With the uppermost fore-limb secured to the hind-limb in the manner we have described, we have the underneath fore-limb suitably exposed for both the higher and lower operations of neurectomy. The position for this operation will be made better still if the lowermost limb (the one to be operated on) is removed from the hobbles and drawn forward by an assistant by means of a piece of rope fastened to the pastern.

Taking what we have described as a general guide, other modifications of thus securing the foot will suggest themselves to the operator to meet the special requirements of the case with which he is dealing.

Regarding the administration of chloroform, no description of the method is needed here, as it will be found fully detailed in most good works on general surgery. Where great immobility is needed, it is one of the most valuable means of restraint we have. Apart from that, its use in any serious operation is always to be advocated, if only on the score of humane consideration for the dumb animal helpless under our hands.

B. INSTRUMENTS REQUIRED.

32

In addition to those required for operations on the softer structures—such as scalpels, forceps, artery forceps, directors, scissors, etc.—the surgery of the foot demands instruments specially adapted for dealing with the horn.

A great deal will depend upon the operator as to whether these are few or many. The average man of resource will deem a smith's rasp and one or two strong drawing-knives amply sufficient, and on no account should they be omitted from the list of those ready to hand.

FIG. 45.—THE ORDINARY DRAWING-KNIFE. The ordinary smith's drawing-knife (Fig. 45) is well known to almost everyone, and is well suited for much of the rougher part of the work. The careful following up of pricks, however, and some of the more special operations demanding removal of portions of the lateral cartilages call for instruments of a more delicate character and peculiar construction. These are to be found in the so-called sage-knife, and the modern (French) pattern of drawing-knife.

FIG. 46. *a, b*, Modern forms of drawing-knife; *c, d, e*, sage-knives. The modern drawing-knife differs from the smith's instrument in being attached to a straight, instead of a curved, handle, and in usually being sharp on both edges instead of only on one. These are made in various sizes (Fig. 46, *a, b*), and the blades flat, curved on the flat, or curved at an angle with the edges of the haft.

The sage-knife, as its name indicates, is a knife with a lanceolate-shaped blade. These also may be obtained in varying forms and sizes (Fig. 46, *c, d, e*). Fig. 46, *c*, is a single-edged, right-handed sage-knife. Fig. 46, *d*, is a left-handed instrument of the same type. The double-edged sage-knife is represented in Fig. 46, *e*.

FIG. 47.—SYMES'S ABSCESS-KNIFE.

It may be mentioned too, in passing, that the ordinary Symes's abscess-knife (Fig. 47) is a most useful instrument when performing the operation of partial excision of the lateral cartilages, its peculiar shape lending itself admirably to the niceties of the operation.

One or two good-shaped firing-irons will also be found useful. They will lighten the labour of tediously excavating grooves with the knife, where that procedure is necessary; and, used in certain positions to be afterwards described, will afford just that necessary degree of stimulus to the horn-secreting structures of the foot, which the use of the knife alone will not.

The man in country practice will also be well advised in carrying to every foot case a compact outfit, such as that carried by the smith. This will consist of hammer and pincers, drawing-knife and buffer. Much valuable time is then often saved which would otherwise be wasted in driving round for the nearest smith.

There are other special operations requiring the use of specially-devised instruments for their successful carrying out. These we shall mention when we come to a consideration of the operations in which they are necessary.

C. THE APPLICATION OF DRESSINGS.

One of the most common methods of applying a dressing to the foot is poulticing. Usually resorted to on account of its warmth-retaining properties, the poultice may also be medicated. In fact, a poultice, strongly impregnated with perchloride of mercury or other powerful antiseptic, is a useful dressing in a case of a punctured foot, or a wise preliminary to an operation involving the wounding of the deeper structures. The poultice may consist of any material that serves to retain heat for the longest time. Meal of any kind that contains a fair percentage of oil is suitable. Crushed linseed, linseed and bran, or linseed-cake dust are among the best.

To prepare it, all that is necessary is to partly fill a bucket with the material and pour upon it boiling water. The hot mass is emptied into a suitable bag, at the bottom of which it is wise to first place a thin layer of straw, in order to prevent the bag wearing through, and then secured round the foot. This is generally done by means of a piece of stout cord, or by straps and buckles fastened round the pastern and above the fetlock.

An improved method of fastening has been devised by Lieutenant-Colonel Nunn:

'A thin rope or stout piece of cord about 5 feet long is doubled in two, and a knot tied at the double end so as to form a loop about 5 or 6 inches long, this length depending on the size of the foot (as at A, Fig. 48). The poultice or other dressing is applied to the foot, and the cloth wrapped round in the ordinary way, the loop of the cord being placed at the back of the pastern (as in A, Fig. 49); the ends of the cord are passed round, one on the inside and the other on the outside, towards the front (as in B, Fig. 49). These ends are then twined together down as far as the toe (see C in Fig. 49). The foot is now lifted up, and the ends of the cord (CC, Fig. 49), are passed through the loop A (as at D, Fig. 49), and then drawn tight. The ends of the cord are now separated, and carried up to the coronet (as at EE, Fig. 49), one on the outside, the other on the inside of the foot. They are then again twisted round each other once or twice (as at F, Fig. 50), and are passed round the pastern once or twice on each side. They are now passed under the cord (E, Fig. 49), and then reversed, so as to tighten up E, and are finally tied round the pastern in the usual manner. The arrangement of the cords on the sole is shown in Fig. 51, which is a view from the posterior part.

F   F   F   F
IG. 48.   IG. 49.   IG. 50.   IG. 51.

FIGS. 48, 49, 50, 51.—ILLUSTRATING LIEUTENANT-COLONEL NUNN'S METHOD OF APPLYING A POULTICE TO THE FOOT.

'The advantages of this method of fastening have been found to be: (1) It does not chafe the skin; (2) if properly applied it has never been known to come undone; (3) it is the only way we know that a poultice can be satisfactorily applied to a mule's hind-foot; (4) horses can be exercised when the poultice is on the foot, which is almost impossible with the ordinary leather boot; (5) the sacking or canvas does not cut through so quickly.'

F   F
IG. 52.   IG. 53.

FIGS. 52, 53.—TWO FORMS OF POULTICE-BOOT.

A further method of applying the poultice is by using one of the poultice-boots made for that purpose (see Figs. 52 and 53).

These have an objection. They are apt to be allowed to get extremely dirty, and so, by carrying infective matter from the foot of one animal to that of another, undo the good that the warmth of the poultice is bringing about. The advantage of the ordinary sacking or canvas is that it may be cast aside after the application of each poultice. Where the boot is kept clean, however, it will save a great deal of time and trouble to the attendant.

While on the subject of poulticing, it is well to remark that in many cases it may be more advantageous to supply the necessary warmth and moisture to the foot by keeping it immersed in a narrow tub of water maintained at the required temperature. By this means the warmth is carried further up the limb (sometimes an important point), and the water can more conveniently be medicated with whatever is required than can the poultice. In fact, it is the author's general practice, where the attendants can be induced to take the necessary pains, to always advise this latter method.

FIG. 54.—SWAB FOR APPLYING MOISTURE TO THE FOOT.

Where a dressing is relied upon by some practitioners on account of the warmth it gives, others, even in identical cases, will depend upon the effects of cold. This may be applied by means of what are called 'swabs.' In their simplest form swabs may consist only of hay-bands or several layers of thick bandage bound round the foot and coronet, and kept cool by having water constantly poured upon them. In many cases the form of swab depicted in Fig. 54 will be found more convenient.

When only one foot is required to be dressed, and a water-supply is available, by far the preferable method is to attach one end of a length of rubber tubing to the water-tap, and fasten the other just above the coronet, allowing the water to trickle slowly over the foot. In cases where a forced water-supply is unobtainable, and the case warrants the extra trouble, much may be done with a medium-sized cask of water placed somewhere over the animal, and the rubber tubing connected with that.

Where the dressing is desired to be kept applied to the sole and frog only, there is no method more satisfactory than the shoe with plates.

FIG. 55.—THE SHOE WITH PLATES. *A*, The plates in position; *B*, the plates separated from the shoe.

FIG. 56.—THE QUITTOR SYRINGE.

The plates are of metal, preferably of thin sheet iron or zinc, and are slipped between the upper surface of the shoe and the foot after the manner shown in Fig. 55. The plates themselves are shaped as depicted in Fig. 55, *a, b, c, a* and *b* curved to meet the outlines of the shoe, and *c* shaped so as to wedge tightly over the posterior ends of the side plates, and between them and the shoe. A distinct advantage of the plate method of dressing is that a certain amount of pressure may be maintained on the sole and frog, a very important consideration in connection with some of the diseases with which we shall later deal.

When dealing with sinuous wounds of the foot, another favourite mode of applying dressings is by means of the syringe, and no better instrument for all cases can be found than that known as a quittor syringe (Fig. 56).

A further mode of applying dressing, and one frequently practised in connection with the foot, is known as 'plugging.' This is almost sufficiently indicated by its name. It consists in rolling portions of the dressing into little cylinders, wrapped round with thin paper, and introduced into a sinus or other position where considered necessary.

D. PLANTAR NEURECTOMY.

As a last resort in the treatment of many diseases of the foot the operation of neurectomy is often advised. It will be wise, therefore, to insert a description of the operation here.

Derivation of the Word.—For many years the operation was known simply as 'nerving' or 'unnerving,' and it was not until 1823, at the suggestion of Dr. George Pearson, that

Percival introduced the word *neurotomy* to signify the operation with which we are now about to deal. The word neurotomy, however, used strictly, means the act or practice of dissection of nerves, and, when applied to the operation as practised to-day, describes only a step in the procedure.

As the operation really consists in cutting down upon, and afterwards excising a portion of the nerve, the modern appellation of *neurectomy*—from the Greek *neuron*, a nerve; and *tome*, a cutting, signifying the cutting out of a nerve or the portion of a nerve—is far more suitable.

According as the nerve operated on is the plantar or the median, the operation is known as plantar or median neurectomy.

History of the Operation.—It is to two English veterinarians that we owe the introduction of the operation to the veterinary world. In 1819 Professor Sewell announced himself as the originator of neurotomy. This claim was disputed by Moorcraft, who appears to have successfully shown himself to be the real person entitled to that honour, he having satisfactorily performed the operation on numerous animals for fully eighteen years prior to Professor Sewell's announcement. It appears that Moorcraft left this country for India in 1808, having practised the operation in more or less obscurity for some six or seven years previous to that. After his departure neurectomy, as introduced by him, either died away in repute, or was not made by him sufficiently public to become a matter of general knowledge. To Professor Sewell, therefore, although not the actual originator of the operation, belongs the honour of making it public to the veterinary profession.

In 1824, five years after Sewell's introduction, we find it practised on the Continent by Girard. We gather, however, from the writings of Percival and Liautard, that both in this country and on the Continent the operation was for several years largely in the stage of experiment. Unsuitable subjects were operated on; the work afterwards given to the animal improperly adjusted to his altered condition; and the bad after-results of the operation almost ignored by some, and greatly exaggerated by others. In fact, some long time elapsed before veterinary surgeons allotted to the operation that measure of credit which the results following it warranted.

The Object of the Operation is to render the foot insensitive to pain, and to give to an otherwise incurably lame animal a further period of usefulness. After the operation, as time goes on, this object may become defeated by the reunion of the divided ends of the nerve. In that case, neurectomy must necessarily be performed again.

The Operation.—Two forms of neurectomy are recognised—the high operation and the low. The low operation deals with the posterior digital branch of the plantar nerve, and the high operation with the plantar itself.

It is the latter operation with which we shall deal first. In our opinion it is that most likely to be followed by satisfactory results. The area supplied by the posterior digital is mainly the posterior portion of the digit. Thus, unless the cause of the lameness is diagnosed with certainty to be situated somewhere in the posterior region of the foot, section of the posterior digital alone will not give total insensibility to pain. Added to that, we may remember this: Below the point at which the digitals branch off from the plantar there is always more likelihood of the part we are attempting to render insensible being supplied by another and adventitious branch, or a branch that, as regards its direction, is abnormally distributed. As a last consideration, we may say that the higher operation is the easier to perform.

Percival, in his works on lameness, has some very sage remarks to make by way of a preliminary, and we cannot do better than quote them here. He says:

'To command success in neurectomy three considerations demand attention:

'1. The subject must be fit and proper; in particular, the disease for which neurectomy is performed should be suitable in kind, seat, stage, etc.

'2. The operation must be skilfully and effectually performed.

'3. The use that is made of the patient afterwards should not exceed what his altered condition appears to have fitted him for.

'The veterinarian who is guided by considerations such as those will find that he has restored to work horses who would otherwise have been utterly useless. A plain and safe argument wherewith to meet the objections to neurectomy is simply to ask the question what the animal is worth, or to what useful purpose he can be put, that happens to be the subject of such an operation.

'If the horse can be shown to be still serviceable and valuable, then he is not a legitimate subject for the operation. The rule of procedure I have laid down is to operate on no other but the *incurably lame horse*; and whenever this has been attended to, not only has success been the more brilliant, but indemnification from blame or reproach has been assured.'

Preparation of the Subject.—But little in the way of medicinal preparation is necessary. When the animal is a gross, heavy feeder, and carries a more than ordinary amount of cupboard, all that is needed is to withhold his usual allowance of food for some time prior to the operation, simply to avoid risk of rupture when casting. If considered advisable, a dose of physic may also be administered.

To the seat of operation, however, careful attention should be given. On the day previous to the operation the hair should be closely removed with the clipping machines, and the skin thoroughly cleansed with warm water and soap. After this, a bandage soaked in a 4 per cent, watery solution of carbolic acid should be wrapped lightly round the limb, and allowed to remain in position until the animal is cast and ready for the operation the following morning. On removing the bandage prior to operating, the part should again be bathed with a cold 5 per cent. solution of carbolic acid and swabbed dry. Attention to these details will serve to leave the wound in that favourable condition in which it heals nicely, and with the minimum amount of trouble.

Preliminary Steps.—By some practitioners the operation is performed with the animal standing, local anæsthesia having been first obtained by the use of cocaine, or an ethyl chloride spray. There is no gainsaying the fact, however, that the operation of neurectomy is a painful one, and that, with most operators, success will be more fully guaranteed with the animal cast and the limb held in a suitable position by an assistant.

The animal is thrown by the hobbles upon the side of the leg which is to be operated on. The cannon of the upper fore-limb is then fixed to the cannon of the upper hind, as described under the section of this chapter devoted to the methods of restraint, and the lower limb freed from the hobbles and drawn forward by an assistant by means of a stout piece of cord round the pastern.

An alternative method of holding the limb is to bind both fore-legs together above the knee by means of the side-line run round a few times in the form of the figure 8, and then fastened off. As in the former method, the lower foot is then removed from the hobble, and again held forward by an assistant. By either method the inside of the limb is operated on first.

FIG. 57.—THE ESMARCH RUBBER BANDAGE AND TOURNIQUET.
Although it is not absolutely necessary, it is an advantage, especially to the inexperienced operator, to apply before operating an Esmarch's bandage and tourniquet (Fig. 57). This expels the greater part of the blood from the limb, and renders the operation comparatively bloodless.

FIG. 58.—RUBBER TOURNIQUET WITH WOODEN BLOCK. The Esmarch bandage is composed of solid rubber, and with it the limb is bandaged tightly from below upwards. On reaching the knee the tourniquet is stretched round the limb, fastened by means of its buckle and strap, and the bandage removed. Those who feel they can dispense with the bandage use the tourniquet alone. For this purpose the form depicted in Fig. 58, and the one in general use at the Royal Veterinary College, is more suitable, on account of its wooden block, which may be placed so as to press on the main artery of supply.

Fig. 59. NEURECTOMY BISTOURY.

Instruments Required.—These should be at hand in an earthenware or enamelled iron tray containing just sufficient of a 5 per cent. solution of carbolic acid to keep them covered. Those that are necessary will be a sharp scalpel, or, if preferred, one of the many forms of bistoury devised for the purpose (see Fig. 59), a pair of artery forceps, a needle ready threaded with silk or gut, one of the patterns of neurectomy needle (see Fig. 60), and a pair of blunt-pointed scissors curved on the flat. It is also an advantage, when once the incision through the skin is made, to employ one of the forms of elastic, self-adjusting tenacula (see Fig. 61) for keeping the edges of the wound apart while searching for the nerve.

FIG. 60. NEURECTOMY NEEDLE.

Incision through the Skin.—We remember that the plantar nerve of the inner side is in close relation with the internal metacarpal artery, and that both, in company with the internal metacarpal vein, run down the limb in close proximity with the inner border of the flexor tendons. Also, we remember that the external plantar nerve has no attendant artery, although, like its fellow, it is to be found in close touch with the edge of the flexor tendons.

Bearing these landmarks in mind, we feel for the nerve in the hollow just above the fetlock-joint by noting the pulsations of the artery, and determining the edge of the flexor tendons. This done, a clean incision is made with the bistoury or the scalpel in the direction of the vessels. The incision should be made firmly and decisively, so that the skin may be cleanly penetrated with one clear cut. If judiciously made, little else in the shape of dissection will be needed.

FIG. 61.—DOUBLE TENACULUM.

It is now that the double tenaculum (Fig. 61) is applied. One clip is fixed to the anterior edge of the wound, and the other carried beneath the limb and made to grasp the posterior edge. If found desirable to keep the edges of the wound apart, and no tenaculum to hand, the same end may be accomplished by means of a needle and silk. In like manner as is the tenaculum, the silk is attached to one edge of the wound, carried under the limb, and firmly secured to the other.

Having made the incision, the wound should be wiped free from blood by means of a pledget of cotton-wool previously soaked in a carbolic acid solution and squeezed dry. At the bottom of the wound will now be seen the glistening white sheath, containing the vein, artery, and nerve. This should be picked up with the forceps, and a further incision made with the bistoury. Care should be exercised in making this second incision, or the artery may accidentally be opened. If an ordinary scalpel is used, the lower end of the sheath should be picked up and the point of the scalpel inserted through it. With the cutting edge of the scalpel turned towards the opening of the wound, the sheath is then slit from below upwards. The second incision satisfactorily made, the wound is again wiped dry, and the nerve seen as a piece of white, curled string in the posterior portion of the wound.

At this stage it is advisable to accurately ascertain whether what we have taken to be the nerve actually is it. This is done by taking it up with the forceps and giving it a sharp tweeze. A sudden struggle on the part of the patient will then leave no doubt in the operator's mind that it is the nerve he has interfered with.

Section of the Nerve.—The neurectomy needle (Fig. 60) is now taken, and, excluding the other structures, passed under the nerve. A piece of stout silk or ordinary string is then threaded through the eye of the needle, the needle withdrawn, and the silk left in position under the nerve. The silk is now tied in a loop, and the nerve by this means gently lifted from its bed. With the curved scissors or the scalpel it is severed as high up as is possible. The lower end of the severed nerve is then grasped firmly with the forceps, pulled downwards as far as possible, and then cut off. At least an inch of the nerve should be excised.

The animal is then turned over, and the opposite side of the limb operated on in the same manner.

The tourniquet is now removed, and the wound is examined for bleeding vessels. If the hæmorrhage is only slight, the wound should be merely dabbed gently with the antiseptic wool until it has stayed. A larger vessel may be taken up with the artery forceps and ligatured, or the hæmorrhage stopped by torsion. On no account, unless it it done to stay hæmorrhage that is otherwise uncontrollable, should the wound be sutured with blood in it. With the wound once dry and clean, it is well to insert three or four silk sutures, but care must be taken not to draw them too tightly. This done, the patient may be allowed to get up. *After-treatment.*—This is simple. Over each wound is placed a pledget of antiseptic cotton-wool or tow, and the whole lightly covered with a bandage soaked in an antiseptic solution. For the first night the animal should be tied up short to the rack, and the following morning the bandages removed. A little boracic acid or iodoform, or a mixture of the two combined with starch (starch and boracic acid equal parts, iodoform 1 drachm to each ounce) should now be dusted over the wounds, the antiseptic pledgets renewed, and the bandage readjusted over all.

At the end of three or four days the bandages may be dispensed with. All that is necessary now is an occasional dusting with an antiseptic powder, and, as far as possible, the restriction of movement. At the end of a week the sutures may be removed, and the animal turned into a loose box or out to pasture.

E. MEDIAN NEURECTOMY.

As a palliative for lameness when confined to the foot, one would imagine that the plantar operation would be all sufficient. There are operators, however, who state that the results following section of the median nerve have been such as to cause them to entirely abandon the lower operation in its favour. If only for that reason a brief mention of the operation must be made here.

The operation was first performed in this country in October, 1895, the subject being one of the out-patients at the Royal Veterinary College Free Clinique.

For five or six years following this date Professor Hobday performed the operation some several hundred times, and was certainly instrumental in bringing the operation into prominence. Though so recently introduced here, it appears to have been practised for several years on the Continent, originating in Germany as early as 1867. In that country a first public account of it was published in 1885 by Professor Peters of Berlin, while in France it was introduced by Pellerin in 1892. In this operation a portion of the median nerve is excised on the inside of the elbow-joint just below the internal condyle of the humerus. Here the nerve runs behind the artery, then crosses it, and descends in a slightly forward direction behind the ridge formed by the radius.

The position of the limb most suitable for the operation is exactly that we have described as most convenient for the plantar excision. The animal is cast, preferably anæsthetized, and the limb removed from the hobbles, and held as far forward as is possible by an assistant with the side-line.

Professor Hobday's description of the operation is as follows:

'A bold incision is made through the skin and aponeurotic portion of the pectoralis transversus and panniculus muscles, about 1 to 3 inches (depending on the size of the horse) below the internal condyle of the humerus, and immediately behind the ridge formed by the radius. This latter, and the nerve which can be felt passing over the elbow-joint, form the chief landmarks. The hæmorrhage which ensues is principally venous, and is easily controlled by the artery forceps. In some cases I have found it of advantage to put on a tourniquet below the seat of operation, but this is not always advisable, as it distends the radial artery. We now have exposed to view the glistening white fascia of the arm, which must be incised cautiously for about an inch. This will reveal the median nerve itself situated upon the red fibres of the flexor metacarpi internus muscle. If not fortunate enough to have cut immediately over the nerve, it can be readily felt with the finger between the belly of the flexor muscle and the radius.'[A]

[Footnote A: *Journal of Comparative Pathology and Therapeutics*, vol. ix., p. 181.]

The nerve exposed, the remainder of the operation is exactly as that described in removing the portion of the nerve in the plantar operation. The wound is sutured and suitably dressed, and a fair amount of exercise afterwards allowed the patient.

F. LENGTH OF REST AFTER NEURECTOMY.

This is placed by the majority of surgeons at about three weeks to a month. Within that period no excessive exertion should be undergone by the patient. A certain amount of quiet exercise, however, is beneficial, facilitating the healing of the wounds, and accustoming the animal to the altered condition of his limb.

G. SEQUELÆ OF NEURECTOMY.

These we shall relate collectively, making no distinction between those following excision of the plantar nerve and those succeeding section of the median. It must be remembered by the surgeon, however, that the unfortunate sequelæ we are now about to describe are likely to be far more grave when following section of the larger nerve.

Liability of Pricked Foot going undetected.—On account of the warning they convey to the surgeon, first place among the sequelæ of neurectomy must be given to accidents following loss of sensation. Take, for example, punctured foot. In any case, in the sense of being unforeseen, it is accidental. In the neurectomized foot it becomes doubly accidental, in that not only is it unforeseen, but that it is for some time indiscoverable. With the foot deprived of sensation, a nail may be picked up, or a prick sustained at the forge, and no intimation given to the attendant until pus has underrun the horn, and broken out at the coronet. What follows, then, is that the hoof as a whole, or the greater part of it, sloughs off.

No neurectomy should be undertaken unless this contingency has been allowed for. The owner should be advised of it by the surgeon, who should at the same time enjoin on his client the absolute necessity of giving to the neurectomized foot daily and careful attention.

Loss of Tone in the Non-sensitive Area.—In addition to the mischief resulting from a wound going undetected, it must be remembered that the loss of tone resulting from the operation gives to every wound (however slight), in the region supplied by the removed nerve, a sluggish and troublesome character. Difficult to deal with as wounds about the foot ordinarily are, they are rendered more so by a previous neurectomy.

Gelatinous Degeneration. This is a condition liable to occur in cases where the operation has been too long deferred, and when considerable structural alteration has already taken place in the shape of diseased bone or tendon, more especially in navicular disease. It consists in a peculiar softening of the structures of the limb, accompanied with enlargement, due to swelling of the connective tissues, the enlargement and softening generally making itself first apparent by a soft, pulpy swelling in the hollow of the heel.

From this onwards the enlargement increases, and lameness becomes excessive, the animal going more and more on his heels, until, finally, no portion of the solar surface of the foot comes to the ground at all.

The case is hopeless, and destruction should be advised.

Reported Case.—'The patient, a brown carriage gelding, was brought to the Royal Veterinary College infirmary in a cart on December 31, the only previous history obtainable being that it had suddenly fallen lame a month before.

'The symptoms presented were excessive lameness of the near fore-limb. On being trotted, the toe was elevated each time the foot reached the ground, progression being entirely on the heels. Separation of the hoof for about 2 inches at the hinder part of the coronet; oedematous swelling from foot to knee, extending during the next three days to the elbow. Great tenderness between the knee and the fetlock; below this no sensation whatever, as a pin was inserted in several places round the coronet without causing any symptoms of pain. On further examination, two unnerving scars were found. No treatment was adopted, and the horse was destroyed on January 6.

'On dissecting the leg, the following appearances presented themselves:

'The limb was very much enlarged, due to thickening of the connective tissue, the skin being removed only with difficulty. The tendons were soft and much thickened. A rupture of the skin at the coronet, just where the skin meets the wall of the foot. Large extravasations of blood at the back of the tendons, situated in the lower half. *External* nerve trunk had become reunited, at the point of junction there being a hard lump about the size of a walnut. *Internal* nerve trunk also had become reunited, and presented a thickened portion at the point of junction, but not so large as that of the outer side, and situated in the lower half of the tendon, about 2 inches higher than that on the external nerve. This nerve trunk was atrophied below the thickening, and had undergone gelatinous degeneration. Judging from the scars on the skin, this side had evidently been unnerved a week or ten days previously to that on the outer side. The band stretching across the back of the perforatus, between the external and internal nerves, appeared on the inside to have become firmly fixed into the tendon.

'On removing the hoof, under the sole there appeared a large quantity of very foetid pus; the laminæ were very much inflamed in patches. There was an enormous thickening of connective tissues in the heel. On cutting longitudinally through the perforatus tendon, there was exposed a large blood-coloured mass, of a gelatinous appearance, situated on the perforatus tendon, the latter being very much thickened, and growing to the navicular bone. The underneath surface of the superior suspensory ligament was much thickened, and firmly adherent to the bone; at the posterior surface of the metacarpus there was a quantity of gelatinous substance. The anterior ligament of the fetlock-joint was thickened; the navicular bone was entire, but showed lesions of navicular disease, being ulcerated. Section through the bone did not reveal anything further. It may be here remarked that the ulcerations were on either side of the central ridge, and not at all on the ridge itself.

'Microscopic examination of the tissue joining the two ends of the nerve together revealed a few nerve fibres; the general appearance was that of granulation tissue, containing capillary vessels, which were fairly plentiful, and comparatively large in size.'[A]

[Footnote A: *Veterinary Record*, vol. iv., p. 386 (Hobday)]

Chronic Oedema of the Leg.—In some cases there is a distinct swelling of the leg some time after the operation. This exposes the limb to the infliction of sores from striking with the opposite foot, with, of course, the difficulty in healing we have just described.

Persistent Pruritus.—This annoying sequel occurs in the neurectomized limb, with or without gelatinous degeneration, and appears to be without a remedy. The itching in some cases is so intense as to lead the animal to constantly gnaw at the top of the foot. As one observer has remarked, the animal may begin literally biting pieces out of his limb. The result of the irritation and gnawing is fatal. Great sloughing of the parts takes place, and the animal has eventually to be slaughtered. v*Fracture of the Bones.*—The sudden loss of sensation in a foot may cause the animal to use violently the limb he has for months past been carefully nursing. It may be that the lameness for which the operation has been performed has been due to disease existing in the navicular bone, and extending, perhaps, to the os pedis. By the disease the bone has already been made brittle, its substance and ligamentous attachments perchance weakened and broken up by a slow-spreading caries, and rarefaction of the remaining bone substance rendered almost certain. In this instance, the free use of the foot, and the application to the diseased structures of an unwonted pressure immediately after the operation results in fracture. With the rupture of the structures we get the elevated toe and soft swelling in the heel, as described in gelatinous degeneration. Treatment, of course, is out of the question.

Neuroma.—A further sequel is the appearance at the seat of the operation of what is termed an 'amputational neuroma.' This is a tumour-like growth occurring on the end of the divided nerve. It is composed of connective-tissue elements permeated by nerve fibres which have grown out from the axis-cylinders of the nerve stump. It may vary in size from a pea to a hazel-nut, and is frequently the cause of much pain. This must be cut down upon and cleanly removed, taking away at the same time as much of the nerve as is possible.

Reunion of the Divided Nerve.—We may say at once that 'reunion' in the popular sense of the word does not take place. At a varying period after section, however, we do get a return of sensation. This is brought about in the following manner: The axis-cylinder of the nerve, still in connection with the spinal cord, swells somewhat, and hypertrophies. The cells of this hypertrophied portion show a great tendency to proliferate and produce new nerve structure. This growing point splits, and gives rise to several fibrils, which are new axis-cylinders. These commence to grow towards the periphery, and, in so doing, grow through the cicatricial tissue that has formed at the seat of the operation.

After passing through the cicatricial tissue (the amount of which tissue, of course, controls the length of time that insensibility remains), the growing axis-cylinders reach the degenerated portions of the nerve below the point of section. It is along the track of the old nerve that the new growths from the stump reproduce themselves.

The fact of the new growths having to pass through the fibrous tissue of the cicatrix before they can gain the course of the old nerve, along which latter their progress of growth is comparatively easy, affords ample illustration that as large a portion as is possible of the nerve should be removed when operating, in order to convey insensibility for the longest time. After reunion, of course, nothing remains but to repeat the operation.

The Existence of an Adventitious Nerve-supply.—While not exactly a sequel of the operation, the fact that it is not discovered until after the operation has been performed warrants us in mentioning it here. It is not an uncommon thing in the lower operation to find that sensation and symptoms of lameness still persist after section of the nerve. In many cases this has been traced to the existence of an abnormal nerve branch. In the higher operation this is not so likely to be met with. That it may occur, however, is shown by the following interesting case related by Harold Sessions, F.R.C.V.S.:[A]

[Footnote A: *Journal of Comparative Pathology and Therapeutics*, vol. xii., p. 343.]

'In June of 1898 I saw a hunter suffering from navicular disease. After carefully examining the leg, I advised the owner to have the operation of neurectomy performed upon him. This he decided to do, and the horse was sent to me about the beginning of July.

FIG. 62.—DISSECTED EXTERNAL METACARPAL NERVE AND BRANCHES. *a*, Metacarpal; *b*, anterior plantar; *c*, extra branch (probably from the internal metacarpal), conveying sensation after division of the external metacarpal.

'The operation was performed in the ordinary way, without any difficulty whatever. The wounds healed nicely, but the horse still continued to go lame. Careful examination showed that there was still sensation on the outside of the foot. Thinking that possibly there might be two external metacarpal nerves, the horse was again cast, the operation being performed slightly lower down. Only the main branch of the external metacarpal nerve could be found. A piece of this was taken out, and the horse let up. On examination, sensation was still found in the posterior part of the outside of the foot. It was very evident that there was some abnormal distribution of the nerve, as sensation was still being conveyed to that part of the foot.

'As the horse was absolutely useless, and would have to be shot unless this piece of nerve could be found, he was again thrown, and after he had been anæsthetized I determined to follow the course of the nerve down, until I found where the accessory branch came from. This I found a little below the fetlock, about 1/2 inch below the point where the anterior plantar nerve is given off from the metacarpal nerve. It was about 1/2 inch below the spot where the anterior plantar nerve passes between the artery and vein of the foot, and it was somewhat difficult to get at it.

'Fig. 62 shows the exact size and distribution of the nerves. After the separation of the accessory branch, sensation was taken from the foot, and the horse went perfectly sound.'

Stumbling.—In addition to the sequelæ we have mentioned, it is urged against the operation of neurectomy that one of the first effects of depriving the foot of the sense of touch is a tendency on the part of the animal to stumble. From the cases we have seen we cannot regard this objection as a serious one. Nevertheless, as veterinarians, with a knowledge of the physiology of the structures with which we are dealing, we must treat the objection with respect, for, after all, we are bound to allow that stumbling, and a bad form of it, would be but a natural sequence of the operation we have just performed. The real fact remains, however, that cases of stumbling, even immediately after the operation, are rare; and that even when they do occur, the animal seems easily able to accommodate himself to the altered condition, and as readily uses the comparatively inert mass at the end of his limb as he did previously the intact foot.

H. ADVANTAGES OF THE OPERATION.

From the prominence we have given to the unfortunate sequelæ of the operation it might possibly be inferred that, while not giving it our absolute condemnation, we regard neurectomy with a certain amount of distrust. That we may contradict any such false impression, we state here that in many cases the operation is the only measure which will offer relief from pain, and restore to work an otherwise useless animal. In support of that we will now quote the recognised advantages of the operation.

That in many cases, when all other methods—surgical and medicinal—have failed, there is an immediate and total freedom from pain and lameness no one will deny. This, if it restores to active work an animal that would otherwise have had to have been cast aside, is ample justification for giving the operation, in spite of its many unfortunate terminations, a real place among the more highly favoured remedial measures to our hand.

'For *Contracted Hoofs*, viewing them in the light of idiopathic disease, or as being the immediate cause of the existing lameness in the uninflamed condition of the foot, and when consequential changes of its organism have taken place which bid defiance to therapeutic measures, *neurotomy* is a *warrantable resource*' (Percival).

'For *Ringbone* neurotomy has been practised with perfect success, after blistering and firing had both failed, notwithstanding the work the animal had to perform afterwards was of the most trying nature' (*ibid.*).

For *Navicular Disease*, when that malady is diagnosed, the earlier neurectomy is performed the better. The greater work given to the diseased bursa and bone, and the return of the contracted heels to the normal, brought about by the greater freedom with which the foot is used, are claimed by many to effect a cure.

Writing of navicular disease, and mentioning his belief in the possibility of the diseased bone effecting its own repair after the operation, Harold Leeney, M.R.C.V.S., says:

'The expansion of the heel, and rapid development of the frog (in this and many other cases) immediately after the operation, has not, I venture to think, attracted so much attention as it deserves, and may have something to do with those cases which appear to be actually *cured*, not merely made to go sound by absence of pain.'[A]

[Footnote A: *Veterinary Record*, vol. xi., p. 297.]

Speaking of the median operation before a meeting of the Central Veterinary Medical Society, Professor Hobday says:[A]

[Footnote A: *Veterinary Record*, vol. xiii., p. 427.]

'For old-standing lamenesses, when due to splints, exostoses, chronically sprained, thickened, and painful perforans and perforatus tendons, or cases of that kind which cause pain by pressing on the adjacent nerve structures, after all other known methods have failed, median neurectomy is the operation which will be most likely to give the animal a new lease of life and usefulness.'

'Of the *Humanity and Utility of Neurectomy* there can be no question whatever, and provided the cases are well selected, and the operation is efficiently performed, the advantages to be derived from it are most striking as well as enduring. But the disadvantages attending the loss of sensation in the foot have been brought forward on many occasions as an argument against neurectomy, and no one can deny that the foot with sensation is better than one without that faculty. But in a long experience of the operation I have never found these disadvantages outweigh the great advantages which have immediately followed it.'[A]

[Footnote A: *Veterinary Journal*, vol. ix., p. 178 (Fleming).]

Beyond these, the direct advantages of neurectomy, are other and more indirect advantages which claim attention.

The most astonishing among them is the fact noted by many writers of repute that exostoses (ringbones, side-bones, splints, etc.) rapidly diminish in size. This is vouched for by such well-known authorities as Zundel and Nocard.

Percival, too, mentions at some length the effect of the removal of pain on the oestral and generative functions, quoting a case of a brood cart-mare by reason of bony deposits being stayed from breeding for some years. Two months after the operation she went to work, and moved sound, her altered condition leading her to breed several healthy foals.

I. THE USE OF THE HORSE THAT HAS UNDERGONE NEURECTOMY.

No operation is of any considerable value to the veterinary surgeon unless he is able to show that after it he has left his patient workable. The alleviation of pain alone, commendable as it is from a humanitarian standpoint, is of no interest to the average owner of horse-flesh, unless with it he sees his animal capable of justifying his existence by the amount of labour performed.

Criticised in this way, is the operation of neurectomy justifiable? Upon that point the opinions of many practitioners, even at the present day, differ. We have already partly answered the objections likely to be raised on this score by stating that the work afterwards allotted the animal should be fixed to suit his altered condition. It may be taken as a general rule that in all cases where the animal's usefulness depends upon his delicacy of touch, as, for example, animals used solely for hacking or hunting, his future usefulness in that special sphere of work will be done away with.

Percival himself, always a strong advocate for the operation, fully recognises this. 'Does the neurotomized horse maintain the same step as before?' he asks. 'To this important question,' he replies, 'I unhesitatingly answer no; he does not. There can be no doubt but that the horse *feels* the ground upon which he is treading, and that he regulates his action in consonance with such feeling, so as to render his step the least jarring and fatiguing to himself, and therefore the easiest and pleasantest to his rider.... Such impressions'—those of touch—'being in the neurotomized subject, so far as regards the feeling of the foot, altogether wanting, a bold, fearless projection of the limb in action will be the consequence, followed by a putting down of the hoof flat upon the ground, as though it were a block, creating a sensation alike unpleasant both to horse and rider.'

Emphatic as Percival is upon this point, there are, nevertheless, others who maintain with equal stoutness that the unnerved animal is positively as safe, if not safer, than the animal who has not been so treated.

'That the tactile sense in the horse's foot is useful, it would be idle to deny; but that it is absolutely essential, even to safe progression, no one who has paid attention to the results of plantar neurectomy will maintain. On several occasions for years I have hunted, hacked, and driven horses which have been deprived of sensation in their fore-feet, and never had an accident with them. Their action has not been impaired by the operation; on the contrary, it has been vastly improved compared with what it had been previous to it. And my opinion has not been single in this respect, as many competent horsemen can give like evidence after long and severe trials of neurotomized horses. The opponents of neurotomy were, probably, not aware that there is in progression a *muscular* as well as a *tactile sense*.'

This latter contention is supported by numerous cases, reported at the time when the operation of neurectomy was at the heyday of its popularity. Two I select from writings of a later period:

Recorded Cases.—1. 'Two of the finest among the many fine horses in the Second Life Guards were so lame from navicular disease, when I joined the regiment, that they were unsafe and unsightly to ride, and were therefore entered on the list to be cast off and sold. One was so crippled that it could scarcely be moved out of its stable. Feeling sorry at having to get rid of such good horses, and anxious to give another blow to the mistaken theory that unnerved animals were unsafe, I obtained the consent of my commanding officer, who patronizes practical conclusions, to perform neurotomy. This was carried out on both horses about eighteen months ago. Within a fortnight they were at their duty, absolutely free from lameness, and with first-rate action, and one of them, from being troublesome and unsteady in the ranks—probably from the pain in its feet—had become quite steady and tractable. Instead of being lame, blundering, and unsafe, both were sound, free in movement, and secure, and, the pain being abolished, they looked improved in condition.

'During the month of July the regiment attended the summer drills at Aldershot, and five days every week for a month these horses carried a weight of about 22 stones each over the roughest and most dangerous ground, nearly always at a fast pace, and for four, five, or six hours each day; and yet they never fell or blundered, and the troopers who rode them had unbounded confidence in their sure-footedness. They returned to Windsor, at the end of the month's severe test, as sound in their paces as when they left, and certainly now offer no indication whatever that they are less safe to ride than any other horse in the regiment. The effects of the relief from pain are also most marked, not only in the altered gait out of doors, but also in the stable.'[A]

[Footnote A: *Veterinary Journal, vol.* ix., p. 178 (George Fleming, F.B.C.V.S.).]

2. 'Some years ago I operated upon a valuable hunter, the property of a gentleman in Kildare, the animal having shown unmistakable symptoms of navicular disease for some months previously, and which had been unsuccessfully combated by the milder forms of treatment for the disease without any benefit. Although the horse went sound, the owner feared to ride him, and sent him to be sold in Dublin, where he was disposed of for a small price, and I then lost sight of him. The following Punchestown Races, to my surprise, amongst a group of horses walking round the paddock previous to saddling for an important race, I recognised my old patient, bandaged, clothed, and trained, ready to take his part in the cross-country contest, and surrounded by a host of admirers willing to back him at any price.

'Having satisfied myself that it was no other than the same animal, my first impulse was at once to find out the jockey who was to ride him, and warn him of his danger by telling him his mount was devoid of feeling in both fore-feet; but the saddling-bell had already rung, and in a few moments more the jockey emerged from the weighing-room and the next view of the horse was his tearing up the course in the preliminary, and "pulling double." I was sorry for the jockey if he felt as I did at that moment, for if he did I fear he and his horse would have parted company at the first fence, as I was certain there would be a smash before the end of the long and difficult three miles of the Kildare Hunt Cup course. It was not until I saw him again in the front rank passing the stand, in the first round, that I breathed freely, and even then I felt very guilty, and, had he come to grief badly, I don't think I should ever have operated on another horse except in such a way as would have left unmistakable traces after it.

'"The old horse wins!" screamed a thousand voices as the competitors safely cleared the last bank (now taken away for a gorse fence) the last time round, and from that moment the operation went up in my estimation a hundredfold, and I almost lost all interest in the finish (and it was a close one, with my patient a good third), resolving I would operate for the future on every animal, young and old, which showed symptoms of navicular disease.

'Neither owner nor jockey knew the horse had been operated on, and he was soon after, on the strength of his performance, sold for a good price to come to England. It is idle to think that all cases are as successful as this was, as experience soon told me; but I consider that, in careful hands, the advantages well outweigh the disadvantages of the operation, and I have selected this instance merely as a practical example.'[A]

[Footnote A: *Veterinary Journal,* vol. iii., p. 254 (W. Pallin, M.B.C.V.S.).]

It is solely with the object of ventilating both sides of the question that we quote the last two cases. In our opinion, the colours in which the results of the operation are there painted are far too rosy. The practitioner who has before him the task of satisfying a client as to what will or what will not be the results of an operation he has suggested will do well to weigh each side of the argument carefully, and endeavour in his explanation to strike the happy mean.

We hold, further, that the animal who has previously been accustomed to fast work, and to work entailing a large call upon the sense of touch when passing over rough and uneven ground, will be far more likely, in his neurectomized condition, to give satisfaction to his owner if put to a slower and a more suitable means of earning his living.

CHAPTER VI
FAULTY CONFORMATION

Under this heading we shall deal with such formations of the feet as depart sufficiently from the normal to render them serious. Faulty conformation may be either congenital or acquired, and acquired gradually as the result of slowly operating causes, or suddenly as the sequel to previous acute disease. Whether congenital or acquired, serious in its nature or comparatively of no account, the veterinary surgeon will often find that the matter of conformation is one which will have a direct bearing on many of his 'foot' cases, and, furthermore, that it is one upon which he will often be called to give advice.

A. WEAK HEELS.

Definition.—That condition of the wall in which, owing to the softness of the horn and the oblique direction of the horn fibres, the heels are unable properly to bear the body-weight, and, as a consequence, curve in beneath the sole. We give the condition first mention, not because of its greater importance, but for the reason that it is frequently the forerunner of the condition to be next described—namely, contracted feet.

Symptoms.—The extreme point of the heel is not affected unless the foot has been greatly neglected, and the condition allowed to develop. Where, however, the foot has been uncared for, curving in of the wall takes place to an alarming degree, and the heels curl underneath the foot to such an extent as to grow over the sole and the bars. By the pressure they exert on the sole corns result, and the animal is lamed.

Causes.—In the main this defect is hereditary. It is seen commonly in connection with flat-foot, and where the horn of the wall is thin and shelly.

Treatment.—In the case of weak or 'turned in' heels no suitable bearing is offered for the shoe in the posterior half of the foot. Any attempt to induce the heels to bear weight is immediately followed by their bending in. It follows from this that the best shoe to be used here is one in which the bearing is confined to the anterior half of the wall, the heels being relieved by being sufficiently pared. As might be expected, this bearing on the anterior half only of the foot is insufficient; pressure must be given the frog. This latter end is best gained by a bar shoe (Fig. 68). With it the anterior portions of the wall, the whole of the bars, and the whole of the frog may be in contact, and the heels only so pared as to take no bearing at all. A few such shoeings sees the defect remedied. In every instance paring of the sole should be discouraged, as it serves but to increase the deformity.

B. CONTRACTED FOOT.

(a) GENERAL CONTRACTION—CONTRACTED HEELS.

Definition. By the term contracted foot, otherwise known as hoof-bound, is indicated a condition in which the foot, more especially the posterior half of it, is, or becomes, narrower from side to side than is normal.

It must be borne in mind, however, that certain breeds of horses have normally a foot which nearer approaches the oval than the circular in form, and that a narrow foot is not necessarily a contracted foot.

The contraction may be bilateral when affecting both heels of the same foot and extending to the quarters, or unilateral when the inside or outside heel only is affected.

In some cases contraction is confined to one foot, while in others it may be noticed equally bad in both. It is a matter of common knowledge that contraction is usually seen in the fore-feet, while the hind seldom or never suffer from it, a fact which, to our minds, seems difficult of adequate explanation. Zundel explains this by stating that contraction is principally *observed* in the fore-feet, by reason of the fact that when lameness arises from it alteration in action will more readily be detected in front than behind. Percival, on the other hand, suggests that the greater expansive powers of the hind-foot, by reason of the impetus of its action, is able to overcome any influence operating towards contraction. It may be, however, that given a cause for contraction, such as the removal of the frog's counter-pressure with the ground by faulty shoeing or excessive paring, the fore-feet, by reason of their being called upon to bear the greater part of the body-weight, are the first to suffer.

Flat feet with weak heels are those most frequently affected, and, as we have already intimated, the condition may exist with or without other disease of the foot.

Depending upon its degree, contracted foot may vary from a simple abnormality, non-inflammatory and painless, to a condition in which it becomes a veritable disease, giving rise to a bad form of lameness, and bringing about a withered and sometimes discharging and cankerous affection of the frog.

Symptoms.—In its early stages contraction is difficult of detection, and where both feet are affected may for some time go unsuspected. With only one foot undergoing change, the early stages may the more readily be marked, for in this case comparison with the other and sound foot will at once reveal the alteration in shape. If lameness in the suspected foot is present, then any lingering doubt will be quickly dispelled.

When far advanced, contraction offers signs that cannot well be missed. The converging of the heels narrows the V-shaped indentation in the sole for the reception of the frog. As a consequence of this, the frog itself becomes atrophied by reason of the *continual* pressure exerted upon it by the ingrowing horn of the wall and the bars. The median and lateral lacunæ of this organ, from being fairly broad and open channels, become pressed into mere crack-like openings (see the commencing of this condition in Fig. 80, and a badly wasted frog in Fig. 74A). As the case goes on, the lateral branches of the frog entirely disappear, and all that is left of the organ is a remnant of its body or cushion, now wedged in tightly between the bars. Following upon the disappearance of the frog, we find that the bars are in contact, or, in some cases, actually overlapping each other at their posterior extremities.

At this stage, perhaps, the whole condition has become aggravated by a foul discharge from the place originally occupied by the frog, and the foot, especially in the region of the heels, has become hot and tender—really a form of local and subacute laminitis.

The long-continued inflammation, although only of a low type, renders the horn of the hoof hard and dry, and only with difficulty will the ordinary foot instruments cut it. This in its turn leads to cracks and fissures in various places, but more especially in the bars and what is left of the frog. Often, too, cracks will appear in the horn of the quarters, and a troublesome and incurable form of sand-crack results.

An animal with contraction advanced as far as this, especially if confined to one foot, goes unmistakably lame. With both feet affected, he ordinarily starts out from the stable in a manner that is commonly called 'groggy.' In other words, the gait is uncertain, and feeling; and stumbling is frequent. Anyone who has had the misfortune to drive an animal with feet in this condition knows full well that every little irregularity in the road at once makes itself felt to the feet, and that the animal, as time goes on, learns to carefully avoid any suspicious-looking group of stones he may see. To drive an animal like this is to keep one's self continually on tenter-hooks, for, sooner or later, the inevitable happens, and the animal comes down.

Up to now we have described the changes of form in the hoof as seen when the contracted foot is viewed from the solar surface. With those changes as evident as we have depicted them, there will be no difficulty in detecting the alterations in the form of the wall.

In addition to a narrowing from side to side there will be noticed an abnormal straightness of the quarters, with a turning in, more or less sudden, of the heels. This effect is given in these cases by the smith maintaining the shoe of a length and width that should normally fit a foot of that particular animal's size and substance. This is probably done with the idea of deceiving anyone examining the solar surface. Viewed from this position, the width of the shoe at the heels gives the impression that it is attached to a foot of normal breadth. This deception is heightened if at the same time has been practised the process of 'opening up the heels.' That expression indicates that the bars have been removed, and the lateral lacunæ of the frog made to continue the concavity of the sole. The arch of the latter is thus made to appear of much greater extent than it really is, and the heels, by reason of their being abruptly cut off when removing the bars, also convey the false impression of being wide apart.

The practitioner unversed in the tricks of the forge will best guard against this by viewing the foot, while on the ground, from behind. From that position he will be able to detect the lowness of the quarters, and the projecting portion of the shoe, that the hoof, by reason of its sudden bending inwards, does not touch.

The 'feeling' manner of the gait before alluded to, together with the disinclination to put the foot firmly and squarely forward, will sometimes lead the examiner to over-look the contraction, and diagnose his case as one of shoulder lameness. In many cases, too, such consequent conditions as 'thrushy frogs' and 'suppurating corns' are often treated with utter disregard of the contraction that has really brought them about. But above all, the disease most likely to be confounded with simple contraction is navicular disease. More than probable it is that many cases of so-called 'navicular' have in reality been nothing more than contraction brought about by one or other of the causes we shall afterwards enumerate—cases where a due attention to the prime cause of the mischief would, in all likelihood, have remedied the lameness.

Changes in the Internal Structures.—It follows as a matter of course that the changes we have described in the form of the hoof itself carry with them alterations in the bones and sensitive structures beneath it. The tissues, as a whole, become atrophied. The os pedis becomes deformed, loses its circular shape, and gradually becomes more or less oval in contour. At the same time, its structure becomes more compact, the cribriform appearance of its anterior and lateral faces more or less destroyed, and the few remaining openings apparently increased in size. This atrophy of the os pedis is best noted at the wings.

In the plantar cushion the effects of the atrophy are noted in the smallness of the organ, in its becoming whiter in colour than normal, and more resistant to pressure.

The coronary cushion is also affected in the same way, where the changes are noted most in its posterior portions.

A further effect of the narrowing of the heels, and their consequent tendency to drop downwards, is the exertion of a continual pressure on the sensitive sole. In course of time, and especially in flat feet, this leads to the appearance of corns.

The navicular bone and bursa and the tendon of the perforans also suffer from the effects of compression. The movement of the tendon is restricted, and arterial supply to the adjacent structures rendered deficient. The tissues of the bone and bursa are insufficiently nourished, and the secretion of synovia lessened. In this way it is conceivable that navicular disease may follow the condition of simple contracted heels.

In common with the other structures, the lateral cartilages also suffer from the continual pressure. Their blood-supply is lessened, their functions interfered with, and side-bones result.

Causes.—Upon the causation of contraction a very great deal has been written, both by early veterinarians and by those of the present day. Many and widely differing opinions have been advanced, but a careful résumé of only a few will lead one to certain fixed conclusions.

We may consider the causes of contraction under two headings—predisposing and exciting.

Predisposing Causes of Contraction.—Among these we will first mention heredity, although it is possible it should not be deemed of so great account as it is by some. That the shape of certain feet, especially those with low heels and abnormally sloping walls, predisposes to contraction no one will deny. So long, however, as the animal goes unshod, so long does the foot maintain a normal condition of the heels. In other words, it is not until the tendency to contraction already there is aggravated by careless shoeing and the effects of work that it operates to any noticeable extent.

The degree of contraction will also be very largely governed by the amount of the development of the frog. With a frog of good size, low down, and taking part in the pressure of the foot on the ground, contraction will be prevented. On the other hand, an ill-developed frog, one wasted by long-continued and spreading thrush, or one robbed of its normal function by excessive paring in the forge, is a common starting-point of the condition we are considering. We have already referred to this in Chapter III., when considering the experiments of Lungwitz in this connection. What we have to bear in mind in these experiments is that the application of a pad to the frog, in such a manner that effective ground-pressure is obtained, results always in a marked expansion of the heels, and that, with counter-pressure with the ground absent, expansion occurs to little or no extent. This is proof positive of the enormous part the frog plays in maintaining an open and elastic condition of the heels—a fact so insisted on by Coleman.

It is worthy of mention, however, that loss of the frog's function does not operate to nearly so serious an extent in horses with high, upright heels as in those with the heels low and excessively sloping.

In illustrating this, Mr. Dollar, in his work on shoeing, mentions the case of a pair of trotting horses of similar age, size, and weight, each having weak fore-heels. In one case the hoofs were flat, in the other upright. The horse with the flat hoofs suffered from contraction, while the other did not.

The reason appears to be that in the animal with upright hoofs the proportion of body-weight borne by the heels is considerably less than in those with the hoofs flat and sloping.

Certain conditions of the horn-producing membranes also predispose to contraction. For example, in horses reared on marshy soils, and afterwards transferred to standing in town stables, we find that a dry and brittle condition of the horn supervenes. This we may regard as a low form of laminitis, brought about by the heat of the material upon which the animal is standing, and the congestion of the feet engendered by his enforced standing for long periods in one position, as opposed to the more or less continuous exercise when at pasture. With the hoof in this condition it loses by evaporation the moisture that normally it should contain, and, as we might expect, a certain degree of contraction of its structure is the inevitable result.

We thus see that contraction brought about in this way is not so much caused by the heat of the stable, as it is by the decreased ability of the horn to retain its own moisture.

On the other hand, it cannot be denied that excessive warmth and dryness combined tend also to an undue abstraction of moisture, even from the horn of the healthy foot; and this explains in great measure how it is that lameness, as a rule, and especially that proceeding from contracted heels, is far more frequent and of greater intensity in the hot, dry months of summer, than in the cooler and more humid atmosphere of winter. It is interesting to note, too, that an alternation of humidity and dryness is far more liable to injure the quality of the horn and tend to its contraction than the long-continued effects of dryness alone. A common illustration of this is to be found in the effects of the ordinary poultice. Everyone knows that when, after a few days' application, they are discontinued, we get as a result an abnormally dry and brittle state of the horn. This is doubtless due to the poultice removing the thin, varnish-like, and protective pellicle known as the periople, and thereby allowing the process of evaporation to act on the water normally contained in the hoof.

Exciting Causes of Contraction.—Among these, first place must undoubtedly be given to shoeing. This does not necessarily imply shoeing more than ordinarily faulty, nor a faulty preparation of the foot, but shoeing as it is generally practised. No ordinary shoe, except a few devised for the purpose, such as the Charlier or the tip, allows the frog to come in contact with the ground. This we take to be the main factor in the causation of contracted heels, especially with a predisposition already present in the foot itself. In the words of Lungwitz: 'Regarded from this point of view, there is no greater evil than shoeing. It abolishes the necessary counter-pressure, and thus interferes with expansion. Bars, sole, and frog cannot perform the functions that naturally belong to them as they would do without the shoe.'

In addition to the evil of the shoe itself, errors of practice in the forge contribute to the causation of contraction. Taking first the preparation of the foot, we find that often the heels are lowered far too much, and the toe allowed to remain too long. This can have but one effect—that of throwing a greater proportion of the animal's weight upon the heels than properly they should bear, with, what we now know to be the consequence of that, a corresponding pushing inwards and downwards of the horn; in other words, contraction.

Excessive paring of the bars, to which we have already partly alluded, is also an active agent in bringing about an inward growth of the horn of the heels and quarters. The bar, or inflexion of the wall at the heel, by means of its close contact with the frog, communicates the outward movements of that organ to the wall of the hoof. With the bar removed, the outward movements of the frog under pressure are naturally rendered of no account, and a proper and intermittent expansion of the wall denied it. The same evil follows, though to a less extent, excessive paring of the sole.

The shape of the bearing surface of the shoe is often to be blamed. Where this is concave—'seated'—and the 'seating' is carried back to the heels, it is easy to see that, when weight is on the foot, there is an ever-present tendency for the bearing edge of the wall to slide down towards the inner edge of the shoe. This tendency, operating on both the inner and outer wall simultaneously, must strongly favour contraction.

A further wrong practice is that of continuing the nailing too far towards the heels. In our opinion this is not now often met with. When it occurs its effect is, of course, to prevent those movements of expansion of the wall which we now know to be normal and most marked at the heels.

It may be remarked of the build of the shoe, or of errors in the preparation of the foot, that neither are of much moment. Neither are they. But when one stays to consider that errors of this description are practised not only once, but each time the horse goes to the forge, and that with some of them—those relating to the build of the shoe—the injury thereby brought about is inflicted not only once, but every day that particular shoe is worn, then it is not to be wondered at that, sooner or later, ill consequences more or less grave result.

Prognosis.—This will depend to a very large extent upon the conformation of the limb, and upon the previous duration of the contraction. Contraction of long standing, where atrophy of the sub-lying, soft structures and the pedal bone may be expected, will prove obstinate to treatment. Especially will this be so if the lateral cartilages have become ossified. Neither may we look for much benefit from treatment if the contraction has occurred in animals with an oblique foot axis and flat hoofs.

On the other hand, if the case is comparatively recent, if the limb is straight and the form of the hoof is upright, and if matters are uncomplicated by side-bones, or other serious alteration in the internal structures, then treatment may be rewarded with some measure of success.

FIG. 63.—TIP SHOE. The dotted portions represent the length of the branches removed.

Treatment.—The greater part of the treatment of contracted foot will almost suggest itself as a corollary of the causes we have enumerated. The normal width of the heels may be renewed, and development of the wasted frog brought about by one of three methods:

1. By restoring the pressure from below to the frog.
2. By the use of an expansion shoe.
3. By operative measures upon the horn of the wall.

1. *By Restoring the Pressure from Below to the Frog.*

This may be accomplished as follows:

(a) *By Shoeing with Tips.*—This method is advocated by Percival, by A.A. Holcombe, D.V.S., Inspector. Bureau of Animal Industry, U.S.A., by Dollar in his work on horseshoeing, and by many others.

Though requiring more care than in fitting the ordinary shoe, the application of a tip is simple. In reality, the tip is just an ordinary shoe shortened by truncating the heels.

Before applying the tip, the horn of the wall at the toe should be shortened sufficiently to prevent any undue obliquity of the hoof, and the foot should be so prepared as to allow the heels of the tip to sink flush with the bearing edge of the wall behind it.

When the foot does not allow of the removal of much horn at the toe, what is termed a 'thinned' tip is to be preferred. Its shape is sufficiently shown by the accompanying figure (Fig. 65).

With the tip the posterior half of the foot is allowed to come into contact with the ground, and the object we are striving for—namely, frog pressure, and greater facilities for alternate expansion and contraction of the heels—is thus brought about.

FIG. 64.—THE TIP SHOE LET IN THE FOOT.

FIG. 65.—THE THINNED TIP.

(b) By Shoeing with the Charlier.—The results brought about by the use of a tip may be arrived at by the application of a Charlier or preplantar shoe, or by a modified Charlier or Charlier tip.

Briefly described, a Charlier is a shoe that allows the sole and the frog to come to the ground exactly as in the unshod foot. This is accomplished by running a groove round the inferior edge of the hoof by removing a portion of the bearing edge of the wall with a specially devised drawing-knife. Into this groove is fitted a narrow and somewhat deep shoe, made, preferably, of a mixture of iron and steel, and forged in such a manner that its front or outer surface follows the outer slope of the wall.

The Charlier should have the inner edge of its upper surface very slightly bevelled, in order to prevent any pressure on the sensitive sole, and should be provided with from four to six nail-holes. These latter should be small in size and conical in shape. The nails themselves should be small, and have a conical head and neck, to fit into the nail-hole of the shoe.

FIG. 66.—THE SPECIAL DRAWING-KNIFE (FLEMING'S) FOR PREPARING THE FOOT FOR THE CHARLIER SHOE.

The modified Charlier, or Charlier tip, perhaps the better of the two for the purpose we are describing, is really a shortened Charlier, and bears the same relation to the Charlier proper as the tip does to the ordinary shoe. It is let into the solar surface of the foot in exactly the same manner as its larger fellow, but it does not extend backwards beyond the commencement of the quarters. By its use greater opportunity for expansion is given to the heels than is done by the Charlier with heels of full length.

FIG. 67.—FOOT PREPARED FOR THE CHARLIER SHOE.

We do not here intend to deal at any length with the arguments for and against the Charlier as regards its adoption for general use. These will be found fully set out in any good work on shoeing.

The point that it is correct in theory it would be idle to attempt to evade; but that it is generally practicable, or that it offers any very pronounced advantages, as compared with the disadvantages urged against it, over the shoes in ordinary use, the limited favour it has drawn to itself, since its introduction in 1865, seems sufficiently to deny.

(c) By the Use of a Bar Shoe.—Where the frog is not excessively wasted benefit will be derived from the use of a bar shoe.

FIG. 68.—BAR SHOE.

The transverse portion at the back, termed the 'bar,' and which gives the shoe its name, is instrumental in bringing about from below that counter-pressure on the frog that we now know to be so necessary a factor in remedying contraction. When the frog, by wasting or disease, is so deficient as to be unable to reach the 'bar,' this shoe must be supplemented by a leather or rubber sole.

In the event of corn or sand-crack existing with the contraction, the shoe known as a 'three-quarter bar' is preferable (see Fig. 103). The break here made in the contour of the shoe allows of dressing the corn, and, in the case of sand-crack, removes the bearing from that portion of the wall. *(d) By the Use of a Bar Pad and a Heelless or 'Half' Shoe.*—The bar pad consists of a shape of rubber composition firmly fixed to a leather foundation, which shape of rubber takes the place of the 'bar' of the bar shoe.

FIG. 69.—RUBBER BAR PAD ON LEATHER.

FIG. 70.—THE BAR, PAD APPLIED WITH A HALF-SHOE.

For habitual use in such cases as prove obstinate to treatment, or where a complete cure was never from the commencement expected, the bar pad is undoubtedly one of the most useful inventions to our hand. The animal's 'going' is improved, the tender frog is protected from injury by loose stones, and greater comfort given to both the horse and the driver.

FIG. 71.—FROG PAD.

FIG. 72.—FROG PAD APPLIED.

(e) By the Use of a Frog Pad and a Shoe of Ordinary Shape.—The shape of rubber on this pad is designed to cover the frog only. Its shape and mode of application is sufficiently shown in the accompanying illustrations.

(f) By turning out to Grass.—Where the expense of keep is no object, a return of contracted feet to the normal may be brought about by removing the shoes and turning the animal out to pasture, thus giving the feet the advantages to be derived from a more or less continuous operation of the normal movements of expansion and contraction. In this case the treatment must extend from three to four, or possibly six months.

2. By the Use of Some Form of Expansion Shoe.

FIG. 73.—SMITH'S EXPANSION SHOE SEEN FROM ITS GROUND SURFACE AND FROM THE SIDE. *a*, The screw, with a fine-cut thread; *b*, nut which travels along it; *c*, a hollow thimble into which the screw passes at one end, the other being cut out V-shaped to catch into a slot (*d*) on the shoe; *e, e*, the grip[A] for the bars, the length and direction of which depend upon the shape of the foot; *f, f*, the counter-sunk rivets forming the hinge (*f*); *g*, the counter-sunk rivet of the expanding piece.

[Footnote A: The inventor of this shoe uses the word 'grip' to denote what, in describing other expansion shoes, we term the 'clip' (H.C.R.).]

(a) Smith's.—For many years past continental writers have been practising this method. So far as we know, however, Lieutenant-Colonel Fred Smith was the first English veterinarian to use a shoe of his own devising, and to report on its effects. This shoe we will, therefore, give first mention.

The above figure, with its accompanying letterpress, sufficiently explains the nature of the shoe. In fitting the shoe, care must be taken to have the hinges (*f, f*) far enough back, or the shoe will have a tendency to spring at the heels, and the grips (*e, e*), which catch on the bars, will have a difficulty in biting. This trouble will be avoided by having the hinges about 1-1/2 to 2 inches from the heels.

After the shoe has been firmly nailed to the foot, the travelling nut *b* is driven forward on the screw *a* so as to cause the grips to just catch on the inside of the bars of the foot. According to the inventor, the amount of pressure to be exerted must be learned by experience, and he says:

'I screw up very gradually until I see the cleft of the frog just beginning to open. I now trot the horse up, and if he goes sound it is certain that the pressure I have exercised will not give rise to trouble. The animal is sent to work to assist in the expansion of the foot. On examining the shoe next day, the grip is found to be quite loose, the foot has enlarged, and the nut is turned once more until the grip on the bars is tightened, the horse being again trotted to ascertain that no injurious pressure is exerted.

'Every day or two I repeat this process, making measurements in all cases before widening the heels. The increase in width of the foot which results is astonishing, 1/4 to 3/8 inch during the first week may be safely predicted, and in a month to six weeks it is impossible to recognise in the large healthy frog and wide heels, the shrivelled-up organ of a short time before.'[A]

[Footnote A: *Journal of Comparative Pathology and Therapeutics*, vol. v., p. 98.]

It is pointed out by the writer of the above (and his observations, doubtless, apply to the use of all other expansion shoes in which the bars are gripped and forcibly expanded) that the whole secret of success lies in avoiding injurious pressure by exerting too great an expansion at one operation. After each manipulation of the expanding apparatus the horse should trot sound and the frog remain cool. Should the foot become hot, and lameness supervene, then tension should at once be relaxed.

Recorded Cases of the Use of the Shoe.—The inventor of the shoe relates two cases of contracted foot treated by these means in which the heels of one, after thirty-nine days' treatment, had increased in width to the extent of 1 inch, and the heels of the other, after twenty-four days', had enlarged 5/8 inch. Of the first case he gives the drawings in Fig. 74.

A represents the foot before treatment; B the same foot after nine days' treatment, when the heels had widened 3/4 inch; and C the same foot at the end of the thirty-nine days' treatment, at which date the frog was an excellent-looking one, and the foot had increased an inch in width.[A]

[Footnote A: *Journal of Comparative Pathology and Therapeutics*, vol. v., p. 100]

FIG. 74.—THE CHANGES IN FORM OF A CONTRACTED FOOT TREATED WITH SMITH'S EXPANSION SHOE

In 1893, at a meeting of the Midland Counties Veterinary Medical Association, the late Mr. Olver said he had applied this shoe to a valuable hunter that had gone so lame that he could scarcely put his foot to the ground. After a fortnight's application, and by the assistance of the double screw in the shoe, the heel was forced out. Then the horse was put to work with the shoe on, and he had hunted the whole of the last season in a perfectly sound condition.[A]

[Footnote A: *Veterinary Record*, vol. vi., p. 143]

F.D. McLaren, M.R.C.V.S., writes:[A] 'I resolved to try one of Captain Smith's shoes in a case where the hoof was badly contracted, and where the frog had entirely disappeared, there being also slight lameness. The roof rapidly expanded, and every other day the nut was moved on a bit to keep the cross-piece tight. I then had the cross-piece bent downwards a little *to prevent the nut pressing on the rapidly-growing frog.*[B] After another fortnight or so, I had a shoe made with clips resting against the inside of the bars,[C] and the next time he was shod these were also dispensed with. It is now a year ago since the animal recovered his frog, and he still has the largest frog in the stable, and the hoof shows no sign of contraction.'

[Footnote A: *Ibid.*, vol. vi., p. 183]

[Footnote B: The italics are mine (H.C.R.).]

[Footnote C: The expanding shoe itself was here evidently dispensed with, and an ordinary shoe with bar-clips used in its stead (H.C.R.).]

(b) De Fay's.—Among other shoes of the expansion class may be mentioned that of De Fay. Like the preceding, it is a shoe with a flat bearing surface, and provided with bar-clips. It is, however, *un* hinged. The requisite degree of periodic expansion is in this case arrived at by a forcible widening of the heels of the shoe, accomplished by bending the substance of which it is made, and for this purpose the instrument illustrated in Fig. 75 is employed.

The foot is first properly trimmed by levelling the heels and thinning the sole on each side of the frog. The shoe is then fixed by nails in the ordinary manner, taking care that the last nails come not too far back, and that the clips rest evenly and firmly on the inside of the bars.

The dilator, hoof-spreader, or vice, as it is variously called, is then applied, its two jaws (*a* and *b*) fitting against the inner edge of the shoe at the heels. Careful note is taken of the width of the hoof as measured on the graduated scale (*e, e*), and the double screw (*g, h*) revolved by means of the wrench (k), until the opening of the jaws thus obtained registers an expansion of 1/12 to 1/8 inch.

The dilatation is repeated at intervals of from eight to ten days, until, at the expiration of a month or six weeks, the amount of total expansion of the heels registers nearly an inch. That the method requires the greatest care may be gathered from the reports of continental writers. They state that frequently the pain and consequent lameness keep the patient confined to the stable for several days.

Numerous and but slightly differing forms of the dilator are on the market. As in principle they are all essentially the same, and are to be found illustrated in any reliable instrument catalogue, they need no description here.

FIG. 75.—DE FAY'S VICE.

(c) Hartmann's.—A further useful expansion shoe is that of Hartmann's (Fig. 76), in that it may be adapted for either unilateral or bilateral contraction. This shoe is also provided with bar-clips, and forcibly expanded at the heels by means of a dilator. The expansion is governed by saw-cuts through the inner margin of the shoe directed towards its outer margin, and running only partially through the inner half of the web (see Fig. 76).

According as the contraction is confined to the inner or outer heel, the saw-cuts, one or two in number, are placed to the inner or outer side of the toe-clip. When the contraction is bilateral, the saw-cuts, one or more in number, are placed on each side of the toe-clip.

(d) Broué's.—This is one of the forms of so-called 'slipper' shoes (see Fig. 77). We have already indicated that the shape of the bearing surface of the ordinary shoe—by its 'seating' or sloping from outside to inside—is sometimes a cause of contraction. In the 'slipper' of Broué this bearing is reversed, and the slope is from inside to outside. In the original form of this shoe the slope to the outside was continued completely round the shoe. Experience taught that the strain this enforced upon the junction of the wall with the sole was injurious, and that the 'reversed seating,' if we may so term it, was best confined to the hinder portions of the shoe's branches.

FIG. 76. This figure illustrates the principle of the Hartmann expanding shoe. *a, a,* The clips to catch the inside of the bars; *b, c,* saw-cuts.

The amount of slope should not be excessive. If it is, too rapid and too forcible an expansion takes place, and pain and severe lameness results. Dollar gives the requisite degree of incline by saying that the outer margin of the bearing surface of the shoe should be from 1/12 to 1/8 inch lower than the inner.

In the case of the Broué slipper, it is the animal's own weight that brings about the widening of the heels, the slope or outward incline of the slipper simply causing the inferior edge of the wall at the heels to spread itself outwards instead of sliding inwards on the bearing surface of the shoe.

FIG. 77.—THE SLIPPER SHOE OF BROUÉ.

(e) Einsiedel's.—Like the 'slipper' of Broué, the Einsiedel shoe depends for its effects upon the slope of the bearing surface.

It differs from the Broué in being provided with a 'bar-clip.' This, in addition to gripping the bars like the bar-clips of other expanding shoes, also assists, under the body-weight, in expanding the heels by the pronounced slope given to its upper surface. The expanding force exerted by the body-weight falls thus, through the medium of the bar-clip, clip, *partly* upon the bars, instead of, as in the Broué, solely upon the wall. We say *partly* advisedly, for, in addition to the slope upon the outer side of the bar-clips, the bearing surface of the heels of the shoe is *slightly* sloped outwards also. The good office served by the bar-clip is the lessening of any tendency to strain upon the white line.

FIG. 78.—THE SLIPPER AND BAR-CLIP SHOE OF EINSIEDEL.

Those we have described by no means exhaust the number of expansion shoes that have been devised. There are numerous others, many of which are composed of three-hinged portions, the two hindermost of which are gradually separated by a toothed arrangement of their inner margins and a travelling bar, the disadvantage of which is that it is liable to work loose. In the majority of this class of shoe the hinges are placed far forward, one on each side of the toe. They there become exposed to excessive wear. In fact, against the bulk of this form of shoe it may be urged that they cannot be worn by the animal at work, that they are expensive, difficult to make, and easily put out of order.

3. *By Operations on the Horn of the Wall.*

(a) Thinning the Wall in the Region of the Quarters.—This is best done by means of an ordinary farrier's rasp. The thinning should lessen gradually from the heel for 2-1/2 to 3 inches in a forward direction. That portion of the wall next to the coronary border, about 1/2 inch in breadth, should not be touched. At this point the thinning should commence, should be at its greatest, and lessen gradually downwards until at the inferior margin of the wall the normal thickness of horn is left. The animal is then shod with a bar shoe and the hoof bound with a bandage soaked in a mixture of tar and grease, in order to keep the thinned portion of the wall from cracking. In this condition the animal may remain at light labour.

When possible, however, it is better to combine the thinning process thus described with turning out to grass. In this case the ordinary shoe is first removed, and the foot poulticed for twenty-four hours to render the horn soft. The foot is then prepared by slightly lowering the heels—leaving the frog untouched—and thinning the quarters in exactly the manner described above.

After this is done, the animal is shod with an ordinary tip, a sharp cantharides blister applied to the coronet, and then turned out in a damp pasture. In this case the object of the tip is to throw the weight on to the heels and quarters. The thinned horn yields to the pressure thus applied, and a hoof with heels of a wider pattern commences to grow down from the coronet. Two to three months' rest is necessary before the animal can again he put to work.[A]

[Footnote A: This is the treatment strongly advocated by A.A. Holcombe, D.V.S., Inspector, Bureau of Animal Industry, U.S.A.]

(b) Thinning the Wall in the Region of the Toe.—This is done with the idea that the tendency of the heels to expand under pressure of the body-weight is helped by the thinned portion at the toe allowing the heels to more readily open behind. Seeing that in the case of toe sand-crack the converse is argued—that contraction of the heels readily takes place and forces the sand-crack wider open—it is doubtful whether this method is of any utility in treating contracted heels.

(c) Grooving the Wall Vertically or Horizontally, and Shoeing with a Bar Shoe.—Marking the wall with a series of grooves, each running in a more or less vertical direction, was suggested to English veterinarians by Smith's operation for side-bones.

The manner of making the grooves, and the instruments necessary, will be found fully described in Section C of Chapter X.

That the method is followed by satisfactory results the undermentioned case will show:

'A mare, which I have had in my possession since she was a foal, has always had contracted feet, which were also unnaturally small.... Lately the mare has been going very "short," and at length her action was quite crippled. At times she was decidedly lame on the off fore-foot. At no time have I been able to detect any sign of structural disease. I thereupon concluded that the lameness was due to mechanical pressure on the sensitive structures, and I determined to try the effects of the above treatment. As this was my first experience of the process, I was careful to carry it out in all its details, as described by Professor Smith. After the bar shoes had been put on, the mare was very lame. I allowed her two days' rest, then commenced regular walking exercise, and she daily improved. After fourteen days there was no lameness, but still short action. I thereupon gave the mare another week's walking exercise, at the expiration of which I drove her a short turn of five miles, which she did quite well, and free from lameness. For three months I kept the saw-cuts open to the coronet, and continued the bar shoes, keeping the mare at exercise, and giving her occasionally a drive. She never liked the bar shoes, and I was glad when I could discontinue them, which I did in the fourth month. When shod with the usual shoes the complete success of the treatment was shown. I have now had her going with the ordinary shoes for the past two or three months, and the improvement in the shape of the feet is very marked; there is no lameness; the mare is free in movement, fast, and spirited, whereas previously she was quite the reverse, and almost unfit to drive.'[A]

[Footnote A: W.S. Adams, M.R.C.V.S., *Veterinary Journal*, vol. xxx., p. 19.]

This method, though but recently introduced to the English veterinary surgeon, is by no means new. According to Zundel, it was recently made known on the Continent by Weber, but was previously known and mentioned by Lagueriniere, Brognier, and Hurtrel d'Arboval.

When the grooving is in a horizontal direction, a single incision is sufficient. This is made 3/4 inch below the coronary margin of the wall, and parallel with it, extending from the point of the heel for 2 or 3 inches in a forward direction. As in the previous method, a bar shoe is applied, and the animal daily exercised. Thus separated from the fixed and contracted portion of the wall below, the more elastic coronet under pressure of the body-weight commences to bulge. The bulging is of such an extent as to cause the new growing hoof from the top to considerably overhang the contracted portion below, and cure of the condition results from the newly-expanded wall above growing down in a normal direction.

This consideration of contracted heels may be concluded by drawing attention to the advisability of always maintaining the horn of the wall in as soft and supple a condition as is natural by the application of suitable hoof dressings.

A useful one for the purpose is that made with lard, to which has been added a small quantity of wax or turpentine.

Especially should a dressing like this be used when the hoof is inclined to be hard and brittle, and where tendency to contraction has already been noticed.

The application of a hoof ointment is also particularly indicated where the foot is much exposed to dampness, where the animal is compelled to stand for long periods upon a dry bedding, or where the bedding is of a substance calculated to have a deleterious effect upon the horn.

This, in conjunction with correct shoeing, will probably serve to avoid the necessity for more drastic measures at a later time.

(b) LOCAL OR CORONARY CONTRACTION.

Definition.—Contraction at the heels, confined to the horn immediately succeeding that occupied by the coronary cushion. Really, the condition is but a somewhat arbitrary subdivision of contracted hoof, as we have just described it in general. For that reason we shall give it but very brief mention.

Symptoms.—In this case the horn of the heels, instead of running down in a straight line from the coronary margin to the bearing surface of the wall, presents a more or less distinct concavity (See Fig. 79, *a, a*).

As is the case with contraction considered as a whole, this deformity may affect one or both heels; and during its first appearance, which is after the first few shoeings, the animal may go distinctly lame.

Causes.—Coronary contraction may occur in hoofs of normal shape immediately shoeing is commenced, and frog pressure with the ground removed. It is far more likely to ensue, however, if the hoof is flat, with the heels low, and the wall sloping. And with those predisposing circumstances it is that the horse goes lame, and not with the hoof of normal shape.

Seeing, then, that this condition is largely dependent upon the shape of the foot, we may, to some extent, regard it as hereditary. Seeing further, however, that it only appears when shoeing is commenced, we may in a greater degree also regard it as acquired. The lesson, therefore, that this and other forms of contraction should teach us is the carefulness with which the shoeing should be superintended in a large stud, or in any case where the animal is of more than ordinary value.

FIG. 79.—HOOF WITH LOCAL OR CORONARY CONTRACTION (AS INDICATED AT THE POINTS *a, a*).

The explanation of the restricted nature of this form of contraction is simple enough. We have only to refer to the lessons taught by the experiments of Lungwitz, described in Chapter III., and the condition almost explains itself. We remember that, briefly, the coronary margin of the wall resembles a closed elastic ring, which yields and expands to local pressure, no matter how slight. We remember also that removal of the counter-pressure of the frog with the ground tended to contraction of the wall's solar edge when weight was applied. Connect these two facts with the experience that this form of contraction more often than not occurs in hoofs with sloping heels, and we arrive at the following:

1. The excessive slope of the heels tends to throw a more than usual part of the body-weight upon the posterior portion of the coronary margin of the wall, with a consequent expansion of that part of the coronary margin implicated.

2. That the shoeing, in removing the counter-pressure of the frog with the ground, is at the same time tending to bring about contraction of the lower portions of the wall at the heels and quarters.

3. That this tendency to contraction will at first appear in the thinner portion of the area of wall named—namely, in that immediately below the bulging coronary margin.

We thus get the appearance depicted in Fig. 79—a contraction *(a, a)* of the heels in the horn below the coronary margin, with the coronary margin itself bulging above, and a hoof of apparently normal width below.

We say 'apparently' with a purpose, for, as actual measurements will show, the wall near the solar edge is really contracting, for reasons which we have just described connected with shoeing. Its 'appearance' of normal width is accounted for thus: The contraction at *a, a* is caused by the dragging inwards of the coronary cushion brought about by the sinking downwards of the plantar cushion, with which body it will be remembered the coronary cushion is continuous. With the constant dragging in and down of the coronary cushion there is given, to the horn-secreting papillæ, studding both the lower third of its outer face and its lowermost surface, a distinct 'cant' outwards. Below the lowermost limit of the coronary cushion, then, by reason of the cant outwards of the coronary papillæ in the situations mentioned, the horn of the wall takes a more outward direction than normal, a fact which lessens in effect the contraction as a whole really going on. It is interesting, too, to note that by this outward cant of the wall below, and the bulging of the coronary margin above it, the contraction *(a, a)* is heightened in effect, and caused to appear greater than really it is.

From what we have said it follows that contraction of the heels, excepting the extreme coronary margin, is existent generally, and not confined solely to *a, a.*

We have, then, in this condition, as we indicated at the commencement, but a phase in the evolution of ordinary contracted heels, for, with the progress of the contraction already existing at *a, a,* and below those points, it is only fair to assume that with it falling in of the at present bulging coronary margin must sooner or later occur, that, though expanded when compared with the wall below it, it will be really contracted as compared with what it was once in that same foot.

We may therefore conclude this section by remarking that factors tending to contraction of the heels in general are equally potent in the causation of contracted coronet alone.

Treatment.—Exactly that described for contracted heels. Bearing in mind that contracted coronary margin is but the onset of contracted heels, and that its first exciting cause is that of removal of the ground-pressure upon the frog, the most careful attention must be paid to the shoeing. The use of bar shoes, ordinary frog pads, or heelless shoes and bar pads, are especially indicated, together with abundant exercise. By these means the normal movements of expansion will be brought into play, and the condition quickly remedied.

C. FLAT-FOOT.

Definition.—By this term is indicated a condition of the foot where the natural concavity of the sole is absent.

Symptoms.—In the flat-foot the inferior edge of the wall, the sole, and the frog, all lie more or less in the same plane. It is a condition observed far more frequently in fore than in hind limbs, and is seen in connection with low heels, more or less obliquity of the wall, and a tendency to contraction. The action of the animal with flat feet is heavy, a result partly of the build of the foot, and partly of the tenderness that soon comes on through the liability of the sole to constant bruising.

FIG. 80. This figure represents the lower surface of a typical flat-foot. It illustrates, too, the commencement of a condition we referred to in Section B of this chapter—namely, the compression of the frog by the ingrowing heels (b) and bars (a).

Causes.—Flat-foot is undoubtedly a congenital defect, and is seen commonly in horses of a heavy, lymphatic type, and especially in those bred and reared on low, marshy lands. It is thus a common condition of the fore-feet of the Lincolnshire shire.

As might be expected, a foot of this description is far more prone to suffer from the effects of shoeing than is the foot of normal shape, and regarded in this light shoeing may be looked upon as, if not an actual cause, certainly a means of aggravating the condition. Directly the shoe—or at any rate the ordinary shoe—is applied, mischief commences. The frog is raised from the ground, and the whole of the weight thrown on to the wall. The heels, already weak and inclined to turn in, are unable to bear the strain. They *turn in*, and contraction commences. This 'turning in' of the heels is favoured by the undue obliquity of the wall. At the same time, the sole being archless, a certain amount of elasticity is lost. The weight is thrown more on to the heels, and the os pedis slightly descends, rendering the flatness of the sole even more marked than before. With the loss of elasticity of the sole concussion makes itself more felt. The animal is easily lamed, bruised sole becomes frequent, and corns sooner or later make their appearance.

Treatment.—Flat-foot is incurable. All that can be done is to pay careful attention to the shoeing, and so prevent the condition from being aggravated. In trimming the foot the sole should not be touched; the frog, too, should be left alone, and the wall pared only so far as regards broken and jagged pieces.

The most suitable shoe is one *moderately* seated. If the seating is excessive, and bearing allowed only on the wall, there is a tendency for the wall to be pushed outwards, and for the sole to drop still further. On the other hand, if the seating is insufficient, or the web of the shoe too wide, and too great a bearing thus given to the sole, then we get, first, an undue pressure upon the last-named portion of the foot a bruise, and, finally, lameness. The correct bearing should take in the whole of the wall and the whole of the white line, and should *just impinge* upon the sole. Above all, the heels of the shoe should be of full length, otherwise, if the shoe is worn just a little too long, its heels are carried under the sole of the foot, and by pressure there produce a corn.

If, with these precautions in shoeing flat-foot, tenderness still persists, a sole of leather or gutta-percha must be used with the shoe.

D. PUMICED-FOOT, DROPPED SOLE, OR CONVEX SOLE.

Definition.—This term is applied to the foot when the shape of the sole is comparable to the bottom of a saucer. When least marked it is really an aggravated form of flat-foot.

Symptoms.—In pumiced-foot the sole projects beyond the level of the wall. The obliquity of the latter is more marked than in the previous condition, and progression, to a large extent, takes place upon the heels. In addition to its deformity, the horn is greatly altered in quality, and, as the name 'pumice' indicates, is more or less porous in appearance, bulging, and brittle.

Causes.—As a general rule, it may be taken that pumiced-foot is a sequel of previous disease, although in its least pronounced form it may occur as the result of accidental or other causes, such as those described in the causation of flat-foot.

Occurring in its most marked form, there is no gainsaying the fact that pumiced-foot is a sequel of either acute or subacute laminitis. As we shall see when we come to study that disease, the dropping of the sole is brought about by distinct and easily-understood morbid processes affecting the sensitive structures. Briefly, these morbid processes in laminitis may be described thus: The accumulated inflammatory exudate, and in some cases pus, weakens and destroys the union between the sensitive and insensitive laminæ. This separation, for reasons afterwards to be explained, is greatest in the region of the toe. The os pedis, loosened from its intimate attachment with the horny box, is dropped upon the sole, and the sole, unable to bear the weight, commences to bulge below.

The altered character of the horn is accounted for by the inflammatory changes in the sensitive laminæ and the papillæ of the keratogenous membrane generally, for it follows as a matter of course that these tissues, themselves in a diseased condition, must naturally produce a horn of a greatly altered and inferior quality.

When following the *subacute* form of laminitis, the changes characterizing pumiced-foot are slow in making their appearance. The animal at first goes short, and the lameness thus indicated gradually becomes more severe, until the animal is no longer able to work. The feet become hot and dry, the hoof loses its circular form, and the growth of horn at the heels becomes excessive. At this stage the appearance of bulging at the sole begins to make itself seen. Later, the outer surface of the wall becomes 'ringed' or 'ribbed,' the rings being somewhat closely approximated in the region of the toe, and the distance between them gradually widening towards the heels. The wall too, especially in the region of the toe, instead of running in a straight line from the coronary margin to the shoe, becomes concave. It is this change, together with the appearance of the rings, that indicates the loosening of the attachment of the os pedis to the wall, and its afterwards backward and downward direction (see Fig. 124).

FIG. 81.—HOOF WITH THE RIBS OR RINGS CAUSED BY CHRONIC LAMINITIS.

As a sequel of *acute* laminitis, these changes make their appearance with more or less suddenness, and are generally complicated in that they owe their occurrence to the formation of pus within the horny box.

Treatment.—Pumiced-foot is always a serious condition. The animal is useless for work upon hard roads or town pavings, and is of only limited utility for slow work upon soft lands. The more serious form, that following acute laminitis, and complicated by the presence of pus, we may regard as beyond hope of treatment.

With the more simple form of the condition, we may do much to render greater the animal's usefulness. The same principles as were applied to the shoeing of flat feet will have to be observed here. Trimming or paring of any kind, save 'straightening up' of the wall, must be severely discountenanced. A broad-webbed shoe, one that will give a certain amount of cover to the sole, is indicated. As in the treatment of flat-foot, however, direct pressure upon the sole must be avoided, and the shoe 'seated.' The 'seating,' however, should not commence from the absolute outer margin of the shoe's upper surface. A *flat* bearing should be given to the wall and the white line, and the seating commenced at the sole.

We have already remarked on the increased growth of horn at the heels. It is in this position, then, that will be found the greatest bearing surface for the shoe, and it is wise, in this case, to have the heels of the shoe kept flat. In other words, the 'seating' is not to be continued to the hindermost portion of the branches of the shoe. By this means there may be obtained at each heel a good solid bearing of from 2 to 3 inches, which would otherwise be lost.

Where the accompanying condition of the horn is bad enough to indicate it, a leather sole should be used, beneath which has been packed a compress of tow and grease, rendered more or less antiseptic by being mixed with tar.

Where the sole is exceedingly thin, and inclined to be easily wounded, and where the hoof, by its brittleness, has become chipped and ragged at the lower margin of the wall, it may perhaps be more advantageous to use, in place of the compress of tow, the *huflederkitt* of Rotten. This is a leather-like, dark brown paste. When warmed in hot water, or by itself, it becomes soft and plastic, and may readily be pressed to the lower surface of the foot, so as to fill in all little cracks and irregularities, and furnish a complete covering to the sole and frog, and to the bearing surface of the wall. When cold it hardens, without losing the shape given to it, into a hard, leather-like substance.

Treated in this way, the animal with pumiced feet may yet be capable of earning his living at light labour or upon a farm.

E. 'RINGED' OR 'RIBBED' HOOF.

Definition.—A condition of the hoof in which the wall is marked by a series of well-defined ridges in the horn, each ridge running parallel with the coronary margin. They are known commonly as 'grass rings,' and may be easily distinguished from the more grave condition we have alluded to as following laminitis, by the mere fact that they do not, as do the laminitic rings, approximate each other in the region of the toe, but that they run round the foot, as we have already said, *parallel with each other.*

FIG. 82.—HOOF SHOWING THE RINGS IN THE HORN BROUGHT ABOUT BY PHYSIOLOGICAL CAUSES.

Causes.—This condition is purely a physiological, and not a pathological one, and the words of its more common name, 'grass rings,' sufficiently indicate one of the most common causes. Anything tending to an alternate increase and decrease in the secretion of horn from the coronet will bring it about. Thus, in an animal at grass, with, according to the weather conditions, an alternate moistness and dryness of the pasture, with its consequent influence on the horn secretion, these rings nearly always appear. The effects of repeated blisters to the coronet make themselves apparent in the same way, and testify to the efficacy of blisters in this region in any case where an increased growth of horn is deemed necessary. From this it is clear that the condition depends primarily upon the amount and condition of the blood supplied to the coronary cushion. Thus, fluctuations in temperature during a long-continued fever, or the effects of alternate heat and cold, or of healthy exercise alternated with comparative idleness, will each rib the foot in much the same manner.

Treatment.—The condition is so simple that we may almost regard it as normal. Consequently, treatment of any kind is superfluous. Where constitutional disturbance is exerting an influence upon either the quality or quantity of the blood directed to the part, then, of course, attention must be paid to the disease from which it is arising.

F. THE HOOF WITH BAD HORN.

(*a*) THE BRITTLE HOOF.

Definition.—As the name indicates, we have in this condition an abnormally dry state of the horn.

Symptoms.—These are obvious. The horn is hard, and when cut by the farrier's tools gives the impression of being baked hard and stony, the natural polish of the external layer is wanting, and there is present, usually, a tendency to contracted heels. With the dryness is a liability to fracture, especially at points where the shoe is attached by the nails. As a consequence, the shoes are easily cast, leading to splits in the direction of the horn fibres. These run dangerously near the sensitive structures, giving rise in many cases to lameness.

Even where pronounced lameness is absent the action becomes short and 'groggy,' and the utmost care is required in the shoeing to keep the animal at work.

Causes.—To a very great extent the condition is hereditary, and is observed frequently in animals of the short, 'cobby' type. In ponies bred in the Welsh and New Forest droves the condition is not uncommon, especially in the smaller animals. Animals who have had their feet much in water—as, for instance, those bred and reared on marshy soils—and afterwards transferred to the constant dryness of stable bedding, are also particularly liable to this condition. It is noticed, too, following the excessive use of unsuitable hoof-dressings, more especially in cases where coat after coat of the dressing is applied without occasionally removing the previous applications.

Treatment.—As a prophylactic, a good hoof-dressing is indicated. It should not consist solely of grease, but should have mixed with it either wax, turpentine, or tar.

Above all, careful shoeing should be insisted on, and the owner of an animal with feet such as these will be well advised if he is recommended to have the shoeing superintended by one well competent to direct it rightly. The foot should be trimmed but lightly, always remembering that in a foot of this description the horn, in addition to being brittle, is generally abnormally thin. Jagged or partly broken pieces should be removed, and the bearing surface rendered as level as possible. The foot should be carefully examined before punching the nail-holes in the shoe, and the nail-holes afterwards placed so as to come opposite the soundest portions of horn. The nails themselves should be as thin as is consistent with durability, and should be driven as high up as possible.

On the least sign of undue wear the shoes should be removed, never, as is too often done, allowing them to remain on so long that a portion breaks away. If, with the laudable idea of not interfering with the horn more than is possible, this is practised, the portion of the shoe breaking off is bound to tear away with it more or less of the brittle horn to which it is attached.

Where the breaks in the horn are so large as to prevent a level bearing for the shoe being obtained, the interstices should be filled up with one or other of the preparations made for this purpose. One of the most suitable is that discovered by M. Defay. By its means sand-cracks or other fractures of the horn may be durably cemented up.

'Even pieces of iron may be securely joined together by its means. The only precaution for its successful application is the careful removal of all grease by spirits of sal-ammoniac, sulphide of carbon, or ether. M. Defay makes no secret of its composition, which is as follows: Take 1 part of coarsely-powdered gum-ammoniac, and 2 parts of gutta-percha, in pieces the size of a hazel-nut. Put them in a tin-lined vessel over a slow fire, and stir constantly until thoroughly mixed. Before the thick, resinous mass gets cold mould it into sticks like sealing-wax. The cement will keep for years, and when required for use it is only necessary to cut off a sufficient quantity, and remelt it immediately before application. We have frequently used this cement for the repair of seriously broken hoofs. It is so tenacious that it will retain the nails by which the shoe is attached without tearing away from the hoof.'[A]

[Footnote A: *Veterinary Journal*, vol. iii., p.71.]

Failing this, the bearing surface may be made level, and fractures repaired by using the *huflederkitt* described in the treatment of pumiced sole.

(*b*) THE SPONGY HOOF.

Definition.—This is the opposite condition to the one we have just described, and is characterized by the soft and non-resistant qualities of the horn.

Symptoms.—Spongy hoof is quite common in animals that have large, flat, and spreading feet—in fact, the two appear to run very much together. It is a common defect in animals reared in marshy districts, and of a heavy, lymphatic type. The Lincolnshire Shire, for instance, has often feet of this description, and, the causative factors being in this case long-continued, render the feet extremely predisposed to canker. The horn is distinctly soft to the knife, and has an appearance more or less greasy. Animals with spongy feet are unfit for long journeys on hard roads. When compelled to travel thus, the feet become hot and tender, and lameness results. A mild form of laminitis, extending over a period of three or four days, often follows on this enforced travelling on a hard road, more especially in cases where the animal is 'heavy topped,' and the usual food of a highly stimulating nature. In fact, it has been the author's experience to meet with this condition several times in the case of shire stallions doing a long walk daily upon hard roads, with the weather hot and dry.

Treatment.—When a horse with spongy feet is shod for the first time, care must be taken to avoid excessive paring of the sole, for already the natural wear of the foot has been sufficient to keep the soft horn in a state of thinness. For the same reason hot fitting of the shoe must not be indulged in for too long a time. That common malpractice of the forge, 'opening up the heels,' must, in this case, be especially guarded against, or the excessive paring of the frog and partial removal of the bars that this operation consists in will lay the foot open to risk of contraction. To begin with, the heels are naturally weak, and, once the bars are removed, there is nothing to prevent them rapidly caving in towards the frog. Even when carefully shod, a foot of this class is readily prone to contract directly the animal is brought into the stable, and the horn commences to dry to excess. An ordinary light shoe should be used, and the nails should be light and thin. They should be driven carefully home, and the 'clinching' made as tight and secure as possible.

G. CLUB-FOOT.

Definition.—Under this name we indicate all cases in which the horn of the wall become straightened from above to below. It will, therefore, include all conformations varying from the so-called 'upright hoof,' in which the toe forms an angle of more than 60 degrees with the ground, to the badly 'clubbed' foot, in which the horn at the toe forms a right angle with the ground, or is even directed obliquely backwards and downwards, so that the coronary margin overhangs the solar edge of the wall.

FIG. 83.—THE CLUB-FOOT.

Symptoms.—Even in its least pronounced form the condition is apparent at a glance, the alteration in the angle formed by the hoof with the ground striking the eye at once, and the heels, as compared with the toe, appearing much too high. When the condition is slight, the wall of the toe is about twice as high as that of the heels, while in the most marked form the toe and the heels may in height be nearly equal (see Fig. 83). When congenital, but little interference with the action is noticed. Such animals, by reason of their 'stiltiness,' are unfit for the saddle, but at ordinary work will perform their duties equally well with the animal of normal-shaped feet. When acquired as the result of overwork, of contracted tendons, or other causes, however, the gait becomes stumbling and uncertain. The body-weight is transferred from the heels to the anterior parts of the foot, and the shoe shows undue signs of wear at the toe.

Causes.—Upright hoof is undoubtedly hereditary, and is even seen as a natural conformation in the feet of asses and mules. When hereditary in the horse, however, it is certainly a defect, and is associated commonly with an upright limb, and a short, upright pastern (see Fig. 83).

Among other causes, we may enumerate sprains or wounds of the flexor tendons, or any disease of the limbs for a long time preventing extension of the fetlock-joint, such as sprains or injuries of the posterior ligaments of the limb, splints or ringbones so placed as to interfere with the movements of the flexor tendons, or, in the hind-limb, spavin, keeping for some months the fetlock in a state of flexion. In the very young animal the condition may be induced by an improper paring of the foot—cutting away too much at the toe, and allowing the heels to remain.

Treatment.—When the condition is congenital, no treatment at all is indicated. It might, in fact, be said that interference would tend rather to minimize than enhance the animal's usefulness; for, in this case, the club-shaped feet are in all probability due to faulty conformation above. In other words, the upright hoof is in this instance but a natural result of the animal's build, with which useful interference is impossible.

Where the upright hoof is a consequence of excessive paring of the toe, or insufficient removal of the heels, the condition may be remedied by directing attention to those particulars, and preventing their continuance. At the same time, a greater obliquity of the limb axis may be given by the use of a suitable shoe. The shoe indicated is a short one, with thin heels and a thick toe. In some cases the abnormality may be remedied by the use of a tip. Whatever method is adopted, care must be taken not to attempt too positive a change in the direction of the limb at one operation. The process must be gradual.

In cases where the abnormality has been brought about by wounds to the flexor tendons, the alteration in the direction of the limb is often so great as to produce 'knuckling over' of the fetlock. This, to a very great extent, may be remedied by the use of a shoe with calkins and an extended toe-piece (see Fig. 84).

FIG. 84.—THE SHOE WITH EXTENDED TOE-PIECE AND HIGH CALKINS.

With this shoe a certain amount of forced exercise is advisable, and at intervals of about two weeks the calkins should be somewhat lowered, until the heels are brought as close to the ground as is possible. In giving directions for this shoe to be made the veterinary surgeon must, when referring to the length of the toe-piece, be guided entirely by the condition of the case. Ordinarily, a suitable length is from 3 to 4 inches. It is necessary also to warn the owner that, by reason of the length projecting, the shoe is liable to be torn off.

Should the 'knuckling over' have become complicated by bony deposits round the seat of the original injury, then a favourable modification of the condition is not so likely to result.

The benefit to be derived from the shoe with an extended toe-piece in a case of excessive knuckling is admirably shown in a brief report of a case, under the title of 'Hooked Foot,' in vol. xiv. of the *Veterinary Record*, p. 716:

'An eighteen months' old filly showed a deformity of the third phalanx, resulting in her walking with the front face of the hoof on the ground. The flexors were apparently all right, and the bending back seemed to be due to contraction of the ligaments of the joint and the sheath of the perforans.

'On the ground of absence of contraction of the flexors, or atrophy and paralysis of the extensors, the surgeon considered the lesion curable by simple orthopædic measures. By means of an elongated toe-piece to the shoe and calkins, which were shortened every fifteen days, the filly was completely cured in seventy days.'

H. THE CROOKED FOOT.

(*a*) THE FOOT WITH UNEQUAL SIDES.

Definition.—The foot thus affected has one side of the wall higher than the other.

Symptoms.—This deformity is the better recognised when the foot on the floor is viewed from behind. In addition to the difference between the height of the inner and outer heel is seen at once a deviation in the normal direction of the horn. That of the higher side is distinctly more upright than that of the lower, and runs from above downwards and inwards towards the axis of the foot, while the horn of the lower side maintains its normal direction of downwards and outwards.

From what we have said before on contracted foot, this bending in of the wall of the upright side will at once be recognised as a form of contraction. It is, in fact, contraction confined to one-half of the foot only, and, as a result, the upright side of the crooked foot is prone to the troubles arising from that condition. Corns are frequent, and atrophy of that half of the frog on the affected side supervenes. With the inflammatory changes accompanying these conditions we find the horn of the affected side deteriorating in quality. It becomes dry and brittle, and extremely liable to sand-crack. At the same time, thrush of the contracted frog begins to make its appearance.

Causes.—More often than not this condition is a result of the conformation of the limb. According as the build above inclines the animal to 'turned in' or 'turned out' toes, so shall we have feet with a wall crooked inwards or crooked outwards; and it may be mentioned here that the evil results inflicted on the foot by ill-shaped limbs above will make themselves the more readily noticed when the animal comes to be shod for any length of time. So long as a natural wear of the foot is allowed, so long does it accommodate itself to the form of limb above. So soon, however, as the shoe is applied, and a more or less equal (and in this case harmful) wear by that means insisted on, so soon does this abnormal change in the height and direction of the horn fibres begin to make itself seen.

While arising in the majority of instances from faulty conformation of the limb, crooked feet may also be brought about by bad shoeing, or by unequal paring of the foot, and, in a few cases, from unequal wear of the foot in a state of nature.

Treatment.—Although it may be taken as a rule that lowering of the higher wall, even if persisted in at every shoeing, will do nothing towards remedying the primary cause (viz., the evil conformation of the limb), yet it will serve to keep the condition within reasonable limits. In this case, while removing so much of the wall as is deemed necessary, care must be taken to leave uncut the sole and the bar. Leaving these intact gives us two natural and very potent protections against the contraction already mentioned as impending.

Where, by reason of the thinness of the horn or other causes, sufficient paring to equalize the tread cannot be practised, then the same end may be arrived at by the use of special shoes. That branch of the shoe applied to the half of the foot with the lower wall should be thickened from above downwards. Or, on the same branch, may be turned up a calkin of sufficient height for the purpose. Of the two methods the first is preferable.

In any case, whether depending upon paring, or upon the use of a special shoe, the animal should be sent to the forge quite often, for it is only by a well-directed, and therefore constant, application of the principles here laid down that improvement may be brought about.

When marked contraction of one-half of the foot is present, it will be best treated with the expanding shoe of Hartmann, already described in the section of this chapter dealing with contracted heels (see Fig. 76).

(*b*) THE CURVED HOOF.

Definition.—The hoof with the wall of one side convex, and that of the opposite side concave. Fig. 85, showing the foot in section from side to side, gives an exact idea of this malformation.

Causes.—As was the case with the condition previously described, this abnormality finds its primary cause in an unequal distribution of weight due to vice of conformation in the limb above, causing one side of the hoof to be higher than the other. As a result of this, the wall that is inordinately increasing in height commences to bulge outwardly (Fig. 85, *a*), while the opposite (Fig. 85, *b*) becomes concave.

The same state of affairs may be occasioned in the forge by leaving one side of the foot too high, and subjecting the other to excessive paring for several consecutive shoeings.

Treatment.—In the main this condition may be regarded as a long-standing and aggravated form of the foot with unequal sides. We may say at once, therefore, that it is not so easily remedied as that simpler defect; that, although identical principles will be followed in its treatment, cure must be a matter of some considerable time.

FIG. 85.—SECTION THROUGH A CROOKED FOOT. *a*, The higher and convex side of the wall; *b*, the lower and concave side of the wall

Again, we must look to successive parings of the wall of the higher side to bring about a gradual return to the normal. At the same time, the tendency to contraction of that side is counteracted by shoeing wide, and, if necessary, giving to the upper surface of that branch of the shoe what we have termed elsewhere a 'reversed seating'—viz., an incline of its upper surface from within outwards.

CHAPTER VII
DISEASES ARISING FROM FAULTY CONFORMATION
A. SAND-CRACK.

Definition.—A solution of continuity of the horn of the foot, occurring usually in the wall, and following the direction of the horn fibres.

Classification.—It is usual to classify sand-cracks according to—

(*a*) *Their Position.*—*Toe-crack* when occurring in the middle line of the horn of the toe, and *quarter-crack* when occurring in the horn of the quarters.

Sand-crack of the frog and sand-crack of the sole may also each be met with. They are, however, of rare occurrence, and are seldom serious enough to merit special attention.

The toe-crack is met with more often in the hind-foot than in the fore, while the quarter-crack more often than not makes its appearance in the fore-foot, and is there, as a rule, confined to the inner side. The reasons for these positions being so affected we shall deal with when treating of the causes of sand-crack in general. It is interesting to note that the portions of wall known as inside and outside toe are seldom affected.

(*b*) *Their Length.*—*Complete* when they extend from the coronary margin of the wall to its wearing edge; *Incomplete* when not so extensive.

(*c*) *Their Severity.*—*Simple* when they occur in the horn only, and do not implicate the sensitive structures beneath; *Complicated* when deep enough to allow of laceration and subsequent inflammation of the keratogenous membrane. Such complications may vary from a simple inflammation set up by laceration and irritation of the sensitive structures by particles of dirt and grit that have gained entrance through the crack, to other and more serious changes in the shape of the formation of pus, hæmorrhage from the laminal vessels, caries of the os pedis, or the development of a tumour-like growth of horn on the inner surface of the wall known as a keraphyllocele.

(*d*) *Their Duration.*—*Recent* when newly formed; *old* when of long standing.

(*e*) *Their Starting-point.*—This last distinction we make ourselves, and, referring to cracks of the wall, term them *high* when commencing from the coronary margin, *low* when starting from the bearing surface.

Causes.—We have already classified sand-crack as a disease arising from faulty conformation. Thus, in just so far as a predisposing build of body may be handed down from parent to offspring, we may regard sand-crack as hereditary. If we do so, however, we must afterwards make up our minds to sharply distinguish between the sand-crack plainly brought about by accidental cause, and that occurring as a result of hereditary evil conformation.

With regard to the latter, we need hardly say that feet with abnormally brittle horn are extremely liable. But with this, as with many other affections of the feet, we shall find it necessary to consider several causes acting in cooperation. In this case, for instance, given the brittle horn, it becomes necessary to further look for exciting causes of its fracture.

We will take conformation first. In the animal with turned-out toes a more than fair share of the body-weight is imposed on the horn of the inner quarter. Here, then, three causes exert their influence together: The horn is brittle; the wall of the inner quarter is thinner than that of the outer; additional weight is imposed upon it. Fracture results.

Take, again, the vice of contracted heels. Here, in the first place, we have a variety of causes tending to bring about the contraction. With the contraction, and its consequent pressure upon the sensitive structures in the region of the quarters and the frog, has arisen a low type of inflammation. The horn of the part has become dry and brittle. The exciting cause of its fracture is found in an excessive day's work upon a hard, dry road, with, perhaps, a suddenly-imposed improper distribution of weight, due to treading upon a loose stone, or a succession of such evil transfers of weight due to travelling upon a road that is rough in its whole extent.

In their turn, too, such defects of the feet as we have mentioned in the last chapter—as, for example, the foot with the pumiced horn, the foot with abnormally upright heels, or that which is upright on one side only, or crooked—each offers a condition which is predisposing to the formation of a sand-crack. In each case it wants but the uneven distribution of the body-weight, which, as a matter of fact, some of these conditions themselves give, to bring about a fracture.

Apart from the predisposition conferred by conformation, must be remembered the simpler predisposing causes leading to brittleness of the hoof. We refer to the after-effects of poulticing, the moving from pasture to stable, the emigration from a damp to a dry climate, or the alternate changes from damp to dry in a temperate region. Each may have a deteriorating influence upon the horn, rendering it liable to the condition we are describing. Excessive dampness alone, especially when the animal is called upon to labour at the drawing of heavy loads upon a rough road, is not infrequently a cause. In this case the wet, together with the constant friction of the sharp materials of which the road is made, serves to destroy the varnish-like periople. The wet gains access to the inner structures of the wall, the agglutination of the horn fibres is weakened, and fissures begin to appear.

Other causes of sand-crack are purely accidental. An animal at fast work over-reaches. The secretion of horn at the injured coronet is interfered with, a diminished supply at an isolated spot being the result. From this point grows down a fissure in the wall.

An injury of the same character may also be sustained in various other ways—treads from other animals when working in pairs, accidental wounding with the stable-fork, blows of any kind, or a self-inflicted tread with the calkin of an opposite foot—each with the same result.

So far as causation is concerned, toe-crack stands in a class almost by itself. It is met with nearly always in a heavy animal in the hind-foot, and is directly attributable to the force exerted in starting a heavy load.

Unskilful shoeing also plays a part in the causation of sand-crack. Removal of the periople by excessive rasping of the wall is most certainly a predisposing cause. Cracks, or their starting-points, may also be caused by using too wide a shoe, or by the use of nails too large in the shank. Also, they may arise from unskilful fitting of the toe-clip, especially in the hind-foot of a heavy animal. It must be admitted, however, that the part shoeing plays in the causation of sand-crack is not a large one; far more depends upon the state of the horn and the animal's conformation than upon the exciting cause.

So far, our observations on the causes of sand-crack have referred to that form occurring in the wall. Sand-crack of the sole or frog we have already said is but seldom met with, and then it is always in connection with some exceptionally deteriorated quality of the horn, as in the case of badly pumiced feet, or occurs as a result of direct injury. Extensive slit-like cuts in this region, when deep enough to lacerate the keratogenous membrane, are sometimes followed by the growth of a fissure in the horn, and what might almost be termed a permanent sand-crack results. Such cuts may be occasioned by sharp flints, broken glass, or other sharp objects picked up on the road, or may result from the animal treading on the toe-clip of a partially cast shoe.

Symptoms.—In every case the fissure, or evidence of its commencement, is a diagnostic symptom. It is well to remember, however, that this may be easily overlooked, especially when the crack is one commencing at the coronary margin. The reason is this: Sand-cracks in this position often commence in the wall proper, and not in the periople. They may, in fact, be first observed as a fine separation of the horn fibres immediately beneath the perioplic covering. A crack of this description may even show hæmorrhage, and have been in existence for some time, without the periople itself showing any lesion whatever. Thus, unless lameness is present, or a more than specially keen search is directed to the parts in question, the sand-crack goes undiscovered, until of greater dimensions.

Further, the fissure may be hidden, either accidentally or of set purpose. It may be covered by the hair, filled in and covered over with mud, or intentionally concealed by being 'stopped' with an artificial horn, with wax, or with gutta-percha, or, as is more common, be hidden by the lavish application of a greasy hoof-dressing.

In this latter connection it is well to warn the veterinary surgeon, especially the beginner, when examining for soundness, to be keenly critical before passing an animal who is presented with feet smothered with tar and grease or any other dressing. More especially should this warning be heeded when examining any of the heavier breeds of animal with an abundance of hair about the coronet.

Referring again to the search for the crack, it is well to know that with toe-crack the fissure is the more readily seen when the foot is lifted from the ground. With quarter-crack, on the other hand, the fissure is wider, and consequently the easier detected with the foot bearing weight.

Although commencing in the insidious manner we have described, the lesion is not thus often seen by the veterinary surgeon. Usually, the animal with sand-crack is brought for his inspection when lameness has arisen from it. In this case the cause for the lameness will reveal itself in the crack, which is now too large to escape observation. The coronet is hot and tender to the touch, and a sensation of warmth is sometimes conveyed to the hand by the horn of the surrounding parts of the wall. It is hardly necessary to say that, with accompanying conditions such as these, the sand-crack is a *deep* one.

Where the lameness is but slight, we may attribute it almost solely to the pain occasioned by the mere wounding of the keratogenous membrane, and to no very extensive inflammatory changes therein. By some authorities this is said to be due to the pinching of the sensitive structures between the edges of the fissure in the horny covering. In our opinion, however, pinching does not occur unless inflammatory exudation into the sensitive structures adjoining the crack has led to sufficient swelling to cause them to protrude. In other words, the movements of the horny box, communicating themselves to the structures beneath, and so occasioning movement in the wounded keratogenous membrane, are quite sufficient to give rise to the lameness without actual pinching of the structures implicated.

The severity of the lameness will vary with the rapidity of the gait, and with the character of the road upon which the animal is made to travel. For instance, many animals in which the lameness is imperceptible at a walk become 'dead' lame at a fast trot. It is sufficiently explained when one remembers the greater movements of expansion and contraction of the posterior parts of the wall brought about by the increase in the rate of progression. The same animal, too, will go distinctly more lame upon a hard than upon a soft surface.

In like manner the lameness from toe-crack also varies in degree with the rate of progression and the character of the travelling, though not to such a noticeable extent as in the lameness from quarter-crack. A greater variation may in this case be brought about by moving the animal on ascending and descending ground. Descending an incline, with a more than ordinary share of the body-weight thus thrown upon the heels, the lameness is most marked. The reason would appear to be that the greater expansion of the wall of the heels thus brought about leads to a proportionate contraction of the wall at the toe, especially at the edges of the crack, thus causing undue pressure upon the exact spot of the wound in the sensitive structures. Ascending—the weight in this case transferred from the posterior to the anterior portion of the foot—the expansion of the heels becomes a contraction, with a corresponding lessening of the contraction at the toe and a distinct decrease in the lameness.

In the case of a deep but recent crack there is always more or less hæmorrhage. This favours risk of infection of the lesion with pus-forming organisms, and so leads to a more or less pronounced lameness, a degree of swelling, heat and tenderness in the coronet above, and a certain amount of surgical fever.

The acute symptoms subdued, but the fissure still remaining, gives us the crack we have classified as 'old.' This may in every case be distinguished from a more recent lesion by the amount of thickening of the overhanging coronet, and the presence of an increased quantity of sub-coronary horn in the region immediately about the crack. The previous inflammatory changes in the adjoining sensitive structures have here led to an increased secretion of horn, and a greater or less deposition of inflammatory connective tissue in the wounded coronary cushion.

Sand-crack of the toe always follows the direction of the horn fibres. That of the quarter, however, may on occasion run a course that is somewhat zigzag, first following the direction of the horn fibres for a short distance, then travelling in a horizontal direction, and finally continuing its course again in a line with the horn fibres, commonly at a point posterior to that at which it commenced.

In a quarter-crack that is old, and when contraction of the heels exists (which in this case it usually does), then will often be found overlapping of the edges of the crack. The expansion of the wall brought about when the body-weight is on the heels, cannot, by reason of the break in it, continue itself anterior to the crack. As a consequence, repeated expansion of the wall posterior to the crack, with the portions anterior to it in a state of enforced quiescence, leads in time to the posterior edge of the crack coming to lie over that of the anterior.

Complications.—The first complication likely to arise in a case of sand-crack is that attending simple laceration of the sensitive structures in a *deep* lesion. With the laceration all the phenomena of a repairing inflammation make their appearance. As a result, there is more or less heat according to the degree of inflammatory hyperæmia, swelling according to the amount of inflammatory exudate, and pain according to the amount of pressure the two foregoing bring to bear on the nerves in the inflamed area.

A second and more serious complication is the greater inflammation set up by the introduction into the crack of foreign substances. Small portions of gravel and flint, both by the irritation set up by their friction and by the infection they carry in with the dirt surrounding them, are responsible for the mischief.

When, from direct communication with the blood-stream, due to extensive hæmorrhage, bacteria from the outside gain entrance, this simple inflammation is further complicated by the formation of pus, or a limited gangrene of the keratogenous membrane.

In cases of great severity the gangrene of the keratogenous membrane spreads until the deeper structures are involved. We then get a necrosis (in the case of toe-crack) of the extensor pedis, and sometimes caries of the os pedis.

In like manner the necrotic changes occurring under these circumstances may invade the deeper structures in the region of quarter-crack. As a result of this, we may have the starting-point of suppurating corn, or necrosis of the lateral cartilage—in other words, cartilaginous quittor.

Commonly accompanying quarter-crack is the condition of contracted heels and atrophied frog. Sometimes described as a complication of sand-crack, it appears to us more rational to rather regard the sand-crack as a result or complication of the vice of contraction.

The overlapping of the edges of the crack before referred to occasionally gives rise to the condition known as false quittor. A probe or a director passed beneath the overhanging ledge of horn reveals sometimes a fissure of 1 inch or considerably more in depth, and quittor is diagnosed. A careful paring away of the overhanging horn, however, reveals the true state of affairs, and exposes to view the original cause of the mischief—a simple fissure in the wall.

A serious complication—one fortunately met with but rarely—is that of keraphyllocele. This is a tumour-like growth of horn, varying in size from the thickness of an ordinary quill pen to that of one's middle finger, growing down from the coronary cushion, and attached to the inner side of the wall of the hoof. With this lameness is always present, and more or less deformity of the hoof results. This condition will be found described at greater length in Chapter IX.

Prognosis.—In the case of sand-crack this should always be guarded. It may be taken as a general rule that cracks commencing from the coronary margin are more troublesome to deal with than those originating below. The reason is not far to seek. They here affect the wall just where the bevel in it for the accommodation of the coronary cushion has rendered it weakest. Not only is it weakest, but being more resilient than the portions below it, it suffers more from the alternate movements of expansion and contraction of the foot than does the horn below.

Although in many cases a cure of the existing crack may be easily accomplished, regard should be paid to the possibility of its recurrence, either in the same position or elsewhere. Really, in offering an opinion as to the future usefulness of an animal so affected, a greater attention should be directed to the animal's conformation than to the crack itself. Where the vice of conformation giving rise to it (as, for example, contracted heels or upright hoof) gives hope of being remedied, then naturally it may be safely said that the liability to sand-crack goes with it.

A like favourable prognosis may be given in the case of cracks occasioned by purely accidental causes.

Ordinarily, however, cracks once commenced tend rather to increase than decrease in size and severity. From being superficial and incomplete, they become complete and deep, with every unfavourable circumstance that an increase in size and depth brings with it.

This much, however, may be promised to the owner. A simple crack, even though originating from the coronary margin, is, in the vast majority of cases, curable. Under a rational treatment its increase in size may be prevented, and a sound wall caused to grow down from the coronet.

Treatment.—The principles governing the treatment of sand-crack are simple enough in themselves, if not always followed by success.

1. *Preventive.*

This, as a rule, does not suggest itself until a crack of greater or less extent has made its appearance. Then, simultaneously with the treatment proper of the lesion, preventive measures should be adopted, to aid both in the healing of the fissure already present, and to ward off the occurrence of others that might be likely to form. The hoof, if abnormally brittle, should be regularly dressed with a suitable ointment (one containing glycerine for preference), and its horn kept as nearly as possible in a normal condition. When the condition of the horn predisposing to its fracture is brought about by excessive wet, then the appropriate preventive measures to be adopted suggest themselves.

With regard to the lesion itself, we may term 'preventive treatment' all those measures having for their object the prevention of increase in the size of the crack. They are as follows:

(a) Blistering the Coronet.—In a simple case, where the crack is superficial and close under the coronary margin of the wall, a sharp cantharides blister to the coronet immediately above it will have the desired effect. An increased secretion of horn is brought about, and by this simple means the crack prevented from becoming longer. Very often this is all that is necessary. In fact, we may say here that, no matter what other treatment is adopted, the simultaneous application of a blister to the coronet is always beneficial. To derive full advantages therefrom, the blistering should be repeated several times at intervals of about a fortnight.

(b) Clamping the Crack.—When the services of a skilled smith are at hand, one of the readiest methods of performing this is to draw the edges of the crack together with an ordinary horse-nail.

On each side of the crack a small horizontal furrow is burned or cut into the wall, leaving the horn for about 1/4 inch on each side of the crack intact. This provides a groove for the ends of the clamping-nail to rest in, and brings them flush with the outer surface of the wall. The nail is then driven carefully home through the crack, and the pointed end grasped by the farrier's pincers. The edges of the crack are then drawn tightly together, and the nail firmly clenched.

FIG. 86.—THE SAND-CRACK FIRING-IRON.

'The horse-nails are prepared in the ordinary way as for driving, with the exception that each is pointed on the reverse side, to prevent puncturing the sensitive structures. Before being used the nails are put in a vice, and the head hammered to form a shoulder, to prevent their being driven too far into the wall, and breaking out the hold.'[A]

[Footnote A: *Veterinarian*, vol. xlviii., p. 100.]

Before driving the nail some operators burn or bore a hole for it. Opinion seems to differ as to whether this is at all necessary.

A method of clamping which, on account of its simplicity, has become greatly popular, is that of Vachette. For this operation is needed the outfit depicted in Figs. 86 and 87.

FIG. 87.—THE SAND-CRACK FORCEPS AND CLAMP.

With the special firing-iron (Fig. 86) an indentation, sufficiently large to admit the points of the clamp (Fig. 87), is made on each side of the crack. The clamp is then adjusted, and pressed home tight by means of the sand-crack forceps (Fig. 87). According to the length of the crack, one, two, or three clamps may be necessary. Another useful clamp, though far more complicated in its structure, is that of Professor McGill (Fig. 88).

FIG. 88.—MCGILL's SAND-CRACK CLAMP.

'The object of this invention is to arrange on a spindle, which is screw-threaded at one end with a right-hand thread and at the other with a left-hand thread, two clips or clamps, free to travel on the thread, there being a nut between the two which can be turned by a spanner. The clips are placed on the hoof, one on each side of the sand-crack, the hoof being prepared to receive the instrument by filing a groove or notch for the clamps to fit into, and by turning the nut on the screw the clamps are brought towards each other, and the crack thus prevented from spreading.'[A]

[Footnote A: *Veterinarian*, vol. lxi., p. 141.]

Still a further useful clamp is that of Koster. This is considerably broader than the clamp of Vachette, and its gripping edges are provided with teeth (see Fig. 89).

As with the clamp of Vachette so with this, a groove is burned into the wall on each side of the crack for the accommodation of the jaws of the instrument, and the clamp itself pressed home by means of a special pair of forceps. This form of clamp holds well, and has the advantage of securing a wider area of horn than that of Vachette or McGill.

FIG. 89.—KOSTER'S SAND-CRACK CLAMP.

Clamping by any method should be advised or undertaken only under certain conditions. The horn should be moderately strong, and the wall should be thick. This practically restricts the use of the clamp to cracks of the toe, and it is there, as a fact, they are found of most benefit. While burning the grooves for the clamp, and while tightening the clamp itself, the animal's foot should be on the ground and bearing weight at the heels, thus insuring the greatest possible approximation of the edges of the crack.

With all methods of clamping an untoward result is sometimes the formation of a fresh crack at the point of insertion of the clamps.

(c) *By the Use of Thin Metal Plates.*—These are of use when the horn of the wall is too thin to allow of clamping, and are therefore of especial use in cracks of the quarters. The plates are made so as to cover the greater part of the length of the lesion, and are fastened to the wall by two or more screws on either side of the crack. It is an advantage to slightly let the plate into the wall by means of fitting it hot. In a complicated crack the plate serves the

71

further useful purpose of holding in position antiseptic pledgets, and so keeping the lesion free from dirt and grit.

(d) By Various Methods of bandaging the whole Circumference of the Wall.—In our opinion this method of attempting to secure immobility of the crack, and so prevent its extension, is not often followed by success. The main objection to the method is that it subjects the whole of the wall to the same pressure, and does not restrict the operation to the point at which it is required. As in the case of the metal plate, however, this method has the advantage that antiseptic dressings may be kept in position in the case of a complicated crack.

FIG. 90.—SAND-CRACK BELT.

The binding of the wall may be accomplished in two ways. The simpler of the two is to merely apply the sand-crack belt depicted in Fig. 90. Beneath this should be applied a compress of tar and tow or other material, and the whole tightened up and kept in position by means of the buckle and strap. This method of binding admits of after-tightening should it unfortunately work loose.

The older method of binding the wall, and one now often practised by the smith, is to use a quantity of so-called 'tar-band' or other stout cord. With this the foot is neatly bound after the manner of a cricket-bat handle, and all movement of the crack apparently restricted. There is always a tendency, however, for such a dressing to work loose, and in the case of a complicated crack it has the disadvantage of permanently hiding from view the changes taking place in the discharge from the fissure.

(e) By wedging the Crack.—This is the exact opposite of clamping. Whereas in clamping we obtain immobility of the crack by keeping it fixed in the position of greatest approximation of its edges, in wedging, the crack is rendered free from movement by maintaining it in that position where its edges are most widely separated. In this case the edges of the crack are pared smooth, the cavity thoroughly cleansed, and a wedge of hard wood firmly driven in so as to fit exactly the fissure.

On the face of it it appears that this procedure would really tend to force open and so lengthen the crack, especially at its coronary extremity. What one should really remember, however, is that the crack *is not made wider* than before, but that it is simply maintained in a position occurring with every contraction of the heels of the foot, when it is normally at its widest. Movement of the edges is thereby stopped, the immediately surrounding structures are rested, and a new growth of horn, free from crack, induced to grow down from the coronet.

This method of treatment only serves to emphasize the fact that, with a sand-crack once formed, it is the constant movement of the parts that tends most to keep it in existence, and not any particularly marked exertion of force.

Some practitioners, with the wedge, apply also a clamp, thus assuring additional firmness and solidity to that portion of the wall under treatment.

The method of wedging is undoubtedly successful, if neatly performed.

(f) By Surgical Shoeing.—A partial rest is given to the affected parts by easing the bearing of the shoe at the point required. This may be done either by removal of part of the wall at the spot indicated, or by thinning the web of the shoe in the same position. The former is the method usually practised. Cessation of movement given in this way is, as we have already said, only partial; for, while the effects of pressure and concussion from below are minimized, the crack is still able to suffer from the movements of expansion and contraction of the foot. Still, as an auxiliary to other treatments, 'easing' of the wall under the affected part should always be practised.

FIG. 91.—THE BEARING 'EASED' BY REMOVAL OF THE WALL.

FIG. 92.—THE BEARING 'EASED' BY THINNING THE WEB OF THE
SHOE.

Figs. 91 and 92 show respectively the manner of 'easing' by removal of the wall, and by thinning the web of the shoe. In this connection it is necessary to point out that on no account should 'springing' of the heels of the shoe be allowed. Fig. 93 illustrates the ill-practice.

In this case, when the entire weight is thrown on to the heels, the portion of wall posterior to the crack is bound to participate unduly in the downward movement, and so tend to widening of the crack at its highest point.

FIG. 93.—THE BEARING 'EASED' BY 'SPRINGING' THE HEEL OF THE
SHOE.

We have already referred to the matter of 'clips.' In no case, whether the crack be at the toe or in the quarters, should a clip be placed immediately below it. If the crack is at the toe, the usual clip should be dispensed with, and a clip at each side made to take its place. At the same time care should be taken to avoid throwing the weight far forward. For that reason a shoe with calkins or with very high heels should be removed, and a shoe with an ordinary flat web substituted.

In the case of quarter-crack, where the constant movement of the parts under expansion and contraction of the foot makes itself most felt, it is wise to apply a shoe with clips fitting moderately tight against the inside of the bars. By this means movement will to a very large extent be curtailed.

Where a marked tendency to contraction is found, as is often the case with quarter-crack, then the shoe with the clips may be rendered more marked in its operation by giving to the outer face of each clip—that face applied to the bar—a slope from above downwards and outwards. In other words, a slipper shoe should be applied and the contraction given equally as much attention as the sand-crack itself.

Where the crack is situated far back in the quarter, and easing of the bearing cannot be accomplished without tending to spring the heels, then the most suitable shoe is a bar shoe. With it the bearing may, of course, be eased in exactly the position required, and the heels still allowed to take their fair share in bearing the body-weight, and thus assist in closing the crack. The bar shoe, if properly fitted, gives us also a bearing on the frog, and aids greatly in counteracting contraction.

2. *Curative.*

(a) The *Application of Dressings to the Lesion.*—In the case of a recent crack, deep, and attended with hæmorrhage, the foot should be thoroughly cleansed. Where possible, a constant flow of cold water from a hose-pipe should be allowed to run over the foot. By this means the inflammatory symptoms will be held in check and pain prevented. Later the shoe may be eased at the required place, and a blister applied to the coronet. This, with rest, will sometimes prove all that is needed.

Should a crack be of old standing, and complicated by the presence of pus, a course of hot poulticing will often prove of benefit. The poultice should be medicated with any reliable disinfectant, and should be renewed, or at any rate reheated, two or three times daily. The crack itself should be thoroughly cleaned after the removal of each poultice, and a

73

concentrated antiseptic solution—such as Tuson's spts. hydrarg. perchlor., carbolic acid, and water, (1 in 10) or liquor zinci chlor.—poured into it. On discontinuing the poulticing, the strength of the antiseptic solutions may be decreased, the parts rested by correct shoeing, and a blister applied to the coronet as before.

If these measures alone should prove insufficient, then the surgeon will either fall back on those we have just related, or proceed to methods next to be described.

(b) Immobilizing the Crack by Means of grooving the Wall.—To our minds, this is as ready and withal as successful a method of dealing with sand-crack as has yet been devised. It may be done in a variety of ways: (1) By two grooves arranged about the crack in the form of a V, as Fig. 94; (2) by a perpendicular groove on either side of the crack, about 1 inch in distance from it, and parallel with the horn fibres, as Fig. 95; (3) by a single horizontal groove at the extreme upper limit of the crack; (4) by drawing two horizontal grooves, one at its upper and one at its lower end (see Fig. 96).

F   F   F
IG. 94   IG. 95   IG. 96

In Figs. 94, 95, and 96 the thick black lines illustrate the positions of the various grooves made with the firing-iron for the purpose of immobilizing a quarter sand-crack.

The points to be observed in carrying out this line of treatment are simple enough. In all cases see that the crack is rendered as clean as possible by the use of suitable dressings, and if an excess of horn is present immediately around it, as in the case of a long-standing and complicated lesion, have it thinned down by rasping.

All that is then needed is one or two moderately sharp, flat firing-irons. The groove is then burned into the horn in the positions indicated, and that portion of the wall containing the sand-crack thus prevented from participating in the movements of the foot. For our own part, we consider the V-shaped incision, or either of the horizontal methods of grooving, preferable to lines running in the direction of the horn fibres. With the latter there is certainly a greater tendency to the formation of new cracks than with either of those we advocate. The V-shaped incision we consider most suitable of all, for the reason that by its means a greater degree of immobility is conferred upon the necessary portion of the wall.

Whichever method is adopted, care should be taken to carry the grooves deep enough into the horn, taking them down as near as possible to the sensitive structures. At the same time, especial care should be exercised in not carrying them too deep at their extreme upper limit, or in that case the liability to the formation of fresh cracks in those positions will be greatly increased. vAfter grooving, a sharp blister should be applied to the coronet every three or four weeks, and the animal, if free from lameness, put to work.

(c) By stripping away a V-shaped Portion of the Wall around the Crack.—This method is only indicated when the crack is greatly complicated by the presence of pus, or by the growth of adventitious horn on the inner surface of the wall. A radical cure is thus obtained, but the animal for a longer time incapacitated from work.

The operation is best performed by first grooving a line to connect the points *a* and *c* (Fig. 97). This should run immediately under the coronary margin of the wall, and should stop short of injuring the coronary cushion beneath. Grooves forming the sides *ab* and *bc* of the triangular piece of horn are next made, and the horn contained within the lines *ab, bc,* and *ca,* carefully removed. The grooves are the easiest made by a cautious use of the firing-iron. The greater thickness of the horn may thus be penetrated, and the grooves afterwards carried to their full and requisite depth by the use of the drawing-knife.

With the removal of the horn the diseased structures are exposed to view. All such should be removed by a free use of the scalpel, and a suitable dressing afterwards applied. A necessary factor in the treatment is the employment of pledgets of antiseptic tow. With these the exposed tissues are covered, and the successive turns of a bandage run tightly over them, so as to exert a moderate degree of pressure. When hæmorrhage has accompanied the operation, this dressing should be removed on the following day, the wound dressed, and the pledgets of tow and the bandage renewed. Any after-dressing need only then be practised at intervals of a week. Repair after this operation is rapid, and takes place both from the exposed podophyllus membrane and from the coronary cushion.

FIG. 97. The dotted lines outline the V-shaped portion of wall to be removed in the treatment of complicated toe-crack.

Fig. 98. The dotted lines indicate the portion of wall to be removed in the complete operation for complicated toe-crack.

(d) By stripping the Wall from the Coronary Margin to its wearing Edge on Either Side of the Crack.—This is merely a more extensive application of the method just described, and is only indicated in a *complete* and *complicated* crack that has refused to yield to other modes of treatment (see Fig. 98).

As in the previous case, a groove is run from *a* to *c*. The grooves *ab* and *de* are then continued to the lowermost edge of the wall, and the whole of the wall within these points removed. To facilitate removal, the white line should be grooved between the points *b* and *d*. After-treatment is exactly the same as that just referred to.

B. CORNS.

Definition.—In veterinary surgery the term 'corn' is used to indicate the changes following upon a bruise to that portion of the sensitive sole between the wall and the bar. Usually they occur in the fore-feet, and are there found more often in the inner than in the outer heel.

The changes are those depending upon the amount of hæmorrhage and the accompanying inflammatory phenomena occasioned by the injury.

Thus, with the hæmorrhage we get ecchymosis, and consequent red staining of the surrounding structures. As is the case with extravasations of blood elsewhere, the hæmoglobin of the escaped corpuscles later undergoes a series of changes, giving rise to a succession of brown, blue, greenish and yellowish coloration.

With the inflammation thereby set up we get swelling of the surrounding bloodvessels, pain from the compression of the swollen structures within the non-yielding hoof, and moistness as a result of the inflammatory exudate.

In a severe case the inflammation is complicated by the presence of pus.

Classification.—Putting on one side the classification of Lafosse (*natural* and *accidental*), as perhaps wanting in correctness, seeing that all are accidental, and disregarding the suggested divisions of Zundel (*corn* of the *sole* and *corn* of the *wall*) as serving no practical use, we believe, with Girard, that it is better to classify corns according to the changes just described.

Following his system, we shall recognise three forms: (1) *Dry*, (2) *moist*, (3) *suppurating.*

The *dry* corn is one in which the injury has fortunately been unattended with excessive inflammatory changes, and where nothing but the coloration imparted to the horn by the extravasated blood remains to indicate what has happened.

The *moist* corn is that in which a great amount of inflammatory exudate is the most prominent symptom. It indicates an injury of comparatively recent infliction.

The *suppurating* corn, as the name indicates, is a corn in which the inflammatory changes are complicated by the presence of pus.

Causes.—The causes of corns we may consider under two headings— namely, *predisposing* and *exciting*.

Predisposing Causes.—By the heading of this chapter we have already intimated that corns are due to faulty conformation of the foot. It is, therefore, merely a description of such shapes of foot as favour their formation that will need mention here.

The wide, flat foot, with low heels, may be first considered. Here the posterior portions of the sole, those portions between the wall and the bars, fall very largely in the same plane as the wearing surface of the bars and the wall. As a consequence, these portions of the sole are more prone to receive injury from stones and rough roads and from the pressure of the shoe.

The low heels, too, favour a more than due proportion of the body-weight being thrown on to the posterior parts of the foot. Two evils, both inclining to the production of corn, result from this. In the first place, the sensitive structures of the posterior portions of the foot are subjected to undue pressure from above; secondly, the posterior half of the foot, by reason of the extra weight thrown upon it, is exposed also to greater effects of concussion than normally it should meet. Added to this we find that the abnormally flat condition of the sole has resulted in a great loss of resiliency. With undue pressure above, and a loss of resiliency and added effects of concussion below, the sensitive structures included between the opposing pedal-bone and the horny sole are bound to suffer more or less bruising each time the foot comes to the ground, especially if the animal is moved at a rapid pace.

Writing here of the effects of pressure and concussion affords a fitting occasion to mention the fact that corns occurring in feet affected with side-bones are always worse than in feet with normal elastic cartilages. The explanation of this is simple, for there can be no doubt that the loss of resiliency in the diseased cartilage is only another aid to undue pressure and concussion. The sensitive structures are pinched between unyielding bone above and practically unyielding horn below.

Feet with high and contracted heels are also predisposed to corn. The contraction in this case interferes with the downward movements of the os pedis during progression, while in a state of rest there is a more or less constant pressure upon the sensitive structures, due to the correct downward displacement of the pedal-bone being opposed by the amount of contraction present. In the contracted foot, too, the nutrition of the vessels supplying the secretory apparatus of the horn is largely interfered with. The horn loses its natural elasticity, fails to respond to the normal movements of the parts within, and aids in the compression and laceration of the sensitive structures.

Weak feet, with horn too thin to withstand the expansive movements continually going on—in other words, feet with weak, spreading heels—are also prone to suffer from corns. In this case the flatness induced by the spreading, and the insufficient protection afforded by the thin horn, both combine to lay the sole open to the effects of concussion and direct injury.

Brittle feet—feet with horn of undue dryness, by reason of the contraction thus brought about—are, again, particularly subject to corn.

So also with long feet. Whether occurring as a natural deformity, or as the result of insufficient paring, bruises of the sole in feet thus shaped are common. The reason for this will be better understood when we come to deal with the shoeing.

Other and minor predisposing causes are those mainly referring to an unnatural dryness of the hoof when animals reared in the country are put to work in large towns. We here really get several predisposing causes combining. A sudden change is made from a more or less moist condition underfoot to one excessively dry. The character of the travelling is wholly altered from occasional work upon soft lands to continual labour upon hard-paved roads. The horn is often exposed to the vicious influences of unsuitable litter, the application of unsuitable dressings, and the deleterious effects of the street mud of our cities. All these play their part in determining a condition of the horn, rendering it open to receive the effects of the more exciting causes which we shall next consider.

Exciting Causes.—Than the shoeing, no more frequent and exciting cause of corn exists. Whatever the predisposing influences may be, it is the shoeing that in nearly every case completes the list, and finally inflicts the injury.

The evils in this connection we shall consider under two headings—viz., (1) the manner in which the foot is pared; (2) the make and fitting of the shoe.

First among the faulty preparations of the foot comes that of excessive thinning of the sole, especially in the regions subject to corn. The farrier addicted to this is not as a rule content to confine his operations to the sole alone. In addition, the frog and the bars also suffer from the too lavish use of his knife. His main object is doubtless that of giving a broad and open appearance to the foot. It follows from this that his operations are confined more to the posterior than the anterior parts of the foot, and that the toe is therefore left too long. This gives us a combination of causes leading to pressure and bruises upon the sensitive structures at the seat of corn.

By this unequal paring of the toe and the heels greater weight is thrown upon the posterior half of the foot. What then happens to the structures thinned as we have described is this: the pared frog, lessened in volume, does not meet the ground. It therefore fails to expand laterally with weight, and cannot assist, as normally it should, in aiding the heels generally in their movements of expansion. The weakened bars and the thinned sole, meeting with no opposition from the frog, give downwards and inwards with the body-weight at the precise moment these movements should be directed mainly outwards. As a further result of non-resistance on the part of the frog, this time in a lateral direction, the bars, the sole, and the wall at the heels all contract at the exact time they should expand. The end result must mean abnormal pressure and bruising of the sensitive structures in that particular region. Naturally, also, the excessive thinning of the horn renders direct injury to the sole from stones or other objects in the road far more probable.

For this one reason alone—the manner in which it favours the production of corn—too great a condemnation cannot be placed upon excessive paring of the sole, the bars, and the frog.

When corns are already present, as they may be from other causes, the same remarks will again apply to excessive paring. It is the custom with many smiths to carefully pare down the discoloured horn in every case of corn they meet with, and at the same time to again weaken the bars and even part of the wall at the heels, with the laudable idea of relieving pressure on the part diseased. After what has gone before, we need hardly say that their well-meant efforts have a precisely opposite effect to the one they intend.

The fitting of the shoe is, perhaps, to a greater extent responsible for the causation of corn than is the paring we have just described.

A few of the evils connected with the shoe may, however, be justly described as unavoidable. We *must* shoe; we cannot shoe and leave a normal foot!

A shoe excessively seated, especially from the last nail-hole backwards, may be regarded as dangerous. In this case, with every application of the body-weight, there is given to the foot a tendency to contract, especially at its lower margin. Result: undue pressure upon the tissues around and the production of corn.

On the other hand, varying with the form of foot, the seating may be insufficient. In the case of flat-foot, or dropped sole, for instance, insufficient seating will lead to undue pressure of the web of the shoe upon the sole, and in that way bring about bruising of the sensitive sole beneath.

Shoes with heels or calks too high, by destroying the counter-pressure of the frog with the ground, serve to bring about a series of changes we have described under contraction, and again result in pinching and bruising of the sensitive structures.

The opposite excess—a shoe thick at the toe and thin at the heels—is blamed by Zundel for causing a like injury. In our opinion, the reason this author gives—namely, that the throwing of greater weight upon the heels leads to bruising of the sensitive structures—can only correctly apply to a *wrongly-applied* shoe of this type, and not to the shoe itself. True, a shoe with a thick toe and thinned heels will throw an undue proportion of the body-weight upon the heels if the foot is not properly prepared for it. A wise man, however, will most certainly so cut down the toe for the reception of this shoe that, with the shoe in position, there will still be maintained a tread that is normal. To our minds harm is far more likely to arise from a shoe of this class through the thinned iron heels of the shoe becoming attenuated under wear to the point of bending, and so inflicting an injury upon the adjoining sole.

Similarly, this last remark with regard to the thinning of the heels of the shoe will apply to a shoe with too broad a web. As the thinning of the shoe proceeds with wear, the inner portion of the thinned branch is bent up on to the sole, and again inflicts the injury.

The matter of bearing is also of importance when considering the causation of corn. In a previous chapter we have already described the correct bearing as that which includes the whole of the lower margin of the wall and the white line, and just impinges on the sole. Any marked deviation from that will, if long continued, be followed by injury to the foot.

With the bearing surface of the shoe too narrow—in contact with the wall solely, or perhaps only a portion of it—it is evident that a large proportion of the foot that should properly bear weight is thrown out of action. A heavy strain is imposed on the white line, and undue descent of the sole and contraction of the heels brought about. Again the result of this is compression and bruising of the tissues around the seat of corn.

With its bearing surface too wide, the shoe immediately exerts direct pressure upon the sole with every movement of the animal. The sole normally is not made to receive this, and harm is bound to result.

Among other ill-fitting shoes we may mention the one with branches too short, and the one with the extremities of the branches too pointed. In the first case, as wear of the shoe proceeds, the thinned end is far more likely to turn in under the seat of corn than is a shoe with branches of ordinarily correct length. It is evident in the second case that the pointed branch, when thinned, is a more dangerous agent than the branch which is nearer the square at its end.

The matter contained in the first half of the foregoing paragraph explains in a large measure the rarity of corns in the hind-feet. Here there is nothing to prevent a shoe with branches of full length being used. The correct bearing is thus maintained, even with a shoe excessively thinned with wear, and the liability to injury from it decreased. An exception is to be found in the case of a feather-edged shoe, such as is used to prevent cutting or brushing. The thinning by wear from above to below of the branch already purposely thinned from side to side leads to the formation of a thin and narrow piece of iron admirably calculated to bend over and injure the sole.

Even with a shoe of correct length, with a flat-bearing surface at the heels, and other conditions favourable to correct application, evil may still result from the shoe itself being made too narrow. As a result of this, the branch of *each* side is set too far under the foot, with consequent injury to the sole. This is, of course, sheer carelessness on the part of the smith. When practised, however, it is not easy of detection, as in all cases the foot is rasped down to cover what has been done. In other words, the foot is made to fit the shoe and not the shoe the foot.

Recognising this close fitting of the shoe as a cause, we are able to explain in some measure how it is that corns should occur with greater frequency in the inner than in the outer heel. There is no doubt that the inner branch of the shoe is nearly always fitted closer than is the outer. In the fore-foot it is also often shorter. Take these two evils and add to them the fact that the inner heel is called upon to bear more of the body-weight than is the outer, and the frequency of corns in the inner heel will no longer be wondered at.

Indirectly, the shoe may still be a cause of corn by reason of the irritation set up by gravel and small pieces of flint becoming firmly fixed between the sole and the web of the shoe. In nearly every case of this description the part to be injured is the white line.

Corns may also result from the animal picking up a stone. The stone becomes firmly wedged in between the inner border of the branch of the shoe and the bar or the frog. With every step the animal takes it becomes wedged more tightly into position. Projecting below the level of the lower surface of the shoe, it imparts the concussion it thus obtains directly to the sole. A bruise—and a bad bruise—is the result.

Finally, it cannot be denied that the work the horse is put to is largely responsible for the causation of corn. In country animals corns are comparatively rare, while in animals in town, almost constantly upon hard paving, they are common. This seems to point strongly to the fact that concussion through constant work upon unyielding roads is a great factor in their production.

Symptoms.—Unless the discoloration of the horn is accidentally discovered by the smith, the simple, dry corn may go undetected. The disturbance excited by it is so small, and the pain occasioned so slight, that the patient may offer no indication of its existence.

Ordinarily, however, the first symptom is that of pain. The animal goes feelingly with one or both feet, in some cases even showing decided lameness. The lameness, however, is in no way diagnostic, and the lesion itself must be discovered before an exact opinion can be pronounced.

As an aside, it is well to observe in this connection that a negative opinion as to the existence of corn should never be given unless the superficial layers of horn have first been removed with the knife.

When standing at rest the animal exhibits signs more or less common to all foot lamenesses. He 'points' the foot—in other words, the limb is slightly advanced, the fetlock partly flexed, and the heels from off the ground. When both feet are affected they are pointed alternately, and the animal often manifests his uneasiness by repeated pawing movements, and by scraping his bedding behind him.

Should the injury run on to suppuration, the lameness becomes most acute. The pawing movements become more pronounced, and there is evident disinclination on the part of the animal to place the foot squarely on the ground. One is then led to manipulate the foot. The hoof is hot to the touch. Percussion causes the animal to flinch, and to flinch particularly when that portion of the wall adjoining the corn is struck. Finally, exploration with the knife reveals the serious extent to which the injury has developed. In a neglected case of this description it is even possible to detect the presence of pus by the amount of swelling and fluctuating condition of the coronet. The suppurative process has advanced in the direction of least resistance, and is on the point of breaking through the tissues immediately above the horn.

Lameness due to corn is oftentimes intermittent. With a simple corn, dry or moist, this intermission is largely dependent on the degree of dryness of the hoof or the road, and also on the character of the road surface. With a neglected, suppurating corn, on the other hand, variation in the degree of lameness, in addition to depending on circumstances such as these, is dependent to a larger extent upon the changes occurring with the suppuration. In this case the time of greatest lameness is immediately before the pus gains outlet. Immediately after its exit at the coronet the animal will go almost sound. Soundness continues so long as the opening at the coronet remains clear. The tendency, however, is for the opening thus made to quickly close again. Pus again accumulates, lameness arises as before, and disappears again with the second discharge of the contents of the sinus now formed.

Pathological Anatomy.—When dealing with their classification we gave in outline the main pathological changes to be met with in corns. It now only remains to give the same matter in slightly greater detail.

In dry corn the changes we meet with are those accompanying blood extravasation. From excessive compression of the parts, or from the effects of direct injury, a portion of the sensitive sole has become lacerated. The escaping blood stains the surrounding soft tissues after the manner of blood extravasation elsewhere. If the escape of blood is sufficiently large, the horn fibres in the immediate vicinity also are stained. It is this stain in the horn that is the direct evidence of the injury, and is itself popularly known as the corn. It may vary in size from quite a small spot to a broad patch as large as half a crown, while its colour may be a uniform red, or a mottled red and white. The microscopic changes in this connection are illustrated in Fig. 99.

FIG. 99.—HORIZONTAL SECTION OF A CORN. The section cut at about the base of the papillæ of the sensitive sole. *a*, papillæ, with horn-cells surrounding them; *b*, interpapillary or intertubular horn; *c*, hollow spaces in the intertubular material filled with blood; *d*, a papilla and its surrounding horn-cells filled with blood.

Ordinarily, this ecchymosis of the horny sole is due to injury of the sensitive sole *immediately beneath* it. It may, however, proceed from injury to the vessels of the laminæ either of the bars or of the wall. In this case the ecchymosis of the horny sole may be explained by the fact that the escaped blood tends to *gravitate* to that position.

When the corn is of long standing, or is due to *repeated* injuries on the same spot, the horn adjacent to the lesion becomes hard and dry, and often abnormally brittle, simply on account of the inflammatory changes thus kept in continuation. This is often seen when attempts are made to *pare out* the corn with the knife.

Should the injury be seated in the sensitive laminæ, then the brittle nature of the horn secreted by the injured tissues makes itself apparent by the appearance of cracks in the wall of the quarter. Why this should occur will be readily understood by a reference to Fig. 100.

FIG. 100.—INNER SURFACE OF THE WALL OF THE QUARTER, SHOWING CHANGES IN THE HORNY LAMINÆ BROUGHT ABOUT BY CHRONIC CORN.

It will here be seen that the injury to the keratogenous membrane has led to great interference with the secretion of horn from the sensitive laminæ. As a result, the regularly leaf-like arrangement of the horny laminæ has been largely broken up. Certain of the laminæ are altogether wanting, while others are broken in their length and rendered incomplete. With this condition there is always more or less contraction of the quarter.

Microscopic examination of the structures involved in such a case reveals the fact that with the contraction is an alteration in the normal direction of the horny and sensitive laminæ.

They become bent backward, and, instead of the regular and normal arrangement depicted in Fig. 32, show the distorted appearance given in Fig. 101.

From the appearances and characters of the blood-stain in the horny sole we are able to deduce evidence relative to the duration and nature of the injury.

FIG. 101.—PERPENDICULAR SECTION OF THE WALL OF A CONTRACTED QUARTER IN A CASE OF CHRONIC CORN. Both the sensitive and horny laminæ are bent backwards, and hæmorrhages have taken place at the base of the sensitive laminæ.

When, for instance, the stain is not to be found in the superficial layers of the sole, but is only discoverable by deep paring, then the injury is a recent one.

Where the stain *is* met with in the superficial layers of horn, and is quickly pared out, then the injury has been inflicted some time before, and has not been repeated. When, as is sometimes the case, layers of horn that are stained are found alternated with layers that are healthy, then we have evidence that the cause of the corn, whatever it may be, is not in constant operation.

Similar indication of the age of the injury is also afforded by the colour of the lesion.

A stain that is deep red is proof that the injury is comparatively recent.

A distinct yellow or greenish tinge, on the other hand, is evidence that the injury is an old one.

In the Moist Corn we have, in addition to the blood extravasation, the outpouring of the inflammatory exudate. In the most superficial layer of the horn this may not be noticeable. As one cuts deeper into the sole with the knife, however, it will be found that the lower layers of horn are more or less infiltrated with the discharge. This gives to the horn a soft consistence, a yellow appearance, and a touch that is moist to the fingers.

With the accompanying inflammation the cells in the neighbourhood of the injury are enfeebled and their normal functions interfered with. We may thus expect a corresponding interference with the growth of horn. This is exactly what happens, and as one cuts deeper still into the horn a point is finally reached when a well-marked cavity is encountered. A pale yellow and usually watery exudate fills it. This cavity points out the exact spot where the force of the injury has been greatest, where death of certain cells of the keratogenous membrane has resulted, and where the natural formation of horn has for a time been suspended.

In the Suppurating Corn, as in moist corn, we have pathological changes due to the tissue reaction to the injury, *plus* the addition of pus organisms. Confined within the horny box we have a discharge that, by reason of the living and constantly multiplying elements it contains—the pus organisms—is always increasing in bulk. This must be at the expense of the softer structures of the foot. Accordingly, as the formation of pus increases, we get pressure upon and final gangrene of the sensitive sole and of the sensitive laminæ of the bars and the wall. With no outlet below, the pus formation increases until finally it finds its way out of the hoof by emerging at the coronet.

This in some instances it may do by confining its necrotic influences solely to the sensitive laminæ of the wall, in which case, if a dependent orifice is quickly made at the sole, the injury to the laminæ is soon repaired by the healthy tissue remaining.

In other cases, however, the necrosis has spread deeper. Caries of the os pedis, of the lateral ligaments of the pedal-joint, or of the lateral cartilages, is a result. When this occurs the exuding discharge from the coronet becomes thinner and more putrescent, and its feel, when rubbed between the fingers, sometimes gritty with minute fragments of broken-up bone. Here, unless operative measures prevent it, necrosis soon spreads deeper still. The deeper portions of the os pedis become affected. The capsular ligament of the joint is penetrated by the suppurative process, and a condition of septic arthritis results. The cavity of the joint becomes more or less tensely distended, according to the amount of drainage present, which in this case is almost nil, with matter in a state of putrescence. As a consequence, the surrounding ligaments become softened and yield, and the articular surfaces displaced. The articular cartilages also suffer, become necrotic in patches, and frequently wholly destroyed. The end result is one of anchylosis of the joint and permanent lameness.

Prognosis.—With the ordinary dry corn a return to the normal may nearly always be looked for. Similarly, with moist corn, and even with careful treatment of the suppurating variety, the same favourable termination may be looked for and promised.

What cannot so safely be assured is that a relapse will not occur. In other words, the extent of the injury, no matter how serious, does not often offer anything that cannot be overcome by Nature and careful surgery; but the conformation of the animal does. A vicious predisposing conformation once there is there always, and although the injury resulting from it may easily give way to correct treatment, the same injury is bound to re-occur when the animal is again put to work.

Although with care suppurating corn, like other cases of suppuration within the hoof, may yield to treatment, the owner of the animal should, nevertheless, be warned that the condition is a serious one, especially should the joint become affected. It may so happen, as sometimes in fact it does, that the animal may die as a result of the infective fever so set up. From no surface in the body can absorption take place quicker than from the synovial membrane of a joint. So soon, therefore, as this membrane comes in contact with septic material, so soon does a severe septic fever make its appearance. The septic matter has gained the blood-stream, and the patient succumbs to septic poisoning.

Apart from death occurring naturally, the changes taking place in the joint in the shape of bony growths or of actual anchylosis may be so severe as to render the animal useless, and slaughter may have to be advised.

Treatment.—We have already said that by far the most active cause in the production of corn is the shoe. It follows from this that it is to the shoeing we must largely look for a successful means of their prevention, and that the treatment of corn in its most simple form is really a matter for the smith, and not for the veterinary surgeon.

The faults in connection with the shoeing we have mentioned fully when treating of the *causes* of corn. From those we learn that a shoe with a flat-bearing surface, or one moderately seated but flat at the heels, is the correct shoe for nearly all feet. The heels of the shoe should not be too high, should not be too short, and should be wide enough apart from each other to insure the wall of the foot obtaining a fair share of the bearing. Finally, even with the present method of shoeing, whenever it is possible to allow the frog to come to the ground, it should be encouraged to do so, and excessive paring either of the latter organ or of the bars or the sole should be strictly discountenanced. Where the sole is thin, or the frog wasted, use a leather sole or a rubber pad. With these precautions, corns may be prevented from occuring even in a foot with a predisposing conformation.

When corn is present, the first treatment usually adopted is that of 'paring it out.' This is advocated by Percival and by many other writers. We cannot say, however, that we agree with it—at any rate, not in the case of simple dry corn.

'Paring it out,' and by that we mean thinning down the sole until close on the sensitive structures, can only be advised in the case of suppurating corn, or in cases where doubt exists as to whether pus is present or not. In the latter case paring becomes necessary as an exploratory means to diagnosis.

When it appears fairly certain, even in the case of a moist corn, that pus does not exist, then paring is to be discountenanced, for the reason that it only tends to weakening of the parts and to assist largely in the corn's recurrence.

Those who advocate it do so for the reason that it relieves pressure on the injured parts.

That it does so directly from below cannot be denied; but that it also favours contraction and compression from side to side is equally certain.

A moderate paring may, however, be indulged in, say, to about one-half the estimated thickness of the sole. Softening of the horn and consequent lessening of pressure may then be brought about by the use of oil, oil and glycerine, tincture of creasote, or by poulticing.

In the case of a moist corn the paring should be stopped immediately the true nature of the injury has made itself apparent. Warm poultices or hot baths should then be used in order to soften the surrounding parts, lessen the pressure, and ease the pain. After a day or two day's poulticing, should pain still continue with any symptom of severity, the formation of pus may be expected, and it is then time for the paring to be carried further, until the question 'pus or no pus?' is definitely settled.

Should the moisture be due simply to the presence of the inflammatory exudate, then poulticing alone will have the desired effect, and the pain will be lessened. With the decrease in pain the poulticing may be discontinued, and the horn over the seat of the injury dressed with some antiseptic and hardening solution. Sulphate of zinc, a mixture of sulphate of zinc and lead acetate, sulphate of copper, or the mixture known as Villate's solution,[A] may either of them be used. Suitably shod, and with a leather sole for preference, the animal may then again be put to work.

[Footnote A: The composition of the escharotic liquid bearing his name was published by M. Villate in 1829 as under:

Subacetate of lead liquid		128 grammes
Sulphate of zinc	[=a=a]	64 grammes
Sulphate of copper	[=a=a]	64 grammes
Acetic acid		1/2 litre

Dissolve the salts in the acid, add little by little the subacetate of lead, and well shake the mixture.]

When dealing with suppurating corn, then, a considerable paring away of the horn of the sole becomes a matter of necessity. The freest possible exit should be given to the pus, and this even when an opening has already occurred at the coronet. Unless this is done, and done promptly, the putrescent matter still contained within the hoof will make further inroads upon the soft structures therein, and later upon the ligaments, and even bone itself.

Having given drainage to the lesion by the dependent orifice in the sole, poulticing should again be resorted to and maintained for at least three or four days. The poulticing may then be discontinued, and the openings in the sole injected with a weak solution of Tuson's spts. hydrarg. perchlor., a 1 in 20 solution of carbolic acid, a solution of copper sulphate, with Villate's solution, or with any other combined antiseptic and astringent. The success of the treatment is soon seen in the cessation of pain and in the decreased amount of discharge from the opening in the sole.

Should pain unfortunately continue, the discharge remain, and a state of fever reveal itself, then it may be understood that the suppurative process has not been checked, that a portion of necrosed ligament, cartilage, or bone still remains, which, surrounded as it is by pus organisms and putrefactive germs, is sufficient to excite a constant irritation and maintain the internal structures in a state of infection. In other words, we have what is known as a quittor.

This will call for deeper operation. The horn of the wall must be removed, and the diseased structures, whether gangrenous keratogenous membrane, necrosed ligament, or carious bone, carefully excised or curetted. This will be better understood by a reference to the chapter on Quittor, where the means for carrying out the necessary operative measures will be found described in detail.

Surgical Shoeing for Corn.—In the case of an ordinary dry corn, where the injury has been definitely ascertained to be accidental, no alteration in the shoeing will be necessary. Where, however, the corn is attended with a more than ordinary degree of inflammation, or where for some reason or other excessive paring has been practised, then it will become needful to shoe with a special shoe. The object to be attained is the removal of pressure from that portion of the wall next to the seat of corn.

The most simple shoe for effecting this is the ordinary three-quarter shoe. The only way in which this differs from the ordinary shoe is that about an inch and a half of that branch of the shoe adjoining the corn is cut off (Fig. 102). If at the same time contraction of the heels exists, then, perhaps, a better shoe is that known as the three-quarter bar (Fig. 103).

Or, if preferred, a complete bar shoe such as that described for sand-crack may be used, and the upper portion of the web in contact with the foot at the seat of corn thinned out so as to avoid pressure on the wall at this point. With this shoe we shall at the same time supply a certain amount of pressure to the frog, and aid in the healthy development of the part indirectly involved in the disease.

The same pressure may also be given to the frog, and protection afforded the sole, by the use of a leather sole, or rubber pad on leather, as described when dealing with contracted feet.

A further method of relieving pressure on this portion of the wall, without removing the wall itself (a practice which should never be advised) is to make certain alterations in the web of the shoe. This may be done in one of two ways.

FIG. 102.—THREE-QUARTER SHOE.

FIG. 103.—THREE-QUARTER BAR SHOE.

In the first, that portion of the bearing surface of the heel of the shoe is 'dropped' about 1/8 inch from the plane of the remainder, so that the shoe at this position does not come into contact with the foot at all (see Fig. 104).

In the second case the shoe is what is termed 'set' at the heel. Here it is the plane of the *wearing* surface of the shoe that is altered. The hinder portion of the required heel is thinned so that its lower surface does not come into contact with the ground. By this means the wall is freed from concussion and pressure. At the same time the upper surface of the shoe is in contact with the wall of the foot (see Fig. 105).

This 'setting' of the shoe is preferable to the method first described. It affords a greater protection to the foot, and does not allow of fragments of stone and flint getting in between the foot and the shoe, and so giving rise to further mischief.

The 'set' portion should be fitted full and long. It is obvious, too, that the animal should not be allowed to carry the shoe too long; otherwise, as the other portion of the shoe wears down to the level of the 'set' heel, pressure on the tender part of the foot will again result.

FIG. 104.—SHOE WITH A 'DROPPED' HEEL.

FIG. 105.—SHOE WITH A 'SET' HEEL.

In applying surgical shoes for corn of long standing, it must be remembered that the protection so afforded must be continued for some time. It is not sufficient to see the lesion itself disappear. In addition to that there is also, in the majority of cases, a certain amount of contraction to be overcome. This can only be done by continuing the use of a leather sole or some form of frog or bar-pad as recommended for the relief of that condition.

C. CHRONIC BRUISED SOLE.

A similar condition to that of corn may be met with in other positions on the sole. It is described by Rogerson as sand-crack of the sole[A], and is invariably met with around that portion of the sole in contact with the shoe.

[Footnote A: *Veterinarian*, vol. lxiii., p. 51.]

The animal is lame, and the shoe is removed in order to ascertain the cause. Nothing at first is noticeable except that the animal flinches when pressure is applied to the spot with the pincers, or the sole is tapped with the hammer.

On removing the sole with the knife, however, a distinct black mark is discovered, which, when followed up by careful paring, is often found to have pus at the bottom.

In this case the injury has resulted, as we have already intimated elsewhere, from causing the animal to wear for too long a time a shoe with too broad a web or insufficiently seated. Or it may have originated with the irritation set up by foreign and hard substances between the web of the shoe and the foot.

In his description of this condition Mr. Rogerson draws attention to the fact that the pus found should not be wrongly attributed to accidental pricking of the foot. He says:

'Considering that the cracks or splits are always found in the immediate vicinity of the nail-holes, a certain amount of discretionary skill is required in order that the lameness may be attributed to its proper cause. This is an instance in which the presence of the veterinary surgeon is imperative, in order to prevent undue blame being attached to the shoeing-smith. Misconception in these cases might very easily arise when parties concerned are disposed to accept an unskilled opinion, sometimes resulting in danger to the proprietor of the forge, not only of losing a shoeing contract, but also of being involved in other ways which would probably prove even more disastrous.

'Horses that stand on sawdust or moss litter are sometimes found with extensive discoloration of the horny sole in front of the frog. Their bedding material collects in the shoe as snow does, and forms a mass, which keeps a continued and uneven pressure upon the sole. A sound foot is not injuriously affected, but a very thin sole is, and so also is a sole which has been bruised by a picked up stone. Even a slight bruise becomes serious if pressure is allowed to remain active over the injured part. Lameness increases, serous fluid is effused between the horn and sensitive part, or even hæmorrhage may take place.'[A]

[Footnote A: Hunting, *Veterinary Record*, vol. xiv., p. 593.]

The Treatment of Chronic Bruised Sole offers no special difficulty. Removal of the cause (in nearly every case incorrect bearing of the shoe) is the first consideration. That done, the lesion may be searched for and treated in the ordinary manner as described for corn. When pus is present it must, of course, be given exit, and an antiseptic solution applied to the wound. Should the sensitive structures be laid bare when allowing the pus to escape, then the wound so made should afterwards be protected with a leather sole and antiseptic stopping.

CHAPTER VIII
WOUNDS OF THE KERATOGENOUS MEMBRANE
A. NAIL-BOUND—BIND OR TIGHT-NAILING.

Definition.—By the term 'nail-bound' is indicated that accident occurring in the forge in which the nail of the shoe is driven too near the sensitive structures. Although involving no actual wound, it is important to consider the condition under the heading of this chapter, in order that it may be distinguished from the graver accident of a 'prick.'

Causes.—Very largely the whole matter of causation turns on the correct fitting of the shoe. The points especially to be noticed in this connection are (1) the position of the nail-holes in the web of the shoe, (2) the 'pitch' of the nail-holes.

Regarding the position of the nails, it goes without saying that the first consideration when 'holing' the shoe should be to punch the holes opposite to sound horn. This remark applies especially to shelly and brittle feet, the type of feet in which tight-nailing most often occurs. The next consideration in this connection is that of punching the holes so that the nail emerges from the upper surface of the web at exactly its correct point of entrance on the bearing surface of the foot. This should be on the white line immediately where it joins the wall. From this position any marked deviation inwards ('fine-nailing,' as it is termed) is bound to give to the nail a direction dangerously near the sensitive structures.

The 'pitch' of the nail-holes should be such that the nail is guided more or less nearly to follow the line of inclination of the wall. Accordingly, the nail-holes at the toe should be 'pitched' distinctly inwards, the inward pitch lessening as the quarters are reached, until the hindermost nail-hole or two is pitched in a direction that is almost perpendicular.

Too great an inward inclination of the nail will, however, give rise to a bind.

It is probable that 'tight-nailing' results more often from fine punching of the shoe than from any fault in the pitch of the hole. Inattention to either detail, however, is apt to bring the mischief about.

Even with a correctly fitted shoe, and with a normal foot, tight-nailing may occur as a result of sheer carelessness on the part of the smith.

Symptoms.—Possibly the animal returns from the forge sound. It is on the following day, as a rule, that evidence of the injury is given by the animal coming out from the stable lame. In a well-marked case the foot is warmer to the hand than its fellow, and percussion over the wall will sometimes reveal the particular nail that is the cause of the trouble. Should the shoe be removed, then the fact that the hole the nail has made is far too close to the sole often points out at once the seat of the mischief.

Treatment. As to whether or not the shoe should be removed is very much a matter for careful discretion on the part of the veterinary surgeon. Where the foot is shelly and brittle even a good smith sometimes finds himself unable to firmly attach the shoe without verging closely on causing the condition we are now describing. The author has known cases where animals with feet of this description have almost invariably returned from the forge, or rather been found the next day, with a suspicion of tenderness. After the lapse of a day or two this has quite often disappeared, and nothing in the meantime been done with the foot. Seeing, therefore, that removal and refitting of the shoe is in this case attended with risk of breaking away portions of the brittle horn, and so rendering the foot in an even worse condition than it was before, it is policy to decline to have the shoes removed unless worse symptoms make their appearance.

In coming to this decision the veterinary surgeon must be guided by noting in the wall the points of exit of the nails. Should the nail adjoining the position already pronounced to be tender have come out at a higher point than the others, it may be assumed that at a lower position in its course through the horn it has gone near the sensitive structures without actually penetrating the horny box, and that in the course of a day or two the sensitive structures involved will accommodate themselves to the pressure thus inflicted.

If, on the other hand, symptoms of tight-nailing show themselves in an animal with good sound feet, then there is no objection to be raised against having the shoe at once removed. Should the offending nail be definitely detected, then the shoe may again be put on, and that particular nail omitted from the set.

B. PUNCTURED FOOT.

(Pricked Foot—Nail-tread—Gathered Nail.)

Definition.—Under this heading we propose describing wounds of the foot occurring in the sole or in the frog, and penetrating the sensitive structures beneath.

Causes.—These we shall consider under two headings:

1. Wounds resulting from the animal himself 'picking-up' or 'treading' on the offending object.

2. Cases of pricking in the forge.

Those occurring under the first heading are, of course, purely accidental. In the majority of cases, the object picked up is a nail; but similar injury may result from the animal treading on sharp pieces of wood or iron, on pieces of umbrella wire, on pointed pieces of bones, broken-off stable-fork points, sharp pieces of flint, etc. The same accident may also occur in the forge as a result of the animal treading on the stumps of nails, from treading on an upturned shoe with the stumps of nails *in situ*, or from treading on an upturned toe-clip. It may also occur from an accidental prick with the stable-fork when 'bedding up,' or from casting part of a shoe when on the road and treading on the nails, in this case left sometimes partly in and partly out of the horn.

'Serious wounds of this description are also met with in animals engaged in carting timber from plantations in which brushwood has recently been cut down. This is, of course, from treading on the stake-like points that are left close to the ground. Hunters also meet with the same class of injury when passing through plantations or over hedge banks, where the hedge has just been laid low or cut down.

'Agricultural horses also meet with severe wounds of this class from treading on an upturned harrow.'[A]

[Footnote A: *Journal of Comparative Pathology and Therapeutics*, vol. iv., p. 2.]

It has been remarked how strange it is that nails should so readily penetrate the comparatively hard covering of the foot. The matter, however, admits of explanation. One knows from common observation how easy it is to tilt a nail with its point upwards by exerting a pressure in a more or less slanting direction upon its head. This is exactly the form of pressure that is no doubt put upon the nail if the animal treads upon it when moving at any pace out of a walk. The foot in its movement forward tilts the nail up, and almost simultaneously puts weight upon it. The great weight of the animal is then quite sufficient to account for its ready penetration.

In purely country districts cases of punctured foot are of far less frequent occurrence than in large towns. In the latter, animals labouring in yards where a quantity of packing is done, or engaged in carting refuse containing such objects as we have mentioned, or broken pieces of earthenware or glass bottles, meet with it constantly.

For the manner of causation of those wounds to the foot occurring in the forge the reader may be referred to the matter under the heading of 'nail-bound.' As in that case so in this the nail may be wrongly directed by improper fitting of the shoe, by the 'pitch' of the hole, or by the position of the hole. The nails may also be wrongly directed as a result of faulty pointing, or by meeting with the stump of a nail that has carelessly been allowed to remain in the substance of the horn.

Often pricking is a result of carelessness engendered by a rush of work. Often it is almost unavoidable on account of the character of the foot that is brought to be shod. Feet with thin horn, especially a thin sole, feet with horn shelly and brittle, each in their way are difficult to shoe.

Sometimes pricking is purely accidental, as in the case of a 'split' nail. The nail as it is driven splits at its point, and continues to split down its centre, one half emerging at the correct spot on the wall, the other half bending inwards, and penetrating the sensitive structures.

Common Situations of the Wound.—In a case of picked-up nail the common seat of puncture is about the point of the frog, either in one of the lateral lacunæ, in the median lacuna, or the apex of the frog itself. In comparison with this puncture of the sole is rare.

Prick sustained at the hands of the smith may, of course, run in either of the following directions: (1) Directly into the position where the horny and sensitive laminæ interleave; (2) between the sensitive laminæ and the os pedis; (3) into the os pedis itself; (4) the nail may bend excessively immediately after entering the horn, and so pass either between the horny and sensitive sole; or (5) between the sensitive sole and the bone.

Classification.—Punctured wounds of the foot may be classified as follows:

Simple or superficial when penetrating no structure of great importance. For instance, a prick that penetrates to the sensitive sole and is not driven with sufficient force to seriously injure the os pedis we may regard as simple. In the same manner a prick to the frog that, although deep, is mainly concerned with penetrating the plantar cushion may also be classed as simple.

Deep or penetrating when driven with sufficient force or in such a direction as to injure structures whose penetration is calculated to give rise either to serious constitutional disturbance or to permanent lameness. In this category we may place injuries to the terminal portion of the perforans, puncture of the navicular bursa, fracture of the navicular bone and penetration of the pedal articulation, and splintering of the os pedis.

Symptoms and Diagnosis.—While discussing the symptoms and diagnosis, we will still continue to consider our subject under the two headings of (1) accidental 'gathering' of some foreign body, and (2) pricks inflicted in the forge.

In a few cases belonging to the former class the veterinary surgeon is fortunate in obtaining a direct history of the injury. The driver has seen the animal go suddenly lame, and has examined the foot for the cause. Either the nail has been found embedded in the horn, or the puncture it has made detected, and the matter has been reported. The foot is then explored and the full extent of the injury ascertained.

In many cases, however, it so happens that no evidence of the infliction of the injury is forthcoming. The momentary lameness occurring at the time of the prick is unreported at the time by the attendant, and the horse for a time goes sound. It is not until the changes set up by the subsequent inflammatory phenomena make their appearance, and lameness results, that attention is called to the foot. When this happens there has, as a rule, been time for pus to form around the seat of puncture—a matter of about forty-eight hours.

The horse is now brought out for the veterinary surgeon's examination, going distinctly lame. If the case is well marked there may then be noted by the man of experience many little signs pointing to the foot as the seat of the lameness. These, though well enough known to the practitioner, are nevertheless difficult to describe. It is, in fact, hard to say exactly in what they really consist, appearing to be as much a matter of intuition as of actual observation.

There is a peculiar 'feeling' characteristic in the gait. The affected foot is put forward fearlessly enough, but is not nearly so rapidly put to the ground. When at rest the foot is almost immediately pointed, and the pain at intervals manifested by pawing movements. It is this extreme liberty of the rest of the limb, as evinced during the pawing movements, that really strikes one. Shoulder, elbow, knee, and fetlock are all easily and painlessly flexed and extended. There is nothing wrong with them; it must be the foot. The short manipulation necessary to test the lameness—viz., the walk and slow trot—is sufficient to raise the animal's pulse and quicken the breathing.

All this is enough, and more than enough, to lead the veterinary surgeon to examine the foot. It is hot to the touch, and at the coronet tender to pressure, possibly in a neglected case fluctuating at the heel. Pain is evinced by the animal withdrawing his foot when percussion takes place over the affected spot. In a bad case one gentle tap is all that is needed. The animal at once snatches away his foot, holds it high from the ground, and makes pawing movements in the air. At that moment, too, his countenance is highly expressive of the pain he is suffering. Again the foot is explored, the injury found, and the pus liberated.

Regarding the manner of exploration of the foot we will take first that case in which the veterinary surgeon is called in early, and in which pus has not yet had time to form. Sometimes the merest cleaning up of the inferior surface of the foot then reveals a distinct stab either in the sole or the frog.

If the accident be recent only a little blood will be found, either liquid, or coagulated about the wound. Later there exudes from the stab a flow of yellow, serous fluid. The opening thus found should be carefully probed, and its depth and situation noted.

At other times the prick is not so readily apparent. The nail or other object has penetrated and afterwards withdrawn itself. The natural elasticity of the horn, especially that of the frog, causes it to contract upon the puncture, and to largely obliterate the hole made. What, therefore, may look to be but a simple injury to the horn alone may in reality be the only evidence of a stab complicating the sensitive structures. It thus behoves the veterinary surgeon to follow up and carefully cut out any unnatural-looking mark in the horn, more especially if the horn is discoloured, or if blood is extravasated into its fibres, or there is moisture exuding from the part.

In some cases of this description the knife in the act of paring comes into contact with the cause of the trouble. Sometimes this is a nail, sometimes a sharp and small piece of flint, so deeply penetrated as to have become quite buried. When met with in this manner, however, the foreign body is more often than not a splinter of wood deeply embedded in the cleft of the frog or in the frog itself.

The fact that multiple punctures may occur should here be remembered, and the remainder of the inferior surface of the foot thinly pared.

On withdrawal of the foreign object blood may immediately follow. Should the former have been fixed in position for some time, however, pus is nearly always found at the bottom of the wound. As a rule, its removal is comparatively easy, but one case recalls itself to the author's mind in which the extraction was a matter of considerable difficulty. The offending object was a large, flat-headed nail, some 2 inches long. This was driven fast into the os pedis, and necessitated the employment of a pair of pincers and the exertion of some amount of force to move it from its position.

In this connection it must be remembered that the penetrating object sometimes breaks off after entering the foot. The fact that this occasionally happens only serves to give point to the advice we have previously rendered—that every stab should be carefully probed, and its exact condition and depth ascertained.

In those cases where percussion has led to the positive opinion that pus really exists, then the exploration must be most searching. There may, or may not, be a suspicious-looking mark to work on. In the latter case, the veterinary surgeon must not be content with confining his paring operations to one spot. The sole should be carefully thinned all round, and the thinning cautiously proceeded with until either small, pin-point hæmorrhages denote that healthy sensitive structures have been reached, or a sudden flow of pus indicates that the injury has been definitely located.

While the symptoms remain much about the same, the diagnosis of pricks received in the forge, as compared with those occurring in the natural manner, is easy. The animal starts to the forge quite sound, and returns, perhaps, with a slight limp. The slight limp in two days' time becomes a decided lameness, and no doubt remains as to what has occurred. The mere fact of the lameness arising immediately after a visit to the forge should be sufficient in the majority of cases to lead one to a correct diagnosis.

Where the opinion has been formed that a prick has been received, then the shoe should be removed.

This operation should always be superintended by the veterinary surgeon himself. After the removal of the clinches, the nails should be drawn one at a time with the pincers, and carefully examined. Often the offending nail may thus be picked out by observing upon it blood-stains, or the moisture from inflammatory exudate or from pus. Further inflammation will also be gathered by occasionally meeting with a nail that has split.

At this stage, too, the veterinary surgeon should have noticed whether or not the smith has previously sent the animal home with what is known as a 'draw back.' He has discovered, immediately after he has done it, that he has pricked the animal. He has then withdrawn the nail, and either sent the animal back with that nail altogether missing from the set in the shoe, or with the hole filled up with a stump.

The shoe once off, the holes made by the nails in the horn should be minutely examined for the presence of hæmorrhage, inflammatory fluid, or pus exuding from them, and also for evidence of their correct placing in the foot. Should fluid matter issue from any one of them, or should it be deemed that one has approached too near the inner margin of the white line, more especially if tenderness exists around it, that hole should be followed up with a 'searcher' or small drawing-knife until diagnosis is certain.

Complications.—Before proceeding to discuss the complications that may arise in the case of pricked foot, we may call to mind that the anatomy of the parts teaches us that the most serious position in which a punctured wound can occur is at the centre of the foot. Here the plantar aponeurosis, the navicular bursa, the navicular bone itself, or the pedal articulation may be injured.

Anterior to this position the most serious mischief that can ordinarily result is stabbing of the os pedis.

Posterior to the position we have named, the only structure to be injured is the plantar cushion.

Anatomically, then, the inferior surface of the foot may be divided into three zones, as follows:

A. *Anterior*, extending from the toe to the point of the frog.

B. *Middle*, extending from the point of the frog to the commencement of its median lacuna.

C. *Posterior*, including everything posterior to the middle zone. This division of the inferior surface of the foot into zones will be somewhat of a guide also when describing the complications next to follow:

(*a*) *Suppuration.*—This is the common complication of most wounds of the foot. When detected, it calls for immediate surgical interference in the shape of removal of the horn of the sole or the frog, as the case may be. This we shall consider further under the treatment.

(*b*) *Separation of the Horny Frog.*—This is a sequel to pus formation in the sensitive structures immediately beneath it, and the condition makes itself apparent by a line of separation between the horn and the skin of the heel of the injured side.

(*c*) *Wounding of the Plantar Aponeurosis.*—This occurs when a moderately-deep penetration of the horn of the middle zone has taken place. It is always most painful, especially when complicated by necrosis. The heel is then persistently elevated, and lameness is extreme, in some cases so severe as to cause the leg to be carried altogether.

In favourable cases the necrosed piece of tendon is sloughed off by the process of suppuration, and escapes with the discharges from the wound. There is then an abatement in the symptoms, and recovery is rapid.

Commonly, however, on account of the non-vascularity of the structure of the tendon, the necrotic spot in it tends to spread. The wound is thus led to become fistulous in character, and the pus forming within it prevented from escaping from the original opening. As a result, lameness and fever persist. There is a gradual increase in the severity of the symptoms, and later fistulous openings appear in the hollow of the heel.

(d) *Puncture of the Navicular Bursa.*—This results from a prick in exactly the same position as that last described, and means that the penetrating object has gone deeper, It may be distinguished from puncture of the plantar aponeurosis alone by the fact that there is an excessive discharge of synovia from the wound. This, as it escapes, is at first clear and straw-coloured. Later it becomes cloudy and flaked with pus, and shows a tendency to coagulate in yellowish clots.

Pain and accompanying fever is most marked, much more so than when the plantar aponeurosis alone is injured.

Should the original wound be insufficiently enlarged, or should its opening become occluded by the solid matters of the discharge, then this condition, like the last, ends in the formation of fistulous openings in the heel. These make their appearance as hot, painful, and fluctuating swellings in that position. Later they break, discharge their contents, and leave a fistulous track behind.

(e) *Fracture of the Navicular Bone.*—Penetration of the substance of the navicular bone, *without* its fracture, adds nothing to the symptoms we have described under puncture of the bursa. That the bone has been reached by the penetrating object may be detected by probing. This, however, must be performed with care, especially if a flow of synovia is absent. Otherwise, the wound, as yet, perhaps, superficial enough to avoid penetrating even the bursa, is made a penetrating one by the probe itself.

Fracture of the navicular bone is fortunately rare.

(f) *Penetration of the Pedal Articulation and Arthritis.*—This we shall consider in greater detail in Chapter XII. It is sufficient here to state that the condition may be suspected when a hot and painful swelling of the whole coronet makes its appearance. There is at the same time a diffused oedema of the fetlock and the region of the cannon, sometimes extending upwards to the whole of the limb.

Of all the complications to be met with in punctured foot this is the one most to be dreaded. The intense pain and the high fever render the animal weak and thin in the extreme. The appetite becomes impaired, sometimes altogether lost, and the patient in many cases appears to die from sheer exhaustion. Added to this is always the extreme probability of the wound becoming purulent, and later the dread of general septic infection of the blood-stream ensuing, and death resulting from that. Even with the happier ending of resolution, anchylosis of the joint and incurable lameness is more often than not left behind. (See Suppurative or Purulent Arthritis, Chapter XII.)

(g) *Ostitis and Caries of the Os Pedis.*—Injuries to the os pedis are met with in the anterior zone of the foot. Evidence that the bone has been injured is not usually forthcoming until after the lapse of some days. One is led to suspect it by the fact that there is no indication of the suppurative process extending further upwards, coupled with the facts that great pain, high fever, and extreme lameness persist, and that there is a continuous discharge from the wound of a copious blood-stained and foetid pus. Used now, the probe reveals the fact that the bone is bared, and conveys to the hand that is holding it a sensation of crumbling fragility.

(h) *Wounding of the Lateral Cartilage and Quittor.*—This occurs as the result of a deep stab in the posterior zone. Ordinarily, wounds in this position are unattended with serious consequences, and the prick has to be a deep and a severe one before the cartilage is reached. What then happens is that a spot of necrosis is formed round the seat of puncture in the cartilage. This, unless met with surgical interference, is sufficient to maintain the wound in a septic condition; it takes on a fistulous character, and a quittor is formed. (See Chapter X.)

(*i*) *Septic Infection of the Limb.*—This we have already once or twice referred to. It simply means that the septic matters from the wound have gained the lymphatics, and finally the blood-vessels of the limb, and set up local lesions elsewhere than in the foot. Although dismissed here with these few words, the condition is a most serious one. Usually, it has resulted from penetration of the pedal articulation and septic infection of the joint. In the vast majority of these cases slaughter is both humane and economical.

Prognosis.—The first consideration in giving a prognosis in punctured foot should be the position of the wound. When occurring in the middle zone, the surgeon's statements should be most guarded, and the dangers attending a wound in that particular position fully explained to the owner. A wound in the anterior position is, as we have said, far less serious, and one in the posterior region of the foot even less serious still.

Whenever possible, the nail or other object causing the prick should be examined. Much of the prognosis may be based upon the estimated depth of the wound, and this, in many cases, it is far safer to calculate from the length of the offending body than from the use of the probe. We need hardly say that in the middle zone the deeper the prick, the more serious the case, and the less favourable the prognosis. As in succession the sensitive sole, the plantar aponeurosis, the navicular bursa, the navicular bone, or the pedal articulation is injured, so with each step deeper of the prick is the severity of the case increased.

The shape of the penetrating object may also be considered. One excessively blunt, and calculated to bruise and crush the tissues, will inflict a more serious wound than one of equal length that is pointed and sharp.

The conformation of the foot should also be regarded. Wounds in well-shaped feet are less serious than in feet with soles that are flat or convex, or in which the horn is pumiced or otherwise deteriorated in quality.

Although unaffecting the prognosis so far as the actual termination of the case is concerned, it may be mentioned that punctured foot is far more serious in a nag than in a heavy draught animal. With an equal degree of lameness resulting in each case, the former will be well-nigh useless, but the latter still capable of performing much of his usual labour.

The temperament and condition of the patient will also in many cases largely influence the prognosis. An animal of excitable and nervous disposition is far more likely to succumb to the effects of pain and exhaustion than the horse of a more lymphatic type. In the case of a patient suffering from a prick to a hind-foot while heavily pregnant, the attempted forecast of the termination should be cautious. More especially does this apply to the case of a heavy cart-mare. Ordinarily, the heavier the breed, the greater the tendency to lymphatic swelling of the hind-limbs. With pregnancy this tendency is enormously increased, and it is no uncommon thing to find a cart-mare in this condition, with legs, as the owner terms it, 'as thick as gate-posts.' A prick to the foot, with the lymphatics of the limb in this state, is extremely likely to end in septic infection of the leg, for there appears to be no doubt but that invasion of the lymphatics with septic matter is favoured by a sluggish stream. Also, in the case of a patient in the advanced stages of pregnancy, it must be remembered that, no matter how great may be the need, one is debarred, for obvious reasons, from using the slings.

Treatment.—*In a simple* case—and by 'simple' here we mean the case in which the injury is discovered early, and pus has not yet commenced to form—our first duties are to give the wound free drainage, and to maintain it in an aseptic condition. The first of these objects is to be arrived at by paring down the horn in a funnel-shaped fashion over the seat of the prick. It is, perhaps, even better to thin the horn down to the sensitive structures for some little distance round the injury. By this latter method pressure from inflammatory exudate is lessened, and the after-formation of pus, if unfortunate enough to occur, the more readily detected, and the less likely to spread upwards. The matter of asepsis may then be attended to.

When the puncture is sufficiently large to admit of it, the antiseptic dressing is best applied by means of the probe. This instrument is thinly wrapped with tow, or other absorbent material, so as to form a small swab. Dipped in a suitable solution (as, for example, Zinc Chloride, Spts. Hydrarg. Perchlor., Carbolic Acid, or any other that suggests itself), the swab is inserted into the prick, and the wound conveniently mopped clean. A further portion of the medicated tow is then pushed partially into the wound, and allowed to remain in position. The foot is subsequently wrapped in a clean bag, and kept free from dirt. This dressing should be repeated twice daily.

If the prick is in a dangerous position, and deep enough to occasion alarm, our precautions to prevent the formation of septic matters within it may be more elaborate. The thinning of the horn and the swabbing of the wound may, as before, be proceeded with. In addition, the whole foot may then be immersed for some hours daily in a cold bath, which bath should be strongly impregnated with one or other of the following salts: Iron Sulphate, Zinc Sulphate, Copper Sulphate, Aluminium Sulphate, Lead Acetate, or Sodium Chloride—better still, a mixture of the various sulphates here mentioned. If preferred, one of the more commonly accepted antiseptics—such as Carbolic Acid, Lysol, Boracic Acid, or Perchloride of Mercury—may be substituted.

By the cold of the bath inflammatory phenomena are held in check, while its added antiseptic prevents the formation of septic discharges. The lameness gradually diminishes, and resolution is rapid. In this way deep and serious, wounds are sometimes easily and successfully treated.

When suppuration has occurred—and this, by-the-by, is by far the most frequent condition in which we find punctured foot—treatment must be prompt and decided. Careful search must at once be made by thinning down the sole, and carefully trimming the frog. On no account should the veterinary attendant rest content with 'digging' in one place, and upon that basing a negative opinion as to the existence of pus. The paring should be carried on, until either pus or hæmorrhage shows itself, in at least three positions—namely, at the most anterior portion of the sole, and in the sole at each side of the frog. In addition to this, the frog itself should be minutely examined for evidence of puncture, or for leaking of pus at the spot where the horn of the heels joins the skin.

In many of our cases, however, this careful search is not so necessary. The accompanying symptoms are so decided as to leave no doubt as to the condition of the case. In such instances paring may often be commenced over the exact position of suppuration as previously ascertained by percussion.

When met with, the track formed by the suppurative process should be followed up in whichever direction it has spread. This will often necessitate the removal of the greater part, if not the whole, of the horny sole.

Having given vent to the pus, and opened up the cavity made by its formation, the foot should be placed in a hot poultice or, preferably, in a hot antiseptic bath.[A]

[Footnote A: At the time of writing this, a certain amount of discussion is going on in our veterinary journals as to whether a hot or a cold bath is the one indicated. It is urged against the application of heat that it favours organismal growth and reproduction, and tends rather to induce the spread of the suppurative process than to overcome it. Those who hold this opinion urge in support of it that cold applications are inimical to the life of the pus organism. At the same time, it must be remembered that in just so far as cold inhibits the growth of the invading germ, so in just the same degree does it adversely influence the functions of the tissues that are to fight against it. To our minds the question thus set up must always remain more or less a moot-point, and while we fully agree that cold undoubtedly checks the growth of septic material, we just as fully believe that warmth serves to place the healthy surrounding structures in a far better condition to maintain a vigorous phagocytosis against it. We thus continue to advise a hot antiseptic poultice, or, better still, a bath.—THE AUTHOR.]

At the end of the third or fourth day the poultice or the bath may be discontinued, and the opening in the sole dressed with any suitable astringent and antiseptic.

The most serious complication arising from this method of treatment is one of excessive granulation of the sensitive sole. This we find to be successfully held in check by a daily application of undiluted Spts. Hydrarg. Perchlor. (Tuson). Should the granulations become very exuberant, then the knife must be called to our aid, and the wound so made afterwards dressed with an astringent.

When the suppuration has under-run the horny frog there should be no hesitation in at once removing all the horn that is visibly separated from the sensitive structures beneath.

When the os pedis is splintered and carious, a portion of the sole round the wound is removed, and the bone exposed. The diseased portion is scraped away either with a curette or with the point of the drawing-knife. In this case the only after-treatment called for is the application of suitable antiseptic dressings.

When necrosis of the plantar aponeurosis has occurred. We have already pointed out the tendency there is in this case for the wound to maintain a fistulous character, and lead to the formation of abscesses in the hollow of the heel. With a wound in this position, as with a wound in any other, the only method of avoiding this termination consists in removing all that is visibly diseased, whether it be soft structures, bone, ligament, or tendon, and giving the wound free drainage.

This can only be done by removing the horny sole and frog, and cutting boldly down upon the structures beneath. The operation is known as resection of the plantar aponeurosis, or the complete operation for gathered nail.

Practised for some years on the Continent, this operation, on account of its gravity, has been avoided by English veterinarians. From reported cases, however, it appears often to be followed by success. That there is a large element of risk in the operation is quite evident, if only from the two facts mentioned beneath:

1. That the close attachment of the plantar aponeurosis to the navicular bursa, and the nearness of both to the pedal articulation, render penetration of a synovial sac or a joint cavity extremely likely.

2. That there is always great difficulty in maintaining strict asepsis of the foot, more especially if it is a hind one.

On the other hand, it may be argued that equal risk to the patient is run in allowing him to remain with a disease (and that disease a progressive one) of the structures so closely antiguous to the navicular bursa and the pedal articulation.

If only for that reason we give the operation brief mention here.

The animal is prepared in the usual way for the operating bed; the foot soaked for a day or two previously in a strong antiseptic solution, the patient cast and chloroformed, and the operation proceeded with.

FIG. 106.—'CURETTE,' OR VOLKMANN'S SPOON.

An Esmarch's bandage should be first applied, and a tourniquet afterwards placed higher up on the limb. The foot is then secured as described in an earlier chapter, and the whole of the horny structures of the lower surface of the foot (the sole, the frog, and the bars) pared until quite near the sensitive structures, or, if under-run with pus, stripped off entirely. An incision is then made in each lateral lacuna of the frog, the two meeting at the frog's point. Each incision thus made should be carried deep enough to cut through the substance of the plantar cushion. A tape is then passed through the point of the frog, tied in a loop, and given to an assistant to draw backwards. The plantar cushion itself is then incised in a direction from before backwards, and pulled on by the assistant, so as to expose the plantar aponeurosis.

Should this be found at all necrotic, it may be taken that purulent inflammation of the navicular bursa and of the navicular bone itself exists. The operator must then proceed to resection of the tendon in order to treat the deeper structures thus affected. At its point of insertion into the semilunar crest the tendon is severed and afterwards reflected. This exposes the inferior face of the navicular bone. Instead of the glistening and clear appearance it ordinarily presents, its glenoid cartilage is found to be showing hæmorrhagic or even purulent spots of necrosis. The terminal portion of the tendon must then be excised.

To effect this a clean transverse incision is made at the extreme upper border of the navicular bone. Here we are in close contact with the pedal articulation, and great care is necessary in making this last incision, in order that the synovial sac may not be penetrated.

All structures showing spots of necrosis should now be carefully removed, either with the knife or with the curette. The knives most suitable for the last stages of this operation are those depicted in Fig. 45 (c, d, and e). The curette, or Volkmann's spoon, we show in Fig. 106.

FIG. 107.—RESECTION OF TERMINAL PORTION OF THE PERFORANS. The horny sole and the horny frog stripped from off the sensitive structures. a, The plantar cushion; b, b, the plantar aponeurosis, or terminal portion of perforans; c, the navicular bone; d, interosseous ligaments of the pedal articulation; e, e, semilunar crest of the os pedis; f, inferior surface of os pedis; g, g, the sensitive laminæ of the bars; h, h, bearing surface of the wall; i, i, the sensitive sole; k, the sensitive frog.

When at all diseased the glenoidal surface of the navicular bone should be curetted, even to the extent of the removal of the whole of the cartilage. A healthy, granulating surface is thus insured.

The above figure from Gutenacker's 'Hufkrankheiten' explains shortly the position of the operation wound and the structures involved, rendering further description unnecessary here.

The operation ended, the dressing follows. Upon this depends very largely the ultimate recovery of the patient, for it is only by careful attention and suitable dressings that effectual repair of the injured structures may be brought about.

A light shoe is first tacked on to the foot, and those portions of the horny sole that have been allowed to remain dressed with Venice turpentine, tar, or other thickly-adherent antiseptic.

The exposed soft tissues are then dressed with pledgets of tow[A] soaked in alcohol and carbolic acid. This dressing must be allowed to remain in position, and is kept there by means of a bandage, or the shoe with plates (Fig. 55) and a bandage over it. No pressure is needed; consequently, the pledgets of tow must not be too thick.

[Footnote A: When using tow in the form of a pad, it is well to remember that many small balls of the material rolled lightly in the palm of the hand and afterwards massed together are far better than one large pad of the tow taken without this preparation. The irregularities of the wound are better fitted, and the whole dressing easier remains *in situ* (H.C.R.).]

In the after-dressing of the wound careful attention must be paid to the granulating surface. Where tending to become too vigorous in growth it should be held in check by suitable caustic dressings. At the same time it must be remembered that the granulating process of repair is always more rapid upon the plantar cushion and fleshy sole than upon the bone, or upon tendinous or cartilaginous structures. As a result of this we have a wound showing various aspects of cicatrization. Healthy granulation may be profuse in one spot, while in another it may be checked either by a flow of synovia from the still open bursa, or by fragments of bone or of tendon still acting as foreign bodies in the wound. These latter may be readily detected by their standing out as dark and uncovered spots in the healthy granulation around, and should be at once removed.

The time that an operation wound of this description takes to heal—and that without complication—is from one to two or three months. Continuation of pain and intensity of lameness are not to be taken as indications of failure. The reparative inflammation in the synovial membrane is quite sufficient to induce pain severe enough to prevent the animal from placing his foot to the ground for some weeks, even though the progress of the case, all unknown, may be all that is desired. So long as a great amount of pain is absent, and so long as appetite remains and swellings in the hollow of the heel fail to make their appearance, so long may the progress of the case be deemed satisfactory.

Recorded Case of the Treatment.—A cart-horse, aged six years, was sent to the Alfort School by a veterinary surgeon for having picked up a nail in the hind-foot. Professor Cadiot, judging the necessity for the complete operation, performed it on January 14, and spared the plantar cushion as much as possible. In consequence of the plantar aponeurosis being extensively necrosed, it was advisable to scrape the navicular bone and a part of the semilunar crest. The wound having been washed with a 1 per cent. solution of perchloride of mercury, it was dusted with iodoform and packed with gauze, and covered with a cotton-wool dressing, kept in position by means of a suitable shoe.

On January 16 there was no snatching up of the limb when the horse was made to put weight upon it; he ate his food well, and his condition improved every day. On January 21 the dressing was removed; the wound appeared pinky and granular, and there was no suppuration. The clot remaining from the hæmorrhage after the operation was removed, the wound was irrigated with a hot solution of sublimate, and then dusted with iodoform and covered with a dressing of iodoform gauze and absorbent wool. At this date the horse could stand on the injured limb. On January 31 a second dressing was made, and the animal almost walked sound. On February 7 the wound had almost closed up, save in its central part, where there was a small cavity, and the lameness had disappeared. On February 15 the wound had completely healed, and its borders were covered by a layer of thin horn. As the animal was sound it was sent to work.

The author directs attention to the rapidity with which a large and complete wound cicatrizes after the operation for gathered nail.[A]

[Footnote A: *Veterinary Record*, vol. XV., p. 226 (Jourdan).]

In the case of Penetrated Navicular Bursa, unaccompanied by the formation of any large quantity of pus, and uncomplicated by necrosis of the aponeurosis, our aim must be to maintain the wound in that happy condition. This is doubtless best done by keeping the foot continually in a cold bath, rendered strongly antiseptic by the addition of sulphate of copper and perchloride of mercury. Should there be intervals when the bath must be neglected, the foot in the meantime must be kept clean by antiseptic packing and bandaging, and a clean bag over all. This treatment should be continued so long as the character of the discharge denotes that synovia is running. If, in spite of our precautions, the discharge becomes purulent, then the track made by the penetrating object should be syringed twice daily with a 1 in 1,000 solution of perchloride of mercury.

During the treatment it will be wise to shoe the animal with a high-heeled shoe. We do not know as yet the full extent of the injury. The navicular bone may be tending to caries; or necrosis of the plantar aponeurosis, all unknown, gradually becoming pronounced. This calls for a relief of tension on the perforans, and is only to be brought about by the high-heeled shoe.

The result of the inflammatory changes in the tendon, aided possibly by the use of the high-heeled shoe, is to afterwards bring about contraction. Where this has occurred, and the animal walks continuously on his toe, the shoe with the projecting toe-piece (Fig. 84) must be applied. When the continual use of the toe-piece appears inadvisable, the shoe devised by Colonel Nunn may be used in its stead (see Fig. 108).

The toe-piece is screwed into the toe of the shoe when the horse is about to be exercised, and forms a powerful point of leverage with which to stretch the contracted tendon, and the shoe, being thin at the heels, admits of this. The advantage of this form of toe-piece over the ordinary form of fixed toe-lever is that it can be removed when the horse is in the stable; while the curved point diminishes the danger of the horse hurting itself—a danger always present if it is on a hind-foot. (See also Treatment of Purulent Arthritis in Chapter XII.)

FIG. 108.—COLONEL NUNN'S SHOE WITH DETACHABLE TOE EXTENSION.

Should a Sinuous Wound remain in the region of the Lateral Cartilage, it should be explored, and its depth and likely number of branches ascertained. Should this exploration denote that the cartilage itself is diseased, or that the wound is not able to be sufficiently drained from the sole, then we know that we have on our hands a case of quittor. The treatment necessary in such a case will be found described in Chapter X.

When the Complication of Purulent Arthritis has arisen, the surgeon has to admit to himself, reluctantly no doubt, that the case is often beyond hope of aid from him. Nothing can be done save to order continuous antiseptic baths and antiseptic irrigation of the wounds with a quittor syringe, and to attend to the general health and condition of the patient. At the best it is but a sorry look-out both for the veterinary attendant and the owner of the animal. Even with resolution incurable lameness results, and the animal is afterwards more or less a walking exhibition of the limitations of surgery, while the owner, unless the animal is valuable for the purpose of breeding, finds himself encumbered with a life that is practically useless. (See Treatment of Purulent Arthritis, Chapter XII.)

In the case of Lameness Persisting after the healing of all appreciable lesions, then neurectomy is followed by good results. The animal, apparently recovered, is for a long time useless. Lameness persists for several months, as if the nail had at the moment of its penetration caused lesions, which doubtless it sometimes does, similar to those of navicular disease. Examination of the foot in this case reveals no lesion, and the pain has evidently a deep origin. The lameness caused by it is subject to variation. Frequently it becomes lessened during rest, and increased by hard work, while sometimes it is very much more pronounced at starting than after exercise.

It is here that neurectomy is called for. The operation does nothing to impede the work of healing going on, and allows free movement of the foot and pastern to take place. At the same time suffering and emaciation cease, and the animal is rendered workable.[A]

[Footnote A: *Veterinary Record*, vol. ii., p. 371.]

C. CORONITIS (SIMPLE). TREAD, OVERREACH, ETC.

1. *Acute.*

Definition.—Under the heading of simple coronitis in its acute form we intend to describe those inflammatory conditions of the skin and underlying structures of the coronet occurring without specific cause. Specific coronitis will be found described in Chapter IX.

Causes.—This condition is almost invariably set up by an injury—either a bruise or an actual wound—to the coronet. By far the most common among such injuries are those inflicted by the animal himself by means of the shoes.

That known as 'tread' is caused by the shoe on the opposite foot, and may happen in a variety of ways. More often than not it is met with in the feet of heavy draught animals, and is there caused by the calkin, either when being violently backed or suddenly turned round. It may also occur in horses with itchy legs, as a result of the animal rubbing the leg with the shoe of the opposite limb. The irritation in this case is nearly always due to parasitic infection (*Symbiotes equi*), and becomes sometimes so unbearable as to render the animal unmindful of the injury he may be inflicting so long as he experiences the relief obtained by the rubbing.

Self-inflicted tread is also sometimes met with when horses are worked abreast at plough. The animal in the furrow, with one foot sometimes in and sometimes out of the hollow, is caused to make a false step, and so brings the injury about.

Animals worked in pairs are further liable to receive a tread from the foot of their companion. This is commonly seen in heavy animals at agricultural labour in fields, where the walking is uneven, and abrupt turning constant. It is not uncommon either in animals at work in vans in town, and is occasionally met with in the feet of carriage-horses.

'Overreach' is the term used to indicate the injury inflicted on the coronary portion of the heel of the fore-foot by the shoe of the hind. Ordinarily, overreach occurs when the animal is at a gallop, and is thus met with in its severest form in hunters and steeplechasers. It can only occur when the fore-foot is raised from the ground and the hind-foot of the same side reached right forward. When the feet separate the injury takes place. In its movement backwards the inner border of the shoe of the hind-foot catches the coronet of the fore, and tears it backwards with it. Quite frequently a portion of the skin is removed entirely, but often it hangs as a triangular flap. The flap in such a case is always attached by its hindermost edge, and indicates plainly enough that the direction of the blow that cut it must have been from before backwards.

Although ordinarily inflicted at the gallop, the same injury may, nevertheless, be caused by allowing a fast trotter, and one with extreme freedom of action behind, to push forward at the utmost limit of his pace. The outside heel is the one most subject to the injury.

While the common form of injury to the coronet is, as we have described, that occasioned by the animal's own shoe, or that of a companion, it is evident that the foot is also open to similar injuries from quite outside sources. Falls of the shafts when unyoking animals from a heavy cart, blows or wounds from the stable fork, wounds resulting from the foot becoming fixed in a gate or a fence, either may equally well set up the mischief.

Apart from severe injury, a particularly troublesome form of coronitis may arise from the condition of the roads. We refer to the conditions attendant on a thaw after snow. The animal is called upon to labour in, or perhaps stand for long periods in, a mixture of snow and water, or snow and mud. That this must have a prejudicial effect upon the structure of the coronet is plain. The circulation of the part, already predisposed to sluggishness by reason of its distance from the heart, is farther impeded by the action of the cold. Small abrasions of the skin, so small as to scarce be noticeable, are in this case freely open to infection with the septic matter the mud contains. Necrosis and consequent sloughing of the skin is bound to follow, and an extensive ulcerous wound, or a spreading suppuration of the coronary cushion is the result.

Symptoms.—We will take first the case in which no actual wound is observable. Here the first indication of the trouble is the appearance of an inflammatory swelling, confined usually to one side, but extending sometimes to the whole of the coronet. Always the part is hot and tender, and with it the patient is lame—so much so, in many cases, as to be unable to put the foot to the ground, the toe alone being used.

In a mild case, uncomplicated by septic infection, these symptoms rapidly subside, and resolution occurs.

Always, however, the presence of septic infection must be suspected and looked for. When this has occurred, the inflammatory swelling becomes larger and more diffuse, and the animal fevered. This is then followed by a slough of the injured part. A portion of the skin first becomes gray, or even black, in appearance, and around it oozes an inflammatory exudate, or even pus. The skin immediately adjoining the spot of necrosis is swollen and hyperæmic, and extremely painful and sensitive. Later, the necrosed portion becomes cast off, and an open wound remains. This as a rule marks the turning-point in the case. The pain and other symptoms rapidly abate, and the wound, with proper attention, is not more than ordinarily difficult to treat.

In the case of an actual wound the symptoms are probably less severe. The injury is, in this instance, the sooner detected, and remedial measures put into operation. In this manner the formation of septic material is often checked, and nothing but the treatment of a simple wound demands attention.

There are, however, complications.

Complications—(a) Diffuse Purulent Inflammation of the Sub-coronary Tissue.—This condition is brought about by the spread into the loose tissue of the coronary cushion of the septic material introduced by the tread. The whole coronet in this instance becomes excessively swollen, hot, and painful, and the dangerous nature of the complication is evident enough when the structure and situation of the parts involved is considered. The amount of tendinous and ligamentous material in the neighbourhood offers a strong predisposition to necrosis, and the necrosis, with its attendant formation of pus, offers a further danger when the close proximity of the pedal articulation and the unyielding character of the horny box is considered with it.

The pus formed in this condition may remain confined to the coronet and break through the skin as an ordinary abscess, or it may, before so doing, burrow beneath the wall, and invade the sensitive laminæ. In this case, whenever portions of the secreting layer of the keratogenous membrane are destroyed, or perhaps only temporarily prevented from fulfilling their horn-producing functions, then corresponding cavities in the horn are the result (see Fig. 109).

(b) Purulent Arthritis.—Only too readily the pus so formed tends to penetration of the articulation and the causation of an incurable arthritis (see Chapter XII.).

FIG. 109.—MESIAL SECTION OF A HOOF ILLUSTRATING THE CONDITIONS FOLLOWING UPON CORONITIS. *a*, Cavity in the horn of the wall; *b*, enlargement of the coronet and the horn of the wall following sub-coronary suppuration; *c*, cavity in the wall following purulent inflammation of the sensitive laminæ; *d*, hollow in the horn of the sole consequent upon suppuration of the sensitive sole.

(c) Necrosis of the Extensor Pedis.—This may arise either as a result of spreading purulent infection of the coronary cushion, or as a result of direct injury immediately over it. The close relation of the terminal portion of this tendon with the pedal articulation, and the incomplete protection from outside injuries here afforded to the joint by the horny box, sufficiently points out the gravity of the condition.

(d) Penetration of the Articulation.—This also may be a result either of the inroads made by pus, or of an actual wound. When occurring from the latter, it is seen more often than not in the hind-foot, being there caused by the calkin of the opposite foot. Where a wound in this position is characterized by an excessive flow of synovia, the condition should be suspected, and, if the wound be large enough, the little finger should be introduced in order to ascertain. Needless to say, the injury is a grave one.

(e) Sand-crack.—Sand-crack is likely to result from tread when an injury is inflicted in the region of the quarter by a severe overreach. Treads, too, especially with the calkin of the hind-shoe, are especially apt to end in this way. In this latter instance the sand-crack usually has its origin in a nasty jagged tear at the top of the wall of the toe.

(f) Quittor.—In one respect any suppurating wound at the coronet may be deemed a quittor. By indicating quittor as a complication of coronitis, however, we denote the more serious form of this disease, in which the wound has taken on a sinuous character, and conducted pus to invasion of the lateral cartilage. It is one of the worst complications we are likely to meet with in this condition, and will be found fully described in Chapter X.

(g) False Quarter.—This complication of coronitis occurs when the injury or after-effect of the formation of pus has been severe enough to destroy outright a comparatively large portion of the papillary layer of the coronary cushion. To this condition we devote Section D of this chapter.

Prognosis.—In giving a prognosis in a case of coronitis, attention should be paid to the manner in which the condition originated, and the extent, when present, of the wound.

When the inflammatory swelling has arisen from bruising alone, without actual division of the skin, when the weather is that of winter, and the swelling showing a marked tendency to spread, then the prognosis must be guarded. As we have seen, this state of affairs is probably ushering in a condition of spreading suppuration of the coronary cushion, and considerable gangrene and sloughing of the skin. We have here no intimation as yet of how far the suppurative process may run, nor what important structures it may involve. Consequently, the guarded prognosis we have mentioned is imperative.

Where an actual wound is to be seen, and where advice is sought early, then a more favourable opinion may be advanced. In this case antiseptic measures, commenced early and persisted in, may prevent the rise of further mischief.

It goes without saying that, should there arise any other of the complications we have mentioned (viz., Arthritis, Necrosis of the Extensor Pedis, Sand-crack, Quittor, and False Quarter), the fact should be pointed out to the owner, and the prognosis regulated thereby.

Treatment—Preventive.—Seeing that at any rate the majority of cases of coronitis result from injuries inflicted by the shoes, we may look at once to that particular for a means of prevention.

Take first the case of 'treads'. There is no doubt that they are most common in animals shod with heavy shoes and with high and sharp calkins. This suggests at once that a preventive is to be found in substituting a calkin that is low and square.

Where the injury is an overreach, and where, on account of the animal's pace and manner of gait it is in risk of being constantly inflicted, the shoeing should be seen to at once.

We have already pointed out that it is the inner border of the lower surface of the toe of the hind-shoe which, in the act of being drawn backwards, inflicts the injury. (See Fig. 110).

In this case prevention may be brought about either by shoeing with a shoe whose ground surface is wholly concave, or by bevelling off the sharp border (see Fig. 110, a, p. 236). When the tendency to overreach is not excessive, prevention may in many cases be effected by simply placing the shoe of the hind-foot a trifle further backwards than would ordinarily be correct, thus allowing the horn of the toe to project beyond the shoe. This at the same time does away with the annoyance of 'forging' or 'clacking,' which, as a rule, accompanies this condition.

While recognising the value of shoeing in these cases, we must not forget that a great deal may be brought about by careful horsemanship. The animal should be held together and kept well up to the bit, but should *not* be allowed to push forward at the top of his pace. With many animals of fast pace and free action overreach is more an indiscretion of youth than any defect in action or conformation, and his powers should therefore be husbanded by the driver until the animal has settled down into a convenient and steady manner of going.

FIG. 110.—UNDER SURFACE OF THE TOE OF A HIND-SHOE. *a*, Marks the portion of the inner margin that inflicts overreach.

FIG. 111.—THE INNER MARGIN OF THE INFERIOR SURFACE OF THE HIND-SHOE BEVELLED TO PREVENT OVERREACH.

Curative.—Although in some cases it is so small as to go undetected, we may take it that in all cases of coronitis there is a wound, with consequent danger of septic infection of the surrounding parts. Therefore, after attention to the shoeing and removal of the cause, the first indication in the treatment will be to render the parts aseptic. This is best done by removing the hair from the coronet and soaking the whole foot in a cold antiseptic solution. After removal from the bath, the coronet may be dressed with a moderately strong solution of carbolic acid or perchloride of mercury. When the injury is slight and recent, such is sufficient to effect resolution.

When marked swelling persists, however, and the increase in heat and tenderness denotes the formation of pus, recovery is not so easily obtained. In this case the application of hot poultices or hot baths is called for. By these means suppuration is promoted and induced to early break through in the most favourable position—namely, the softened skin of the coronet. The pus so escaping is always more or less blood-stained, and contains both large and small pieces of broken down and decomposed tissue. After discharge of the pus, the cavity remaining should be mopped out with an antiseptic solution, and a pledget of antiseptic tow or other material left in position. All that is then needed is constant dressing in a suitable manner. We prefer in this instance washing some three or four times a day with hot water until a perfectly clean wound is obtained, and, after the washing, painting the raw surface with a strong solution (1 in 200, or 1 in 100) of perchloride of mercury.

When the abscess we have described as forming is extremely large, or where it is more than ordinarily slow in 'pointing,' the likelihood of its having burrowed for some distance below the upper margin of the wall must be suspected. Here it is sometimes wise to thin the wall with the rasp immediately below the point of greatest swelling of the coronet. This will serve to lessen pressure on the sensitive structures beneath.

Immediately the abscess contents have found exit at the coronet, the cavity formerly occupied by the pus should be explored. If to any extent it is found then to have 'pocketed' beneath the upper border of the wall, a counter-opening should be made where the horn of the wall has been thinned with the rasp.

When it so happens, either from extensive bruising or from the action of excessive cold, that we have or suspect the condition of sloughing, then the first indication is to aid the live tissues to throw off the necrosed portion. In spite of what is sometimes urged to the contrary, a hot poultice is, perhaps, the best means of bringing this about. Directly the necrosed piece is shed, a wound remains which, so far as treatment is concerned, may be regarded exactly as that left by the formation of pus. Hot water applications, some three or four times daily, will serve both to cleanse the wound and also to maintain vitality in the tissues immediately surrounding it. After each washing, the use of a strong antiseptic solution to the wound is again beneficial.

In the case of an actual wound, whether, as in overreach, affecting the coronet alone or involving destruction of part of the wall, or, as in the case of toe-tread, penetrating the pedal articulation, the treatment to be followed is simple enough, in theory, if not always easy to carry out. It consists solely in maintaining a rigid asepsis of the parts until healing is well advanced or complete. The whole foot, including the coronet, should first be thoroughly washed in warm water. At the same time there should be used some agent that will tend to remove the natural grease of the parts. In this manner cleansing will be rendered more thorough, and penetration of the antiseptic solution to be afterwards applied made the more certain. The most ready way of effecting this is to use the ordinary stable 'water'-brush, and plenty of a freely-lathering soap.

This done, the foot should be rinsed in cold water, and afterwards constantly soaked in a cold antiseptic bath. Where it is inconvenient or impossible to have the constant bathing carried out, a dry antiseptic dressing may be tried in its stead. In this case the foot should first be thoroughly washed and dressed as before. Afterwards an antiseptic powder in the shape of a mixture of iodoform 1 part, boracic acid 10 parts, should be freely dusted on the wound, a pledget of carbolized tow or cotton-wool placed over it, and the whole maintained in position with a bandage previously soaked in a 1 in 500 solution of perchloride of mercury. Once on, this dressing should be allowed to remain until healing is complete. Should the animal manifest pain, however, by constantly pawing, or should swelling and heat of the parts be suspected, the bandage should be removed, and the condition of the wound ascertained.

An excellent example of the value of this method of treatment is that given below:

'I call to mind a valuable hunter in my practice a few seasons since, who, whilst hunting, we suppose, struck himself in the way we suggest. He not only removed the superior portion of the inner heel, but tore about 3 inches of the hoof from the top nearly to the bottom. This was clapped back by the owner, tied with a handkerchief, and the horse removed home. When the handkerchief was removed, I confess I did not think the horse looked at all like hunting again. The heel was fairly pulled down, the portion of the hoof that was hanging to it I could easily have wrenched off. The parts were fomented, however, with warm water which was slightly carbolized. I then removed a great portion of the heel and the lateral cartilage, which was split; placed the portion of hoof again on the laminæ, smothered the wound with iodoform pulv., covered it with cotton-wool packing, and all the boracic acid I could get it to hold. A piece of linen bandage was then tightly wrapped a few times round, and the lot enclosed in a plaster-of-Paris bandage. I did not undo it for a fortnight, when, to my great pleasure, the heel and hoof presented a highly satisfactory appearance. I did it up in much the same way for another ten days, then put the sand-crack clamps into the hoof and fixed it to the sound part. The hoof remained in position while the new horn grew from the top, and the horse hunted again the same season.'[A]

[Footnote A: *Veterinary Record*, vol. ix., p. 501 (Bower).]

Sequels.—Either of the complications we have mentioned—as, for instance, Arthritis, Sand-crack, or Quittor—may persist and remain as sequels to the case. In addition to these, there may be left behind a cavity in the horn of the wall (see Fig. 109), or a loss of the horn-substance of the wall proper, as that depicted in Fig. 112, or described under the heading of False Quarter.

Fig. 112.—HOOF WITH A CAVITY IN THE SUBSTANCE OF THE WALL FOLLOWING UPON 'TREAD' TO THE CORONET.

The treatment of Arthritis, Sand-crack, Quittor, False Quarter, and Seedy-toe, will be found in the chapters devoted to their consideration.

2. *Chronic.*

Definition.—Coronitis in which, owing to the persistence of the cause, inflammatory phenomena continue, resulting in the growth of large fibrous tumours about the coronet.

Causes.—In many cases it is possible, of course, that abnormal large growths in this position may have an origin similar to that of neoplasms elsewhere—that is to say, an origin as yet undiscovered. There is no doubt, however, that the majority of the huge enlargements about the coronet have their starting-point in one or other of the diseases to which the foot is liable, in which the cause remains, and a low type of inflammation persists.

In chronic and neglected suppurating corn, in untreated quittor, and in long-standing complicated sand-crack, for instance, we have conditions in which pus and other septic matters find ready entrance into the sub-coronary tissues. Should either of these be neglected, or should the pus formation from the onset take on a slow but gradually spreading form (in other words, should either of these cases run a chronic rather than an acute course) then, with the persistence of the inflammatory phenomena so caused, is bound to result a steady and increasing growth of inflammatory fibrous connective tissue. This, as it grows, becomes in its turn penetrated by the ever-invading pus, and, under the stimulus thus caused, itself throws out new tissue. And so, constantly excited, the tumour-like mass tends to steady increase in size, until enlargements are formed which one may sometimes truly term enormous.

Symptoms.—The appearance of the growth is, of course, immediately evident. Usually these swellings are slow in forming, so that the size of the enlargement depends entirely upon its age. We may thus meet with growths of this description, varying in weight from 4 or 5 pounds to the almost incredible size of 33-1/2 pounds. In the majority of cases a discharging sore is to be found upon it—in some cases several. Explored, these sores reveal their true nature. Their lip-like openings, and the ready manner in which they may be searched by the probe, show them to be sinuses.

In a few cases, however, the outer surface of these tumours is intact. When this is the case, it is possible that the growth is a true fibroma—that is to say, a non-inflammatory new growth of fibrous connective tissue. On the other hand, it may have resulted from one or other of the causes we have enumerated, and its exact diagnosis have been impossible until operative measures had been proceeded with. In this case, small and encysted foci of inspissated pus scattered more or less throughout the growth indicate its true nature.

Pain as a rule is absent, and, unless the growth, on account of its size, interferes with progress, the animal walks perfectly sound. Here the patient may, without offending the dictates of humanity, be put to slow work.

Treatment.—In very many cases, possibly on account of the decreased circulation and vitality of the parts, these growths occur in aged animals. Here treatment is not economic, and may for that reason be put out of the question. Further, the growths are more common in heavy cart animals of a lymphatic type than in those of a lighter breed. Couple this with the fact that the tumour is often unattended with pain, and we see that the animal is still able to perform his accustomed labour. Here, again, treatment is contra-indicated.

For still another reason surgical treatment, which is the only treatment likely to be of benefit, must not be undertaken rashly. A large and open wound is bound to be left behind. So large is it in many cases that the complete covering of the exposed surface with epidermal growths from the circumference cannot possibly be looked for. There is then left a large and horny-looking scar, which is an even worse eyesore than was the original enlargement.

When the patient is a young and otherwise valuable animal, however, and when the case, judged either by the size of the swelling or its outside appearance, promises a fair measure of success, operative measures may be determined on.

In this case the author's practice has been, after casting the animal, to apply a tourniquet to the limb and proceed to excision. A lozenge-shaped incision, extending to near but not quite the circumference of the swelling, should be made with a large knife right through the skin and deeply into the growth. The whole is then removed, proceeding in an excavating manner under the thickened skin at the margin. Hæmorrhage, though proceeding from several apparently large vessels in the structure of the tumour, and oozing generally over the whole of the outer surface, is rarely profuse enough to interfere with the operation, and is easily controlled by cold water douches and the application of the artery forceps to one or more of the larger vessels. The operation completed, the larger bleeding-points should be secured by exerting torsion with the artery forceps, and the surface oozing stayed by frequent dashing with cold water.

When the hæmorrhage has sufficiently ceased, an ordinary flat firing-iron should be passed over the whole of the cut surface, and an effectual eschar formed.

Following this, and *before removing the tourniquet*, the wound should be filled with pledgets of carbolized tow, and the whole tightly secured by a stout and broad linen bandage of not less than 6 yards in length.

Reported Case.—'The patient, a middle-aged cart mare, had a pair of fore-feet the like of which I never saw. As the result of long-standing and imperfectly-treated quittor all over the seat of side-bone on the outer side of each fore-foot, beginning pretty far forward, and extending to the heel on the inner side, filling up the hollow and reaching nearly to the fetlock, was a big, bulging, hard, calloused enlargement or tumour standing out 3 or 4 inches all round, covered with thick horny skin and stubby hair, and having on its surface the small openings of several sinuses leading deeply down to the ossified and diseased cartilage underneath. And yet with all this diseased undergrowth the mare, strangely enough, walked and trotted sound. I was told that this mare had been troubled with suppurating corns and quittor, that many unsuccessful attempts had been made at cure, but that, getting worse instead of better, these tumours had formed.

'After casting and anæsthetizing, a strong rubber tourniquet was placed above the knee and the operation commenced. With a surgeon's amputating knife all the big fibrous mass which I could safely remove was cut and sliced off, and the coronet and pastern reduced as nearly as possible to its natural dimensions. The diseased cartilage, or side-bone, gave some trouble, a considerable portion having to be cut and scraped, and the sinus in it gouged out; but its complete removal did not appear to be called for.

'There was little if any hæmorrhage until release of the tourniquet, when the whole broad surface became deluged with blood, three or four small arteries spurting and veins flowing in all directions, so much so that I was glad to refix the clasp, and with the firing-iron seal up the vessels, searing gently all over the surface.

FIG. 113.—CHRONIC CORONITIS FOLLOWING 'TREAD.'

'A good dusting with antiseptic powder, a thick pad of carbolized wool, and two long calico bandages wound tightly round, completed the work.

'The other, the near-leg, was then dealt with in the same way.'

'The mass removed weighed a little over 9-1/2 pounds—5 pounds from the off-foot and 4-1/2 pounds from the near. Its structure was fibrous tissue, almost as firm and hard as cartilage, and with no appearance of malignancy.

'The after-treatment consisted simply of fresh dry dressings—copper, sulphate, zinc sulphate, and calamine, equal parts—applied every third or fourth day, after first bathing the feet in a shallow tub of warm antiseptic water.

'At the end of eight or ten weeks a fairly presentable appearance existed. The greater part of what had been raw surface was covered with healthy skin, and the remainder had become dry and horny.'[A]

[Footnote A: *Veterinary Record*, vol. xiv., p. 201 (C. Cunningham, M.R.C.V.S.).]

A further form of chronic coronitis is that shown in Fig. 113.

This condition is commonly the result of a severe and jagged tread with the calkin, and takes the form of an ulcerous and excessively granulating wound. As time goes on the granulations become hard and horny-looking, and their fibrous tissue as hard and unyielding as tendon or cartilage.

These if treated in the early stages with repeated dressings of caustic, or, if very exuberant, the use of the knife, usually yield to treatment. If neglected until the condition depicted in the figure is arrived at, then treatment, as a rule, is of no avail. Neither is treatment of any use if any great loss of the coronary cushion has occurred.

D. FALSE QUARTER.

Definition.—False quarter is the term applied to that condition of the horn of the quarter in which, owing to disease or injury of the coronet, the wall is grown in a manner that is incomplete.

Symptoms.—This condition of the foot appears as a gap or shallow indentation, narrow or wide, in the thickness of the wall, with its length in the direction of the horn fibres. By this we do not mean that the sensitive laminæ are bared and exposed. Horn of a sort there is, and with this the sensitive structures are covered. Running down the centre of the incomplete horn is usually a narrow fissure marking the line of separation in the papillary layer of the coronary cushion, which, as we shall later see, is responsible for the malformation.

On either side of the indentation, as if wishing to aid further than ordinarily it should in bearing the body-weight, the horn takes on an increased growth, and stands above the level of the horn surrounding it. It may, as perhaps it really is, be regarded as a form of hypertrophy, brought about by the increased work that the loss of substance in the region of the false quarter puts upon it.

So long as the sensitive structures are protected the animal remains sound. Sometimes, however, from the effects of concussion or of the body-weight, a fissure appears in the narrow veneer of horn that covers them. Into this, which, of course, is but a form of sand-crack, gravel and dirt penetrate, and so set up inflammatory changes in the keratogenous membrane. As a result suppuration ensues, and the animal is lame.

Causes.—False quarter may result from any disease of the foot that involves destruction of a portion of the coronary cushion. As we may see from a reference to Chapter III., it is from the papillæ of this body that the horn tubules of the wall are secreted. Destruction of any portion of it necessarily results in a corresponding loss of horn in that position. The disease occasioning this more often than any other is perhaps quittor. It may also result from suppurating corn, from a severe tread or overreach, or from the effects of a slowly progressing suppurating coronitis.

Treatment.—A radical treatment of false quarter is not to be found. Once destruction of the secreting layer of the coronary cushion has occurred, the appearance of the fissure in the wall will always have to be reckoned with. A false quarter, therefore, not only renders the horse liable to occasional lameness, but also renders weaker that side of the hoof in which it occurs.

The only method of treatment that can be practised, therefore, is that of palliation. Seeing that the trouble the veterinary attendant will have to deal with is loss of a portion of the weight-bearing surface, his attention is immediately directed to the shoeing. As with sand-crack, so with false quarter, the frog and the bars must be called upon to take more of the body-weight than commonly they do with the ordinary shoe. The indication, then, is a bar shoe. At the same time, the bearing of the wall on the shoe on either side of the fissure should be eased by slightly paring it, and the hypertrophied horn on the outer surface of the wall removed with the rasp.

In cases where penetration of the sensitive structures has occurred, complicated with the formation of pus, the same treatment as for complicated crack is to be followed. The foot should be poulticed for several days with hot antiseptic dressings, and thorough cleansing of the infected parted brought about. Afterwards strong solutions of suitable antiseptics should be applied daily until such time as the horny covering has renewed itself. This done and the bar shoe applied, the fissure may be plugged with any effectual stopping. Either a mixture, such as Percival's, of pitch 2 parts, tar 1 part, and resin 1 part, melted and mixed together, or one of the artificial hoof-horns may either be used with advantage.

E. ACCIDENTAL TEARING OFF OF THE ENTIRE HOOF.

Causes.—Seeing that this accident to, and consequent severe wounding of, the keratogenous membrane nearly always occurs in but one way, it is worthy of special mention. So far as we are able to ascertain, it is an accident peculiar to horses continually engaged in shunting operations either in pits or station-yards. At the moment the animal is released from the waggon he has been pulling, and should turn to the right or the left in order to allow it to pass him, the shoe either becomes wedged in between two converging rails, or is trapped by the wheel of the waggon. Either the approaching waggon with the added weight its impetus gives it then pushes the animal suddenly away, leaving a part of his foot still fixed to the rails, or the animal himself, feeling securely held, makes a sudden effort to release himself, and draws his foot cleanly out of the imprisoned horny box.

The author calls to mind a case in which entire removal of the horn of the foot of an ox occurred through the passing over it of the wheel of a heavily-laden cart. It is therefore quite conceivable that the same accident might occur to the horse. As a matter of fact, we find one case on record where one-half of the horny box was thus removed.[A]

[Footnote A: *Veterinary Record*, vol. xiii., p. 129.]

So far as we are able to gather, it is more a result of imprisonment of the shoe than of the foot. It appears, further, to be always a result of the animal being newly shod, and the clinches firmly secured; so much so that it would be probable, with imperfectly secured clinches, that the animal would draw the hoof from the clinches and the shoe rather than the foot from its horny covering.

Therefore, as the author of one of the cases we shall afterwards relate suggests, it should be proposed as a preventive that the shoe-nails of animals regularly engaged in work on the metals should not be clinched in the regulation manner, but should have their points merely screwed off, and the nails afterwards rasped level with the wall.

These cases are particularly interesting as illustrating the rapid manner in which a new hoof is afterwards formed, and the way in which the exposed sensitive laminæ take their share in adding to, though not forming the bulk of, the horn of the wall.

From the cases we are able to record it will be seen that this accident need not be looked upon as fatal, nor the injury itself beyond hope of repair. Dependent largely upon the temperament of the animal, the amount of pain that is caused, and the way in which the animal bears it, recovery may be looked for. Even from the very commencement of the accident, however, the pain may be so acute and the animal so violent with it that slaughter becomes necessary.

Treatment.—This consists in applying an antiseptic and sedative dressing to the injured parts (for example, Carbolized Oil and Tincture of Opium, equal parts) and afterwards bandaging.

From the only data we are able to work on, it appears that this dressing should be repeated daily, the bandage being removed, each time, the foot well bathed in warm water, and the dressing and bandage afterwards replaced. On first sight, it would appear that once cleansed and bandaged the dressings might be left *in situ* for several days. Seeing, however, that suppuration, if once set up, would add further to the intense pain the animal is already suffering, and considering the always constant exposure of the foot to infection, it is perhaps wise to persist in daily changing of the dressings.

At the same time, the general health of the animal should be attended to. Suitable febrifuges should be administered, either in the shape of a dose of physic, or salines and liq. ammonia. acetatis; and the pain, if appearing unbearable, allayed by doses of choral and hypodermic injections of morphia.

Recorded Cases.—1. 'A short time ago I was called to see a horse which had had his hoof torn off in a railway "point." When I arrived at the stable the injury had been done two hours, and the horse had been led from the railway to a loose-box nearly half-a-mile off. On going to this box I was surprised and horrified to find the poor animal mad with pain, rolling and dashing himself about. When on his back he would struggle and kick the walls with the injured foot, as though unconscious of pain. Not one moment was he still, and as I could see that the sensitive structures were much damaged by his violence, I obtained a gun and put him out of his pain.

'The accident happened in this way. The horse was employed in shunting coal-waggons, and had just drawn four loaded trucks up to a point at which they diverged to the left, and the horse, being unhooked, ought to have turned to the right. Here, unfortunately, the near fore-foot became wedged in between two converging railway plates, one of which formed a part of the waggon-way, on which the trucks were running. The horse was a big animal, and freshly shod with heavy shoes, on which a toe-piece and calkins were used. The shoe was roughly but strongly nailed on with eight nails, the clinches of which were all firm. This shoe was fitted wide at the heels, and when the foot was fixed in the points (toe downwards) it protruded over the face of the rail. When the trucks reached it they pressed it down, and, the horse leaning forward, the hoof was drawn off like a glove. The hoof was almost as clean inside as if taken off by maceration—only towards the toe was a small portion of the coffin-bone and some torn laminæ left inside the hoof.

'As soon as possible after the accident, so I was told, the foot was bound up with tow and a bandage; then a sack was cut up and placed over all, and the horse slowly led to his loose-box. He "carried" the leg all the way, limping along on the three sound ones. Almost immediately after reaching the box he lay down, but only for a short time. The standing position was not long maintained—profuse perspiration set in, and the alternations of position became more rapid and violent, till plunging and rolling were added to the other signs of excruciating pain. I was also told that the groaning of the poor animal was almost constant, and at times so loud and prolonged as to amount to a shriek.

'I have no experience of a similar case, and I should not have supposed that this accident would have caused such acute suffering and violent symptoms. I think I have heard of such cases making a complete recovery; but I feel sure that, in this case, I only anticipated death by, at most, a few hours.'[A]

[Footnote A: *Veterinary Record*, vol. iv., p. 127.]

2. 'The case I am about to give you an account of, being one of rare occurrence, I thought would not prove uninteresting to the members of the Veterinary Medical Association. It is an instance of complete removal of the hoof by mechanical force.

'Our patient was a brown mare, five years old, the property of Messrs. Crawshaw and Co., railway contractors on the Sheffield and Manchester line.

'On June 20 the mare was, as usual, working on the line, drawing one of the waggons for the removal of soil from one place to another, and, as was the custom, the pace is generally increased at about the distance of from sixty to eighty yards from where the unloading takes place, in order to add to the velocity, so that the contents of the waggons might roll down so great a precipice. It was at this increased action, when the mare was being removed from the waggon, that she stepped between the ends of two iron rails, sufficiently apart to admit the foot only, when one end of the rail inserted itself between the sole and toe of the shoe, the other at the top and in front of the crust.

'The mare, finding herself fixed, endeavoured to disengage herself, and, in doing so, got in front of the waggon, which, coming at a great pace, forced her down into the pit, leaving behind the off fore-hoof, which was only removed from its situation between the two rails by a large hammer, it being so firmly wedged in. The shoe and hoof were bent in a very peculiar manner, as the accompanying cuts will show, the inside heel being completely raised from above the level of the frog, not one of the nails being unclenched, or in the slightest degree having given way to so large an amount of force imposed upon them, although the toe of the shoe was raised from the sole by the rail being immediately under it (see Fig. 114). The mare had been shod the day before, and, having a good sound foot, the shoe was firmly put on.

'Being a mile from home, she was with some difficulty made to travel that distance. On her arrival, my preceptor, Mr. Taylor, was immediately sent for, who found her, as I have before stated, with the off fore-foot hoofless.

'Proceeding to examine the foot, he ascertained that it had bled considerably, which, however, was stopped by bandages to the foot and a ligature round the coronet. The laminæ on one side and a small portion of the sensitive sole, though not to any great extent, were lacerated. The coffin-bone was not at all injured. The bleeding having nearly ceased, she was put into slings, the foot carefully washed with warm water, and immediately bound up with pledgets of tow saturated with the simple tincture of myrrh and tincture of opium, of each equal parts.

FIG. 114.—HOOF TORN FROM THE FOOT BY ACCIDENT.

'The dressing was ordered to be allowed to remain on all night, and on the following morning to be removed. The foot was then bathed, as before, in warm water, and the application of the tinctures repeated night and morning. The medicine internally given was castor oil, with tinct. opium, and this, in a diminished dose, was ordered the next morning. Blood was also abstracted from the jugular vein, to the amount of 6 quarts, so as to allay the inflammatory fever set up. The food consisted of bran and linseed, with small portions of hay and water. The mare being in a highly excited state, and suffering such severe pain, the opinion Mr. Taylor gave was that, should she get over the first four days (which appeared quite uncertain), he had no doubt of her ultimately getting well, and also that she would have a perfect hoof formed. It was now left for the owners' consideration, whether they thought the mare worth her keep till such took place, the time mentioned by Mr. Taylor being four or five months. She was seen again the fourth day after the accident, and was then found to be perfectly tranquil and feeding well; her pulse, which at the first visit could not be counted, was now not more than 65 beats in the minute. On removing the dressings, the foot presented a very favourable appearance, the treatment therefore varied only in the application of a linseed-meal poultice over the former dressings of tinctures of opium and myrrh, confining the whole in a soft leather boot. Diet as before, in addition to which give a few oats. Should the bowels become constipated, repeat the castor oil without the opium.

'*June* 28.—The animal was again seen, and appeared to be going on very favourably. The poultices were directed to be discontinued, and the parts dressed every other day with sol. sulph. cupri, as the granulations were getting rather luxuriant.

'*July* 6.—To-day she was found to have gone on so well, having two days before been removed from the slings, that it was thought justifiable to turn her out, protecting the foot with a boot, and ordering the dressings to be repeated.

'*July* 23.—She was seen by me in the field, where I had the boot removed, and so much had she improved, that not less than 2 inches of crust, proceeding from the coronary ring, had been formed, and the foot looked remarkably healthy.

'It will be seen that the accident occurred on June 20, a fortnight after which time I observed the horny crust to be forming from the coronet, and the insensitive laminæ at the same time, in which on every visit an increase of growth was perceptible, and it soon attained a thickness exceeding that of the other hoof, but which at the same time presented a more upright appearance. It was not until three weeks after our first visit that any formation of new sole or frog was to be seen. Of the two the sole was the first, being secreted by the sensitive sole, the growth proceeding from the heels. In like manner the insensitive frog was being produced by the sensitive.

FIG. 115.—HOOF TORN FROM THE FOOT BY ACCIDENT.

'During the last week in October the mare, having her foot protected with a bar shoe plated at the bottom, and so formed as to open without necessity of removing the shoe, in order to facilitate the applications of the tinctures, was put to light work, which has since been gradually increased, and she now performs her usual labour equal to any other horse.

'The growth of the wall or crust and insensitive laminæ is not yet quite complete, nor is the sole, there being wanting about an inch of the horny substance of it, the entire completion of which I should rather doubt, as I mentioned in my former communication that the sensitive laminæ and a small portion of the sole were lacerated, and it is in these parts that the imperfections exist.

'The yet imperfectly-formed wall not admitting of the insertion of nails all around it, the shoe is held on partly by nails and partly by a strap attached to it bound round the coronet.'[A]

[Footnote A: *Veterinary Record*, vol. iv., p. 182 (B. Cartledge).]

3. 'This case is related by Mr. A. Rogerson, F.R.C.V.S. It occurred to an animal regularly engaged in shunting, and happened through the corner of the shoe becoming "trapped" between a line of metal and the wheel of a truck. It is particularly interesting on account of the photograph accompanying it, and which we here reproduce in Fig. 115.

'The photograph shows plainly the manner in which the holding of the "clinches" on the left side of the hoof has resulted in drawing it off from the foot. Had these clinches, as Mr. Rogerson suggests, been left unfastened, then the accident in all probability would not have occurred. The animal was destroyed.'[A]

[Footnote A: *Ibid.*, vol. xiii., p. 2.]

CHAPTER IX
INFLAMMATORY AFFECTIONS OF THE KERATOGENOUS APPARATUS
A. ACUTE. ACUTE LAMINITIS.

Definition.—The term 'laminitis' is used to indicate a spontaneous and diffuse inflammation of the whole of the sensitive structures of the foot, more particularly the sensitive laminæ. Usually it occurs in the two front feet, often in all four, and occasionally in the hind alone.

Causes.—In dealing with the causes of laminitis, we will first dispose of those coming under the heading of *traumatic.* Correctly speaking, however, lesions of the laminæ thus occurring do not present the same symptoms, nor run an identical course with the disease we now purpose describing, and for which we would prefer to entirely reserve the term 'laminitis.' The fact, however, that traumatic causes are detailed in other works on the same subject compels us to give them mention here.

Strictly traumatic causes giving rise to a limited inflammation of the sensitive laminæ are violent blows upon the foot, either purely accidental, or self-inflicted by violent kicking.

A similar limited laminitis is to be found in the conditions we have described under 'Nail-bound and Punctured Foot.' It is met with also in the injuries resulting from tread and overreach, and in the tissue-changes accompanying corn.

The tenderness following upon excessive hammering in the forge, or of too long an application of the shoe in hot-fitting has also been described as laminitis.

With either of the conditions we have mentioned, it goes without saying that there is either a simple congestion or an actual inflammation, localized or general, of the laminæ of the injured foot. In neither case, however, can the resulting mischief be closely compared with the lesions attending an attack of laminitis proper, a disease which appears to have an almost specific cause, and to run a course peculiarly its own.

The specific cause we have indicated as existing can, in the present state of our knowledge, be only vaguely described as a poisoned state of the blood-stream. This, as clinical evidence teaches us, may result from a variety of causes.

Among these, by far the most common is that state of the circulation induced by excessive feeding with too stimulating or too irritating a diet. In any case, where the use of old oats as a staple diet is departed from, and where the quantity and manner of using the substitute is left to the discretion of careless or unskilled attendants, trouble is likely to ensue. The food more prone, perhaps, than any other to bring about an attack is wheat improperly prepared—that is, uncooked or unground. So much so is this the case that one full meal of this provender to an animal unused to it is sufficient to lead to a train of symptoms often ending fatally.

Beans, peas, barley, rye, new maize, or even new oats, are all liable, if carelessly used, to have the same effect.

It is the laminitis following feeding on new oats that has caused us to apply to the food the adjective 'irritating.' Here, more often than not, the peristaltic action of the bowels is found to be abnormally in evidence, and the excessive use of the diet is always accompanied by a more or less fluid discharge of the intestinal contents.

In addition to the foods we have mentioned, many others might be enumerated, more especially the numerous 'made-up' feeding materials now on the market. Many are composed of substances that may be regarded as absolutely opposed to the correct feeding of a horse, and their use can only be followed by this and other evil results.

Another most fruitful cause of laminitis is a severe and continued inflammatory condition of the system elsewhere. It is the laminitis known to veterinary surgeons as 'metastatic,' and perhaps the two most notable examples of it are the laminitis following a prolonged attack of pneumonia, and the 'Parturient Laminitis' occurring as a concomitant of septic metritis.

Parturient laminitis it is that offers us the most striking illustration of the truth that a poisoned state of the blood-stream is a sure factor in the causation of an attack. From the direct evidence of our senses (namely, manual exploration of the infected womb, and the stench of the exuding discharge) we know that we have in the interior of the womb matter in a state of putrescence. From the experience of previous post-mortems we know, further, that the putrescent matter thus originating often gains the blood-stream, and forms foci of septic lesions elsewhere—liver or lung. When, therefore, during an attack of septic metritis a condition of laminitis supervenes, we are justified in attributing it to the escape of septic matter from the already infected uterus.

In the same category of laminitis from metastasis may also be placed the laminitis occurring as a result of an overdose of aloes. The enteritis thus set up is often followed by laminitis, and that of a serious type.

Prolonged and excessive work upon a hard road is also apt to induce an attack. When this occurs it in many cases resolves itself into a case of cruelty. (See reported case, No. 1, p. 279.)

Laminitis from this cause was frequent among coach and carriage horses in the pre-railroad period, and resulted from attempting to obtain from the animal a faster pace and a greater number of miles than he was physically capable of giving.

In our day, however, it is more often a result of gross feeding, combined with only that amount of work which the horse, if ordinarily fed, would be easily able to perform. An excellent example of this is the laminitis occurring in the Shire stallion when commencing his rounds of service in the spring and early summer. At this season these animals are constantly supplied with a more than sufficient supply of a highly stimulating and nutritious diet. In this case the blood is already in that state in which it is predisposed to the disease. Add to this the unwonted exercise—for during all the winter the animals are idle—and congestion of the venous apparatus of the extremities is not to be wondered at.

Passing from these, the more common, we may consider other and less frequent causes of the disease. Congestion of the laminal blood-vessels and consequent laminitis occurs when animals are made to maintain a standing position for prolonged periods, as, for instance, when making sea voyages. A long and painful disease of one foot, necessitating the whole of the weight being borne by the other, ends often in laminitis of the second member. It may thus occur as a sequel to quittor, complicated sand-crack, suppurating corn, and punctured wounds of the feet.

Laminitis has also been known to occur as a result of septic infection of the blood-stream consequent on the operation of castration. (See recorded case, No. 2, p. 281.)

A sudden lowering of the surface circulation at a time when the animal is excessively perspiring is also said to favour an attack, as also is the giving to drink of cold water to an animal just in from a long and tiring journey. Also, according to Zundel, 'the influence of the season cannot be denied, and it is during the summer months that laminitis is more frequent, while it is rare in winter, as well as in the spring and autumn.'

Further, laminitis has been described as occurring when the animal is at grass, and when all causes—at any rate, active ones—have appeared to be absent. (See reported case, No. 3, p. 282.)

Regarding heredity, we may safely say that, as a cause of laminitis, it may be almost totally disregarded. That a bad form of foot, either a flat-foot or a foot with heels contracted, and already thus affected with a mild type of inflammation, did not offer a certain predisposition, we should not like to assert. There must, however, be an exciting cause—namely, a poisoned condition of the blood-stream. This latter cannot, of course, be in any way regarded as hereditary.

In short, the dietetic cause is by far the most common, and, in prosecuting inquiries as to the starting-point of an attack, the veterinarian's attention should be directed in the main to that particular.

Symptoms.—Laminitis is always ushered in by a set of symptoms indicative of a high state of fever. The pulse is raised from the normal to as many as 80 or 90 a minute, muscular tremors are in evidence, the respirations are short and hurried, and the temperature rises to 105°, 106°, or 107° F. The visible mucous membranes are injected, that of the eye, in addition to the hyperæmia, often tinged a dirty yellow. The mouth is dry and hot, the urine scanty, and the bowels frequently torpid. As yet, however, the walk is sound.

Called in during this early stage, the veterinarian is often puzzled as to the exact significance of the symptoms. Enteritis, lymphangitis, or pneumonia he knows to be often heralded in the same manner. In this connection, Zundel says: 'Laminitis, in most instances, is preceded by certain general symptoms, such as are premonitory of the invasions of ordinary inflammatory diseases, but of an uncertain significance.'

So far we agree with him, but to what we have already said we would add that, even in this early stage, there is an additional symptom, unmentioned by Zundel, which often leads one to an exact diagnosis. The feet are in turn lifted a short distance from the ground, and almost immediately replaced. This movement ('paddling,' we may term it) is constant, the animal appearing to obtain ease in no one position for more than a few moments at a time.

Seen but a few hours later, when the swelling caused by the hyperæmia and outpouring of the inflammatory exudate has led to compression of the sensitive structures within the horny box, the symptoms presented admit of no misreading, save by the most casual and careless observer. The patient now stands as though fixed to the ground. The pulse is hard and frequent, the respirations tremendously increased in number, the body wet with a patchy perspiration, and the countenance indicative of the most acute suffering. Only with difficulty, and often only at the instigation of the whip, can the animal be induced to move. This he does by throwing his weight, so far as he is able, on to the heels of the feet affected, and putting the feet slowly forward in a shuffling and feeling manner. The feet themselves give to the hand a sensation of abnormal heat, percussion upon them with the hammer is followed by painful attempts at withdrawal, while any effort we may make to remove one foot from the ground is useless, so great an aversion does the animal show to placing a greater weight upon the opposite foot.

According as the front-feet alone, the hind-feet alone, or all four feet are affected, the symptoms will vary.

With all four feet diseased, the animal stands with the two front-feet extended in front of him, while the hind-limbs are at the same time propped as far beneath him as is possible. The horse is, in fact, standing upon the extreme hindermost portions of the feet.

Why the animal should thus distribute his weight is easily explained. Standing in the normal position, the body-weight is borne by the sensitive laminæ, the sole, of course, sharing in the burden, but the laminæ taking by far the greater part of the pressure thus exerted. With the vessels of the laminæ gorged with blood, and the laminal connective tissue infiltrated with a profuse inflammatory exudate, the most excruciating pain is bound to result by reason of the compression of the diseased tissues within the non-yielding structures. In some little measure the suffering animal may afford himself relief by partly removing pressure from the fore-parts of the hoof. When placing the body-weight behind, the pressure, instead of falling upon the highly sensitive laminæ, is directed to the follicular and fatty tissues of the plantar cushion: from there, with only a small portion of the sensitive sole intervening, to the horny frog, and from thence to the ground.

The same distribution of weight also places the foot in a position of greatest expansion, thus, by giving greater room to the diseased parts, again affording relief of pressure on the inflamed lamina, while it at the same time relieves of weight the foremost portions of the sensitive sole.

With the fore-feet alone attacked, the animal affects exactly the same position of standing as that just described. The fore-feet are again extended, and the hind propped far beneath him. The fore extended, in order to obtain the relief occasioned by standing on the heels; the hind in this case carried forward in order to take a greater share of the body-weight, and thus relieve the congested members in front.

With the hind only attacked, then the fore and the hind feet are more closely approximated than in the normal position. The reason, of course, is that the hind-feet are carried forward in order to be placed upon the heels, while the fore are taken backwards to relieve the hind of the body-weight.

In like manner the movements of the animal will vary with the feet affected. With only the front-feet diseased the animal is, comparatively speaking, comfortable. The hind-feet take the weight, and the animal stands for long periods together, resting alternately first one fore-foot and then the other, moving often in a circle of which his body is the radius, and his hind-limbs the centre. If urged to move forward, then immediately his countenance and movements manifest the pain to which he is put. Only with reluctance does he cause the fore-feet to take weight. They are shuffled forward quickly one after the other, so that weight may not be placed upon them for one instant longer than is necessary, and the hind-limbs immediately brought again with two short, awkward movements beneath the body. Progress thus takes place in a succession of movements 'half hobble,' 'half jump.'

Painful though this may appear, progress is still more difficult when the hind-feet alone are diseased. Afraid that, in placing his fore-members freely forward, he will add to the pain in his hind, the walk takes place in a series of extremely short steps, with the feet more or less closely approximated. The gait is thus rendered extremely awkward, and Zundel, by saying that 'the animal appears as if treading on sharp needles,' most fitly describes it.

Movement with all four feet affected, though less awkward in appearance, is doubtless more painful than in either of the other conditions. Here the animal can hardly be induced to shift his position at all. Only by flogging, and that severe, can he be made to go forward. When so induced to move, the agonizing pain to which the patient is subjected may be gathered by noting his countenance and manner of progression.

With each movement forward, muscular tremors affect the limbs; each step is short, jerky, and convulsive; the respirations and pulse are almost immediately greatly quickened, and the lower lip is hung pendulous, and moved almost unconsciously up and down with a flapping noise against the upper. A patchy perspiration breaks out about the body and quarters, and the tail is outstretched and quivering. At the same time the lines of the face become drawn, the commissures of the lips pulled upwards, the eyes staring and haggard, the eyelids puckered, the nostrils extended, and the whole expression indicative of the intense and agonizing pain of the disease.

One can perhaps better give one's client some vague idea of the patient's suffering by likening the pain to the throbbing sensation of a festered finger-nail. Tell him that each hoof of the horse is similarly, or, if anything, more delicately, constructed, that in each foot the same process of 'festering' is going on, and that upon them the animal has perforce to stand.

As one might expect, the position of greatest ease is the decumbent. Strange to say, though, in many cases of laminitis the animal persists in maintaining a standing posture. Once down, however, one has sometimes the greatest difficulty in persuading him again to rise. The lying position is so long maintained that bedsores begin to make their appearance, and the animal rapidly loses flesh, not only by reason of the fever and the pain, but by giving to rest the time he should normally give to feeding.

Difficulty in rising is greatest when all four feet are affected; is *nearly* as great when the hind-limbs only are in trouble, but is least when the disease exists alone in the two fore-feet.

THE COURSE OF THE DISEASE AND ITS PATHOLOGICAL ANATOMY.— As with most inflammations of any severity, so with this we may consider the pathological changes taking place in the foot under three headings: (a) The period of Congestion; (b) the period of Exudation; (c) the period of Suppuration.

(a) *Congestion.*—In the early stages of laminitis there is a state of engorgement of the vessels of the keratogenous apparatus generally, but more particularly the laminal portion of it. With the hoof removed at this stage the sensitive laminæ are found to be swollen, dark red in colour, and affording a distinct feeling of increased thickness when pressed between the fingers, Incised, there escapes from the cut surface a large flow of dark venous-looking blood. At this stage hæmorrhages of the laminal vessels occur. The escaping blood infiltrates the surrounding connective tissue, and in many cases destroys the union between the horny and sensitive laminæ. This change is most noticeable in the region of the toe and the commencement of the quarters, the os pedis appearing as though pushed backwards by the escaping fluid collected between the wall and the bone. In severe cases, fortunately but rarely seen, the blood so escaping continues to infiltrate, and separate the tissues until it is seen to be freely oozing at the region of the coronet. (See reported case, No. 1, p. 279.)

(b) *Exudation.*—The period of exudation marks the outpouring of the inflammatory fluid. This, even more than the hæmorrhages attending the stage of congestion, tends to destroy the intimacy between the sensitive and the horny laminæ, leading finally to their complete separation at the region of the toe. Fig. 116 illustrates this state of affairs after laminitis has existed for a week. The sensitive and horny laminæ are here shown to be distinctly separated from each other, a well-marked cavity existing between them, which cavity is greatest in extent at the toe of the os pedis. With the sensitive structures thus detached from the wall, it is evident that very much that formerly held the os pedis in normal position has been destroyed. What then happens is that the whole of the body-weight is placed upon the sole. Never intended to bear the strain thus imposed, it naturally sinks. With the sinking is a corresponding 'dropping' of the pedal bone—in fact, of the whole of the bony column. Seeing that the structures *above* the hoof are still normally adherent to the bones, it follows that they must, as the os pedis sinks, be carried with it. As a consequence we get a marked depression at the coronet (see Fig. 117, *a*), which depression may be often noticed after the second or third week of a severe attack of the disease.

FIG. 116.—LONGITUDINAL SECTION OF A FOOT WITH LAMINITIS OF EIGHT DAYS' STANDING. The separation between the sensitive structures and the hoof is indicated by a dark line. The cavity is filled with exudate. It will be noted that as yet there is little change in the position of the os pedis.

Here, again, though to a greater extent than that caused by the hæmorrhage alone, the os pedis appears to be pushed backwards, the space at the toe between the bone and the horny box being closely filled with the yellow, slightly blood-stained exudate. This condition is well depicted in Fig. 117.

FIG. 117.—LONGITUDINAL SECTION OF A FOOT WITH LAMINITIS OF FOURTEEN DAYS' STANDING. *a*, The depression at the coronet caused by the dropping of the bony column within the horny-box: *b*, a portion of the sensitive sole pushed downwards and forwards by the descending os pedis.

With the descent of the os pedis we get in many cases a penetration of the horny sole (see Fig. 117), leading always to serious displacement of the sensitive sole (see Fig. 117, *b*), and often to caries of the exposed bone.

The backward displacement of the os pedis may be accounted for in two ways. Firstly, the greater vascularity of the membrane covering its front leads to a greater outpouring of inflammatory fluid in that particular position. Here, therefore, loss of adhesion with the wall is greatest, while into the cavity so formed is poured a large quantity of a fluid that is practically incompressible. The os pedis *must* be pushed backwards. Secondly, the manner in which the animal distributes his weight—namely, upon the heels—is calculated to aid in the bone's backward movement, for with his feet in this position tension upon the extensor pedis is relaxed, while that upon the flexor perforans is greatly increased.

(c) *Suppuration.*—Should the animal survive the pain and exhausting calls made upon his system by the accompanying fever of the foregoing conditions, the case ends either in resolution or suppuration. When suppuration occurs it is found, as a rule, at the sole, leading to almost entire separation of the sensitive and horny structures. The pain, if possible, is even worse than in either of the foregoing stages, and relief for the suffering patient is only obtainable by the natural exit of the pus at the coronet, or by giving it escape with the knife at the sole. As a rule, suppuration in laminitis is rare, and then only occurs when the disease has been of some several days' duration. It has been the author's experience, however, to meet with it in a case but three days' old. This particular animal had laminitis restricted to the hind-feet. The condition was diagnosed and pus liberated at the sole of one foot during the third day of the lameness. The animal was cast on the fourth day, and pus obtained from the sole of the opposite foot.

Complications.—In a moderate case, carefully treated, laminitis terminates at the end of three or four days in resolution. The general symptoms of fever gradually subside, the appetite returns, and the walk becomes easier. Cases thus terminating fortunately leave behind them no change of serious importance, either in the sensitive tissues or in the horny envelope. Should resolution, however, be longer delayed, then the case, although eventually terminating successfully so far as soundness in gait is concerned, leaves more or less evidence behind in the shape of rings about the wall and alterations in the build of the sole.

When the happy ending of rapid resolution is denied us, then, in addition to the condition we have described as suppuration, we may meet with one or other of the following complications:

(*a*) *Metastatic Pneumonia.*—This complication is not uncommon, and, when occurring, more often than not ends fatally. It may be accounted for indirectly by the greater work the lungs are called upon to perform in carrying out the increased number of respirations occasioned by the general fever and pain, and directly by the poisonous materials circulating in the blood-stream.

(*b*) *Metastatic Colic.*—This may be either a subacute obstruction of the bowel or an enteritis accompanied by an offensive purge.

A striking case of the former is related in the *Veterinary Journal* (vol. xvi., p. 180) by H. Thompson, of Aspatria. Here no evacuation of the bowels occurred for three days, and the pains of laminitis were added to by the usual pains of intestinal obstruction.

The colic of enteritis is in some cases caused by the nature of the food, giving rise to laminitis. In our opinion, however, it is more often occasioned by the drastic action of the aloes nearly always resorted to in the treatment of the disorder. As does the pneumonia, the enteritis thus brought about nearly always has a fatal termination.

(c) *Gangrene of the Structures within the Hoof.*—This complication is the one most to be dreaded. It occurs as a result of the great pressure exerted by an excessive exudation, and doubtless affects first the laminæ and softer structures. Once commenced, however, it rapidly extends to death of the other structures (ligament, tendon, and even bone), and gives a fatal ending to the case.

That gangrene of the tissues ("mortification" as our older writers called it) has occurred is soon made evident to the veterinarian by the symptoms shown by the patient. The agonizingly acute pains suddenly subside, the feet are placed firmly and squarely to the ground, and the animal walks with ease. Perhaps but the night before the patient is seen racked with excruciating pain; the morning sees the astounding change of apparent absolute recovery. Too well, however, the eye of the experienced veterinary surgeon sees that such is not the case. Even before proceeding to take a record of the other symptoms, he knows that it is but the commencement of the end. Methodically, however, he notes the other conditions. The pulse he finds small and imperceptible, save at the radial. The thermometer registers a subnormal temperature, the extremities are cold, and cold sweats bedew the body. To the same experienced eye the countenance of the animal is almost suggestive of what has occurred. The drawn and haggard expression, to which we have previously referred, becomes more marked, and the angles of the lips are drawn back in what has been described by some writers as a 'sardonic' grin.

We can best express what the whole look of the animal's countenance indicates to us by saying that it gives us the impression that the animal himself knows that some serious change, and a change fatally inimical to his chances of life, has taken place in his feet.

It may be that in some odd cases, although it has not yet been our lot to meet with them, gangrene may terminate in the casting off of one or more hoofs. Needless to say, there can still be but one termination to the case.

(d) *Periostitis and Ostitis.*—This complication is referred to by other writers under the term of 'Peditis.' It signifies, of course, that the periosteum and the bone have become invaded by the inflammatory process. It is our opinion that these two conditions, even including an actual arthritis, always exist, even in an attack of laminitis that ends favourably. We do not claim, however, to be able to relate any means, save that of post-mortem examination, by which it may be singled out from the other changes occurring in the foot. The high fever and pain occasioned by the inroads of the inflammation into the other sensitive structures serves to effectually mask whatever evidence of it we might otherwise obtain. It may be sometimes only small in degree, but we feel confident that inflammation, at any rate of the *outer* layer of the periosteum, is in laminitis constant even, we repeat, in a mild case.

FIG. 118.—SHOWING CHANGES IN THE OS PEDIS WITH LAMINITIS OF LONG STANDING, (a, Viewed from the front; b, viewed from the side.) The porous condition of the bone, which is here shown, is a result of a rarefying or rarefactive ostitis. This specimen also illustrated (what the photograph cannot show) an accompanying condition of condensation of bone, or osteoplastic ostitis. (For a fuller description of the changes occurring in these forms of ostitis, see Chapter XI.)

When the case is a serious one we have ample evidence to show that ostitis exists, and exists in a severe form. The bones become vastly altered in shape, a process of absorption leads to the formation of large, irregular cavities within their substance, and what of the bone is left is rendered hard and ivory-like (condensed) near what was the original centre, while the edges and other portions show often a tendency to become brittle and porous.

Fig. 118 illustrates the effects of a severe ostitis in pedal bones removed from hoofs with laminitis of several weeks' standing.

(*e*) *Chronic Laminitis.*—The most common complication—or, perhaps, rather we should term it 'sequel'—to acute laminitis is the chronic form of the disease. For this condition we have reserved a separate section of our work. It will be found described in Section B 1 of this chapter.

Diagnosis and Prognosis.—One is almost tempted to state that the diagnosis of laminitis offers no difficulty. In the very early stages, however, it may, as we have already indicated, be mistaken for the oncoming of Enteritis, Lymphangitis, or even Pneumonia. The paddling of the feet may help us. If this is absent, however, nothing but a most careful examination, or, if necessary, the withholding of our opinion until the following visit will prevent a blunder being made.

Even when well established, laminitis has been mistaken for paralysis, for tetanus, for rheumatic affections of the loins, or even for some undiscovered affection of the muscles of the arms and chest. This latter is no doubt suggested to the uninitiated by the reluctance the animal shows to move the muscles *apparently* of that region, and led the older writers to give to the disease its name of 'Chest-founder.' It is only fair to add, however, that these blunders in diagnosis are nearly always committed by persons without a veterinary training.

Thus warned, the veterinary surgeon of average ability should have no difficulty in establishing a distinction between the diseases we have enumerated as likely to be confounded with it, and the one this chapter is describing.

The prognosis in laminitis should, in our opinion, always be guarded. No advice given in a work of this description can be of any real use, for every case must be judged entirely on its merits. The severity of the symptoms, the cause of the attack, the complications, and the idiosyncrasies of the patient, have all to be taken into account. These the veterinarian must be left to judge for himself.

Treatment.—The treatment of acute laminitis in its early stage must be based upon the fact that we have to deal with a congested state of the circulatory apparatus of the whole of the keratogenous membrane. This fact was well enough known to the older veterinarians. It is not surprising, therefore, to learn that jugular phlebotomy was at once resorted to as the readiest means of relieving the overcharged vessels of their blood. As a matter of fact, bleeding from the jugular is still advocated by modern authorities. We cannot say, however, that we unhesitatingly recommend it. Mechanically, of course, the removal of a large quantity of blood is bound to result in a lowering of the pressure in the vessels. The effect, however, is but transient. Blood removed in this way is again quickly returned to the vessels so far as its fluid matter is concerned, and the pressure, removed for a time, is again as great as before. With the other and more vital constituents of the blood-stream—namely, the corpuscles—restoration is not so rapid. We have, in fact, a weakened state of the system, in which it is probable it will not so successfully combat the adverse conditions the disease may induce.

With these prefatory remarks, we may advise bleeding under certain conditions. The quantity removed must be moderate (7 to 8 pints), and the pulse and other conditions must show no signs of weakness or collapse.

Local bleeding, either from the toe or the coronet, is also advised. In the former situation the sole is thinned down until a sufficient flow is obtained, while at the coronet scarification is the method adopted. Bleeding locally, however, is far less effectual than the jugular operation. Neither must it be forgotten that wounds in these situations, more particularly at the toe, are extremely liable, especially with the existing poisoned state of the blood-current, to take on a septic character. What might possibly have remained a comparatively simple inflammation is induced by the operation itself to terminate in the more complicated and serious condition of suppuration.

Other means of combating the congested state of the membrane are principally those of local applications. With many veterinary surgeons warm poulticing is still largely advocated and practised. We do not believe in it. Warmth, as a means of removing local congestion, can only be successful when applied *widely* round the congested area, and so dilating surrounding bloodvessels and lymphatics. Applied to the congested area itself, and to that alone, it is almost worse than useless.

With the foot, both around and below it, a surrounding area is denied us. The only vessels we are able to dilate with the warmth, and so enable them to carry off the fluid from the congested foot, are those in the limb above. That poulticing cannot be successfully there applied is self-evident. Apart from that, it is an open question whether poultices may not do actual harm in inducing suppuration in cases where, probably, it would not otherwise occur.

For these reasons we hold to the opinion that when a local application is determined on it should be a cold one. Various methods of applying cold are in vogue. Cold swabs are perhaps most in favour. They must, however, be *kept* cold. When a suitable water-course, pond, or other expanse of shallow water is at hand, then the animal may be kept standing therein, or preferably walked about in it. When suitable apparatus is obtainable, a constant stream over each foot from a rubber hosepipe is most beneficial.

Astringent baths, containing solutions of alum, of copper sulphate, of iron sulphate, or of common salt, or composed of a mixture of two or more of the salts mentioned, may also be used with advantage. In addition to the fact that such solutions are for a time below the temperature of simple water, we have the advantage that they have also a more or less antiseptic property.

While on the subject of the relief of the congestion, we must not forget to mention a treatment which we ourselves have practised with considerable success—namely, that of forced exercise. It appears to have been first brought into prominence by Mr. Broad, of Bath, and the two terms 'Forced Exercise and Rocker Shoes' and 'Broad's Treatment' have come to be synonymous.

The Broad shoe is a shoe with a web of quite twice the thickness of the animal's ordinary shoe, and has this web gradually thinned from the toe backwards until at the heels the shoe is at its thinnest (see Fig. 119).

The excessive thickness of the shoe serves two purposes. It allows of the requisite amount of slope being given to the web, and so enables the animal readily to throw himself back on to his heels, a position in which, as we have already indicated, he obtains the greatest ease. It also minimizes to some extent the effects of concussion.

FIG. 119.—SEATED ROCKER BAR SHOE (BROAD'S) FOR TREATMENT OF LAMINITIS.

With forced exercise, as practised by Mr. Broad, this shoe is first applied, and the animal afterwards made to walk upon soft ground, or even upon the roadway, for a half an hour to an hour and a half three times a day.

For our own part, we consider the shoe to be almost if not quite superfluous, so far as its influence upon the progress of the disease is concerned. We therefore dispense with it, and have the animal exercised in his ordinary shoes. To do this, the patient has sometimes to be severely flogged into taking the first few steps. After that progress gradually becomes easier.

It has been said to be cruel. In so far as we knowingly, and of set purpose, occasion the animal pain, cruel it undoubtedly is; but it is cruelty with an aim that is truly benevolent, and the object of our benevolence is the animal upon whom the cruelty is practised.

One word of advice is needed. The forced exercise must be commenced early. In the later stages, when the stage of congestion has passed from that to the acuter stages of the inflammation and the outpouring of the inflammatory exudate, then forced exercise cannot be safely commenced. The loss of adhesion between the pedal bone and the horny box, which we know to be then existent, negatives its advisability.

By many it is advised to always remove the shoes. From what we have already said, it will be seen that this is not our practice. But one argument in favour of so doing appears to us to carry weight, and that is that 'dropping' of the sole is probably prevented from becoming so marked. That condition, however, is entirely dependent upon the changes occurring within the horny box. It is bound to occur with the animal shod or unshod, and to reach a stage when only contact with the ground prevents its further descent. The complication then sometimes following—namely, penetration of the sole by the bone, is not prevented by having the shoes removed. It may, in fact, be thus rendered more likely.

Internal treatment consists in the exhibition of suitable febrifuges and the administration of a dose of aloes.

With regard to the wisdom of the latter proceeding, opinion seems to be divided. Personally, we hold an open mind concerning it. This much is certain: in many cases of laminitis—those cases which have their origin in overfeeding with an irritating food—there is already a strong predisposition to enteritis. The administration of aloes in this case is extremely apt to induce a fatal super-purgation. Aloes is, again, contra-indicated when the laminitis is a result of excessively long journeys, and the patient is already greatly exhausted. Neither can it be advocated in the laminitis occurring as a sequel to septic metritis or to pneumonia.

On the other hand, when the disease has occurred as a result of long standing in the stable and an overloaded condition of the bowels, or where one full meal of some constipating food, such as whole wheat, pea or bean meal, wheat or barley meal, has occasioned the attack, then a dose of aloes at the commencement of the treatment is productive of good.

Suitable febrifuges are found in potassium nitrate, potassium chlorate, sodium sulphate, or magnesium sulphate, either of which or a mixture of two or more of them, the animal will readily take in his drinking-water.

The administration of sedatives is also indicated. In this connection aconite will be found most useful. More especially in the early stages of the disease, when pain is excessive and the temperature high, will its good effects be noticed. This also the animal will often take in his drinking-water. We have been in the habit of so prescribing the B.P. tincture in 1/2-dram doses three times daily. By its use the temperature is rapidly lowered, the pulse reduced in number and in fulness, and the pain in some instances perceptibly diminished. With others hypodermic injections of morphia and atropine have given equally satisfactory results.

Needless to say, good nursing is a *sine quâ non*. During the first stages of the fever a light and easily digested diet should be allowed—bran-mashes, roots and grass when obtainable, and a carefully regulated supply of water. The animal should be warmly clothed and the box well ventilated, even to the opening of the doors and windows. Only in this way is pneumonia as a sequel sometimes prevented. The patient's comfort should be attended to in providing him with a suitable bed. Anything in the shape of long litter should be avoided. When nothing else is at hand, litter that has already been broken and shortened by previous use is best. With this the box floor should be thickly covered, and matting of the material prevented by constant turning. A good bed for the horse with laminitis is peat-moss mixed with short straw. This, without being dragged into irregular heaps, remains springy and elastic with but little attention. Better than all, however, especially with good weather, is an open crewyard. Here the animal has an abundance of fresh air, has a bed that is always soft, and has plenty of room in which to get up and down with some degree of ease.

Leaving the dietetic and medicinal, we may consider other treatments of laminitis that come more particularly under the heading of operative.

The first matter that here demands our attention is that of allowing the exudate to escape at the sole. If after the expiration of three or four days pain and other symptoms of distress continue, then it may be judged that the inflammatory exudate has made its appearance. Operative measures allowing of its escape, though not giving absolute ease, do undoubtedly relieve the more marked expressions of suffering, and should be at once determined on. To do this completely it is necessary to cast the animal. The sole is then thinned at the toe with the drawing-knife until the sensitive structures are reached. A flow of yellow and sometimes blood-stained discharge is immediately obtained, and the sole itself found to be underrun to a considerable extent. An opening sufficiently large to admit of free drainage (about the size of a half a crown-piece) is made, the wounds antiseptically dressed, and the hobbles removed.

If showing an inclination to do so, the animal should then be allowed to remain and rest. In one instance in which we so operated (a case of laminitis in the hind-feet alone), the relief given was at once manifested. For three days previously the animal had remained standing in agonizing pain. On the fourth he was cast, and the discharge—partly inflammatory exudate, and partly a sanious foetid pus—liberated. The hobbles were removed, and the animal allowed to remain down while our attention was drawn to another case. This attended to, we walked back to the field where, our first patient was lying. His breathing, but a short time before distressedly short and catching, was now so slow and deeply regular that for one brief moment the thought flashed across our mind that he was dead. He was in a *profound* sleep.

Other operators sometimes give the exudate escape while making the grooves in what is now known as 'Smith's Operation.'

In this operation the hoof is so grooved as to allow of its expansion, so relieving the pressure on the sensitive structures within it. Incidentally, the inflammatory exudate is given exit.

FIG. 120.—DIAGRAM OF HOOF SHOWING THE POSITION OF THE THREE GROOVES MADE IN THE TREATMENT OF LAMINITIS.

The animal is cast, the shoes removed, and three vertical grooves made in the wall. The first is cut down the centre of toe, extending from the coronet to the ground surface. The second is made to the right of this, and the third to the left, each following the direction of the horn fibres, and each distant about 2 inches from the first (see 1, 2, and 3, Fig. 120).

Each of the grooves must run completely from the coronary margin to the ground surface, and each should be carried through the substance of the horn until the horny laminæ are reached. This done, the underneath surface of the foot is grooved at the white line (see curved groove 4, Fig. 121) in such a manner as to entirely isolate the two pieces of horn *a* and *b* from the remainder of the hoof.

Expansion of the horny box is thus brought about, while at the same time the semicircular groove at the toe is made deep enough to allow of the escape of the exudate.

If thought wise by the operator, the two pieces of horn *a* and *b* may be isolated, and the exudate given exit by making the fourth groove in the position of the dotted lines in Fig. 120—that is to say, at the lowermost portion of the sensitive structures. By this means the sole will be left intact.

FIG. 121.—LOWER SURFACE OF FOOT SHOWING POSITION OF THE GROOVES MADE IN THE TREATMENT OF LAMINITIS.

Fuller instruction for making the grooves and the instruments required will be found described in Section C of Chapter X.

The animal should be afterwards shod, and the bearing on the portions *a* and *b* of the wall removed. Almost immediate relief is afforded the patient.

Recorded Cases.—1. 'On the evening of September 28 last, I was called rather hurriedly to attend a posting-horse which had just arrived from a twenty-one miles' journey, and was said to be "very ill." I lost no time in proceeding to the spot, and found my patient "very ill" indeed. No need for long consideration as to diagnosis; the symptoms showed at once that I had an uncommonly severe case of acute founder before me. On examination I found the pulse was 120, the respirations 100, and the thermometer 106° F. The poor brute could not move, the fore-legs were well out before, and the hind-legs thrown back behind; in fact, he was, as one might say, propping himself up with his four legs!

'On examining his feet, I discovered what I had never either seen or heard of before—namely, *blood freely oozing out* at the coronet of all four feet; if anything, the hind-feet were the worst, and, showing that this bloody discharge at coronets had commenced during progression and before he was stabled, the inside of the thighs were all shotted over with blood, which had been thrown up by his feet while he was trotting or walking. He was completely soaked all over with perspiration.

'My prognosis could not well be otherwise than unsatisfactory. I resolved, however, to do all I could to relieve the poor suffering brute. As a matter of course, jugular phlebotomy was utterly impracticable; so, to relieve the pressure in the feet, I had him (after, with extreme difficulty, removing the shoes) bled, or rather opened, at all four toes, and hot poultices applied. On opening the off-side toe, in both hind and fore feet, I found an escape of very dark-coloured blood, with a great many bubbles of gas, thus showing that the destructive process was fairly established in the two bony extremities mentioned. The near fore and near hind feet showed no signs of gas-bubbles on being opened at the toe.

'I gave a laxative in combination with a diffusible stimulant, and ordered doses of aconite and potassium iodide; I also applied strong sinapisms to each side, immediately behind the shoulders. After three hours I found my patient rather easier; respiration about 90, and temperature 104°; willing to take a little water, and even attempted to take some hay. Ordered continued applications of hot water to the poultices at feet, and clothed him up for the night. Next morning there was little improvement; respirations over 80, and temperature 103.5°. Continue same treatment. Second morning, horse apparently easier; temperature 102.5°, but very difficult respiration; laxative had operated during the night; ordered diffusible stimulants. About two hours and a half after my last visit, the horse turned round in his stall and dropped down dead!

'*History of the Horse.*—He belonged to an extensive horse-hiring establishment; was purchased a short time before for £60—a long price for a post-horse—had recently suffered and been off work from some "severe cold"; was taken out, and did forty-seven miles of a journey the day *before* I saw him; on forenoon of the day on which he was attacked he did two or three short turns, and then twenty-one miles of a journey in the afternoon, during which he became so ill as scarcely to be able to conclude the twenty-one miles; this was the last turn he was to do. He was a grand stepper, and no doubt was pushed a little during this final journey, as the driver intended, after a short rest, to finish off with the twenty-six miles between this and home. With the short turns on the second forenoon, this would have been over 100 miles in less than two days, with a horse just out of a *severe cold*.'[A]

[Footnote A: *Veterinary Journal*, vol. xvii., p. 314 (A.E. Macgillivray).]

2. 'Whilst attending a patient on a farm on September 5 last my attention was called to a cart-horse, five years of age, that had been castrated in the standing position by a travelling castrator about ten days previously.

'I found the animal presenting the following symptoms: Head down, blowing hard, very dull, and disinclined to move, temperature 105° F., hard, rapid, slightly irregular pulse, membranes injected, appetite lost; scrotum, sheath, and penis tremendously swollen, castration wounds unhealthy, and exuding a thin, reddish-brown discharge of a most foetid odour.

'The next day well-marked symptoms of laminitis were present. I finally ceased attending him about the middle of October, and at the end of that month he was turned out for the winter.'[A]

[Footnote A: *Veterinary Record*, vol. xiv., p. 649 (Charles A. Powell).]

3. 'On July 8 an interesting case of laminitis came under my notice. The subject was a mare, eight years old, which had been running on the common here for some months, and was taken up on the night of July 2 by a boy, who did not observe anything amiss with her. The following morning, on the owner going to the stable, he found the animal in great pain, and at once sent for me. I discovered her to be suffering from laminitis, and saw her again in the evening, when she was much worse. The attack proved to be a most severe one.

'The owner informed me that she had not been allowed any corn for two months, and that she had no distance to travel on the road from the common.

'Though on such a poor pasture, the mare was very fat; she had never been unwell before this attack.

'This is the first case I have seen of laminitis occurring when the animal was on grass.'[A]

[Footnote A: *Veterinary Journal*, vol. ix., p. 176 (W. Stanley Carless).]

B. CHRONIC.

1. CHRONIC LAMINITIS.

Definition.—A low and persisting type of inflammation of the sensitive structures of the foot, characterized by changes in the form of the hoof, and incurable pathological alterations within it.

Causes.—Chronic laminitis more often than not is a sequel to the acute form we have just described. With an attack of acute laminitis that defies treatment, and does not end in resolution in from ten days to a fortnight, then the chronic form may be expected.

The brittle horn, convex sole, and other changes we have described under Pumiced Foot may, however, be regarded as a chronic laminitis, and this condition, as we have already indicated in Chapter VI., may run a course slow and insidious from the onset.

Symptoms.—When the disease arises without previous acute symptoms, the first thing noticeable is an alteration in the gait. The animal begins to go feelingly, especially when first moved out from the stable. Our opinion is asked as to the cause of the lameness, and an inspection is made. With the changes in the form of the hoof as yet wanting, we have nothing to guide us, and other causes for the lameness suggest themselves, probably corns. Evidence of these is not forthcoming, and we in all probability withhold our opinion until a later visit. On the second or a subsequent call we are perhaps lucky enough to find our patient down. Diagnosis is then rendered easier. Made to rise, the animal stands in the attitude we have described as indicative of laminitis. We have him walked and trotted out. The symptoms of tenderness disappear, and the animal soon goes fairly sound. He is, in fact, workable—that is, by anyone who is careless as to the comfort of his beast.

When following an acute attack, we have the most marked symptoms of pain and distress, somewhat abating after the second or third week. The walk, however, is still painful, and, for a short time after rising from the ground, even difficult.

In short, in both cases we have the horse going on his heels, with a walk that is painful, and with symptoms of pain that are most apparent when moved on after a rest.

Later, the changes in the form of the hoof begin to appear. It seems to have lost its elasticity, and is seen to be dry and chippy, and to have become denuded of its varnish-like outer covering.

In addition, it is of largely altered shape. The toe, by reason of the animal walking on his heels, and by reason of an increased growth of horn, becomes elevated, so that the front of the wall, instead of forming an obtuse angle with the ground, comes to run very nearly horizontal with it. The horn of the heels, as compared with that of the toe, takes on an increased growth. The same thing we have already indicated as happening at the toe, though in lesser degree. Taken together, this increased growth of horn at the toe and at the heels has the result of lengthening the diameter of the foot from before backwards, the transverse diameter remaining more or less normal. The hoof thus loses its circular build, and comes to approach nearer an elongated oval.

[FIG. 122.—FOOT BADLY DEFORMED AS A RESULT OF CHRONIC LAMINITIS. At this stage, too, the pathological 'ribbing' of the hoof is observable. The outer surface of the wall becomes marked with a series of ridges encircling the hoof from heel to heel (see Fig. 81, which illustrates a moderate deformity of the hoof occurring after laminitis). In the badly laminitic hoof, however, this deformity is largely increased, until in some cases the shapeless mass can hardly be likened to a foot at all (see Fig. 122).

The inferior or solar surface of the foot also offers certain changes for our consideration. The first thing that strikes one is the convexity of the sole. This, as we have already pointed out, is due to descent of the os pedis, and the highest point of the convex portion is that immediately in front of the apex of the frog. Here the horn is sometimes found to be quite yielding to the finger, is excessively thin, and is more or less granular and inclined to break up under manipulation. As a consequence, any rough use of the drawing-knife, or an accidental wounding with sharp flints or stones, leads to exposure of the sensitive structures and local gangrene.

With the horn of the sole thus deteriorated by reason of excessive and continued pressure upon the parts secreting it, it is not surprising to find that, in many cases, actual penetration of it with the os pedis occurs. It is the anterior portion of the inferior margin of the bone that makes its appearance, and shows itself as a small semicircular white or dark gray line on the sole.

FIG. 123.—SOLAR ASPECT OF FOOT WITH CHRONIC LAMINITIS, SHOWING ITS ABNORMAL OVAL SHAPE FROM BEFORE BACKWARDS, AND THE EXCESS OF HORN GROWING FROM THE WHITE LINE IN THE REGION OF THE TOE.

Exposure of the bone is soon followed by its necrosis, in which case the wound takes on an ulcerating character. From it there is a discharge of pus, black in colour and offensive in smell, and, protruding from the opening, are excessive granulations of the remains of the sensitive sole.

The 'white line,' so apparent when a normal foot is cleaned with the knife, can no longer be sharply distinguished from the surrounding horn, while in some cases the horn composing it takes on an abnormal growth at the toe (see Fig. 123). This adds still further to the abnormal lengthening of the antero-posterior diameter of the foot already mentioned.

In other cases horn in this position is altogether wanting, and in its place is a well-defined cavity, into which the blade of a knife can be readily passed. This cavity is bounded in front by the original wall of the hoof, and is here lined by a degenerated and hypertrophied growth of the horny laminæ. Posteriorly the cavity is bounded by the front of the os pedis, and is lined by a thin growth of horn secreted by the keratogenous membrane covering the bone. Superiorly the cavity is quite narrow, and extends to near the lower surface of the coronary cushion, while inferiorly, at its open portion, it is often 1/2 inch to 1 inch wide. Laterally it extends on each side of the toe to the commencement of the quarters.

FIG. 124.—LONGITUDINAL SECTION OF A FOOT WITH LAMINITIS OF THREE WEEKS' STANDING. On the anterior face of the cavity, in front of the os pedis, are thickened horny laminæ. Due to the sinking of the bony column, the os pedis has perforated the horny sole.

Exploration with a director, or with the blade of a scalpel, removes from the opening a dry detritus. This is composed of the solid constituents of the escaped blood, the dried remains of the inflammatory exudate, and broken-down fragments of cheesy-looking horn. The size to which the cavity may sometimes extend is illustrated in Fig. 124. The thickened horny laminæ forming the anterior boundary of the cavity are here depicted, together with commencing perforation of the horny sole by the os pedis. It is this cavity which, when opened at the bottom and discharging its mealy-looking contents, is known as seedy-toe, for a further description of which see p. 293.

The lameness occurring with chronic laminitis does not always persist. As time goes on the sensitive structures accommodate themselves to the altered form and conditions of the horny box. In certain situations—namely, where pressure is greatest—the softer structures become atrophied, and sometimes even wholly destroyed; while in other positions the changes in form of the hoof tend to increase in size of its interior, with a consequent diminution of pressure upon, and increased growth of the structures within it.

Pathological Anatomy.—In detailing the changes to be observed in chronic laminitis, we take up the description where we left it when dealing with the pathological anatomy of the acute form. The alterations to be met with are best observed by taking a foot so diseased and making of it two sections—one longitudinal, from before backwards; the other horizontal, and in such a position as to cut the os pedis through at its centre.

These sections will expose to view the cavity formed by the pouring out of the exudate, and its full extent may be noticed by examining the sections alternately. Taking the horizontal section first, it will be seen that the hollow space extends wholly round the toe, and as far back as the commencement of the quarters. In the latter position one is able to observe laminæ still in their normal positions and condition. At the toe, however, the horny and secretive laminæ are widely separated, and the space between them filled with a yellow, semi-solid material, the remains of the inflammatory exudate and new horn secreted by the keratogenous membrane. The laminæ, both horny and sensitive, are greatly enlarged. This is a hypertrophy, resulting from the continued effects of the inflammation, and leads in time to the formation of laminæ quite three or four times their normal size. It is this hypertrophy of the laminæ and the pressure of the exudate that causes the bulging and increased growth of the horn at the toe (see Fig. 125), and contributes towards the oval formation of the foot we have mentioned before.

FIG. 125.—LONGITUDINAL SECTION OF A FOOT WITH LAMINITIS OF SEVERAL YEARS' DURATION.

In the longitudinal section the first thing noticeable is the change in position of the bones, more especially in that of the os pedis. The circumstances we have mentioned before—pressure of the exudate upon it in front and tension of the perforans on it behind— have caused it to assume a more upright position than is normal, so much so that in a bad case the front of the bone becomes quite vertical. This vicious direction the other bones of the digit follow (see Fig. 125).

Consequent upon the displacement of the bone, the plantar cushion, by reason of the continued pressure thus put upon it, becomes atrophied, while its hinder half is, as it were, squeezed into taking up a position more posterior and higher in the digit than normally it should. The horn-secreting papillæ covering its inferior face thus become directed backwards sooner than downwards, in which way we account in some measure for the noticeable increase of horn at the heels.

Treatment.—Chronic laminitis is incurable. Treatment must therefore be directed towards the palliation of such conditions as are present, with the object of rendering the the animal better able to perform work. When perforation of the sole has occurred, with the attendant formation of pus and necrosis of the os pedis, it is doubtful whether treatment of any kind is advisable. There are on record cases of this description, where careful curetting of the exposed and necrotic portions and the after application of antiseptic dressings, held in position by a plate shoe or a leather sole, has been followed by good results, and the animal restored for a time to labour. In our opinion, however, early slaughter is the most economical course to adopt, and certainly the wisest advice to give to the ordinary client.

When perforation of the sole is absent, and when serious alteration in the shape of the horny box has not occurred, then the most simple treatment is to put the animal straight away to slow work, with the feet protected by suitable shoes.

Here, again, the most useful shoe is the Rocker Bar (Fig. 119). The broad web and deep seating gives ample protection to the convex sole, and with the ease in distributing his weight that this shoe affords the animal is able to perform slow work on soft lands with some degree of comfort.

Should the growth of the horn at the toe and at the heels be unduly excessive, then our attention may be directed towards reducing it to some approach to the normal. This is accomplished by removing with the rasp and the knife those portions indicated by the dotted lines in Fig. 127. Here it will be seen that the bulk of the horn removed is that protruding at the toe. After this the animal should again be suitably shod. In this connection it should be noted that the fact of the animal walking largely on the heels tends to a forward displacement of the shoe. This must be prevented by providing each heel of the shoe with a clip, after the manner shown in Fig. 128; or, in the case of a bar shoe, supplying it with a clip at the centre of the bar.

FIG. 126.—DIAGRAM ILLUSTRATING THE ABNORMAL GROWTH OF HORN AT THE TOE AND HEELS OF THE FOOT WITH CHRONIC LAMINITIS.

FIG. 127.—THE SAME FOOT AS IN FIG. 126. The dotted lines show the excess of horn removed preparatory to shoeing.

Among other treatments to be noted we may mention one or two to be found chiefly in Continental works on this subject.

The method of Gross consists in thinning down with a rasp about 1-1/2 inches of the horn of the wall immediately below the coronet, the thinned portion extending from heel to heel. The groove made is filled with basilicon ointment,[A] and the coronet stimulated with a cantharides ointment, In this way there is induced to grow from the coronet a new wall of nearly normal dimensions.

[Footnote A: Basilicon ointment is made by heating together resin 8 parts, beeswax 8 parts, olive oil 8 parts, and lard 6 parts. Allow to cool without stirring.]

By other operators (Bayer, Imminger, Meyer, and Gunther) this treatment has been modified by enlarging upon it and removing the whole of the adventitious horn.

FIG. 128.—THE SHOE WITH HEEL-CLIP.

This is done by means of the drawing-knife and the rasp, the ugly-looking pumiced foot being carefully cut and trimmed until, so far as outward appearances are concerned, it is perfectly normal. This done, the whole foot is treated with a suitable hoof ointment, and a shoe applied that affords protection to the sole without imposing pressure upon it. The shoe indicated is either an ordinary shoe with an unusually broad and well-seated web, or the seated Rocker Bar of Broad. With either it is well to additionally protect the sole by means of a leather or rubber pad and tar stopping, or by using the Huflederkitt described on p. 148. In every case the nails must be kept well back in order to avoid the weakened and degenerated horn at the toe, and to take advantage of the greater growth of horn at the heels.

The wisdom of thus removing the whole of the adventitious horn may be questioned. Although a foot of a nearly normal shape is obtained, it must be remembered that the grave

122

alterations within it are unchanged, and that in certain positions the operation must have carried us nearer the sensitive structures than is advisable.

All other treatments failing, the operation of neurectomy has been advised. This we do not think wise. One would imagine that, with degenerative processes already going on in the foot, the tendency to gelatinous degeneration, always to be looked for in neurectomy, would be increased. This, as a matter of fact, is the case, and is borne out by the statements of those who have tried this method of treatment. In many cases the lameness even is not got rid of. Even where it is, the operation is afterwards followed by a great tendency to stumble, by sloughing of the hoof, or by a marked increase in the adventitious horn, and a consequent greater deformity of the foot.

Sooner than risk neurectomy, it seems to us wiser to give a trial to the operation advocated by M.G. Joly, namely, that of ligaturing one of the digital arteries on each affected foot. This operation is performed in the same position as is the higher operation of plantar neurectomy, and may be either internal or external. The vessel is exposed, and a double ligature, preferably of silk, placed on it. The artery is then divided between the two ligatures. The immediate effect of the operation is to cause a considerable diminution in the arterial pressure, and so lessen the intensity of the ostitis in the os pedis. Its consequences are not so serious as those of neurectomy, and it decongests tissues which neurectomy congests.

In cases related by M. Joly this operation, practised both in conjunction with removal of the excess of horn and without it, has resulted in a marked improvement in the gait, the animal going to work one month after the treatment, and remaining sound for some time afterwards.

2. SEEDY-TOE.

Definition.—A defect in the horn of the wall, usually at the toe, but occurring elsewhere, resulting in loss of its substance in either its internal or external layers (see Figs. 129, 130, and 131).

Causes.—The most common factor in the causation of this defect is undoubtedly disease of the sensitive laminæ. We have, in fact, just given an excellent example of the formation of a seedy-toe in the sections of this chapter devoted to laminitis (see pp. 265 and 286). The cavity here formed by the outpouring of the inflammatory exudate and the separation of the sensitive and horny laminæ persists. It becomes filled with the dried remains of the exudate and perverted secretions from the horny and sensitive laminæ (see p. 287). As yet, however, the cavity is closed below, and its existence only surmised. Later, with successive visits to the forge, the layer of solar horn forming its floor is cut away, and the cavity exposed to view. Its mealy-looking contents are removed, and the case reported by the smith.

Although occurring in this way with an acute attack of laminitis, it must be remembered that seedy-toe may arise without previous noticeable cause. The first intimation the owner has is a report from the forge that seedy-toe is in existence. To refer to cases so arising a probable cause is far from easy. At one time it was believed to be due to parasitic infection of the horn. Others have blamed the pressure of the toe-clip, excessive hammering of the wall, or pressure from nails too large or driven too close. Others, again, say that seedy-toe may result from a prick in the forge, from hot-fitting of the shoe, from standing on a dry and sandy soil, or from the use of high calkins on the front shoes. In these cases—cases with an insidious onset—we are inclined to the opinion that the disease of the horn commences from below, and that the sensitive laminæ become implicated later. Holding this view, one must account for the commencing disease of the horn by giving, as causes, firstly, those factors (as, for instance, alternate excessive dampness and dryness) leading to disintegration of the horn tubules; secondly, the penetrating into and between the degenerated tubules of parasitic matter from the ground; and, thirdly, the final breaking up of the horn, and spread of the lesion under the invasion thus started.

FIG. 129.—DIAGRAM ILLUSTRATING POSITION OF SEEDY-TOE (INTERNAL). 1, The horn of the wall; 2, the horn of the sole; 3, the cavity of the seedy-toe; 4, the os pedis; 5, the keratogenous membrane.

Symptoms.—Lameness sometimes attends seedy-toe, and sometimes does not. This is an important point to be carried in mind by the veterinary surgeon who is accustomed in his practice to have many animals pass through his hands for examination as to soundness. An animal with advanced seedy-toe—a condition constituting serious unsoundness—may walk and trot absolutely sound, and may give no indication, either in the shape of the wall or the condition of the sole, that anything abnormal is in existence. Later, however, after the veterinary surgeon has passed him, the purchaser lodges the complaint that the horse has a bad seedy-toe, which, so he is told, must have been there for some time. In this case, culpable though he may appear, there is every excuse for the veterinary surgeon.

Once the cavity is opened at the toe in the neighbourhood of the white line, then diagnosis is easy. A blunt piece of wood, the farrier's knife, or a director may be easily passed into it, sometimes as far up as the coronary cushion (see Fig. 129). Issuing from the opening is seen occasionally a little inspissated pus; more often, however, the dry, mealy-looking detritus to which we have before referred. This form of the disease we may term 'Internal Seedy-Toe.' for, plainly enough, it has had its origin in chronic inflammatory changes in the keratogenous membrane.

FIG. 130.—EXTERNAL SEEDY-TOE COMMENCING AT THE PLANTAR BORDER OF THE WALL.

FIG. 131.—EXTERNAL SEEDY-TOE COMMENCING ON THE ANTERIOR FACE OF THE WALL.

Disease of the horn and loss of its substance may, however, also commence from without. A report on this condition, under the title of 'External Seedy-Toe,' is to be found in vol. xxix. of the *Veterinary Journal,* from which we borrow Figs. 130 and 131.

In Fig. 130 it will be seen that the disease commences at the plantar surface of the toe, and extends upwards and inwards. The same condition may also appear anywhere between the coronet and the ground, gradually extending into the substance of the wall, as shown in Fig. 131. According to the writer, Colonel Nunn, the progress of the disease in this latter case appears to be faster in a downward than in an upward direction. This, however, is more apparent than real, as the rate of growth of the horn downwards detracts from the progress of the disease upwards, although it spreads over the horn at the same rate.

Before concluding the symptoms, we may again allude to the fact that, although usually occurring at the toe, the same condition may be met with in other positions— namely, at either of the quarters. In appearance and in other respects it is identical with that occurring at the toe.

When the animal is lame and the existence of seedy-toe is surmised, or when the cause of the lameness is altogether obscure, a little information may perhaps be gathered from noting the wear of the shoe. If the animal has been going lame for any length of time as a result of disease in the sensitive laminæ, then the shoe will be greatly thinned at the heels, and the toe but little worn.

Treatment.—As with diseased structures elsewhere, the most rational treatment, when possible, is that of excision. The entire portion of the wall forming the anterior boundary of the cavity is thinned down with the rasp and afterwards removed with the knife, wholly exposing the hypertrophied, but usually soft layer of horn covering the sensitive structures.

These hypertrophied portions are also removed, and every particle of the dust-like detritus cleaned away. After-treatment consists in dressing the parts with a good hoof ointment, protecting them, if necessary, with a pad of tow and a stout bandage. It may be that the removal of a large portion of the wall may for some time throw the animal out of work. Acting on Colonel Fred Smith's suggestion, this may be avoided by having made a thin plate of sheet-iron, slightly larger in circumference than the portion of horn removed, and shaped to follow the contour of the foot. This made, it is sunk flush with the wall by hot-fitting it, and kept in position by several small steel screws fixed into the sound horn, just as in the treatment for sand-crack (see p. 174). This will serve the useful purpose of maintaining in position any dressing that may be thought necessary, of acting as a support to the horn left on each side of the portion removed, and of keeping the exposed structures free from dirt and grit.

Practical points to be remembered in fitting plates of this description to the feet are: The plate must never quite reach the shoe, or it will participate in the concussion of progression, and so loosen the screws that hold it in place. For the same reason, that portion of the sole adjoining the piece of horn removed must have its bearing on the shoe relieved. The screws holding the plate should be oiled to prevent rusting, and should take an oblique direction in order to obtain as great a hold as possible on the wall.

When excision is deemed unwise or unnecessary, treatment should be directed towards maintaining the cavity in a state of asepsis. To this end it should be thoroughly cleaned of its contents, and afterwards dressed with medicated tow. The ordinary tar and grease stopping is as suitable as any. This, together with the tow, is tightly plugged into the opening and kept in position by a wide-webbed shoe. Instead of the tar stopping and the tow, there may be used with advantage the artificial hoof-horn of Defay (see p. 152). Before using this the cavity should again be thoroughly cleaned out, and should in addition be mopped out with ether. The latter injunction is important, as unless the grease is thus first removed, the composition will fail to adhere to the horn. With the cavity thus cleaned and prepared, the artificial horn, melted ready to hand, is poured into it and allowed to set.

In every case, no matter what else the treatment, the bearing of the horn adjacent to the lesion should be removed from the shoe. Whether practising the method of plugging the cavity or that of excision of the wall external to it, attempts to quickly obtain a new growth of horn from the coronet should be made. To further that, frequent stimulant applications should be used. Ointment of Biniodide of Mercury 1 in 8, of Cantharides 1 in 8, or the ordinary Oil of Cantharides, either will serve.

3. KERAPHYLLOCELE.

Definition.—By this term is indicated an enlargement forming on the inner surface of the wall. In shape and extent these enlargements vary. Usually they are rounded and extend from the coronary cushion to the sole, sometimes only as thick as an ordinary goose-quill, at other times reaching the size of one's finger. Often they are irregular in formation and flattened from side to side.

FIG. 132.—A PORTION OF THE HORN OF THE WALL AT THE TOE REMOVED IN ORDER TO SHOW A KERAPHYLLOCELE ON ITS INNER SURFACE.

Causes.—Keraphyllocele is very often a sequel to the changes occurring at the toe in laminitis. Probably, however, the most common cause is an injury upon, or a crack through, the wall. It may thus occur from excessive hammering of the foot, from violent kicking against a wall or the stable fittings, and from the injury to the coronet known as 'tread.' It may also occur as a sequel to complicated sand-crack, and to chronic corn.

That fissures in the wall are undoubtedly a cause has been placed on record by the late Professor Walley, who noticed the appearance of these horny growths following upon the operation of grooving the wall.[A]

[Footnote A: *Journal of Comparative Pathology and Therapeutics*, vol. iii, p. 170.]
This gentleman had a large Clydesdale horse under his care for a bad sand-crack in front of the near hind-foot, and, as the lameness was extreme, he adopted his usual method of treatment—viz., rest, fomentations, poulticing, and the making of the V-shaped section through the wall, and subsequently the application of an appropriate bar shoe to the foot, and repeated blisters to the coronet. In a short time the lameness passed off, and the horse was put to work. A few days later the animal met with an accident, and was killed.

On examining a section of the hoof it was found that a vertical horny ridge corresponding to the external fissure had been formed on the internal surface of the wall, and that a well-marked cicatrix extended upwards through the structure of the hoof at the part forming the cutigeral groove; furthermore, *a similar ingrowth had been taking place in the line of the oblique incisions made for the relief of the sand-crack.*

This case has an important bearing on the operation of grooving the wall, which operation we have several times in this work advocated for the relief of other diseases. It teaches us that the incisions should not be carried so completely through the horn as to interfere with and irritate the sensitive laminæ, and so set up the chronic inflammatory condition leading to hypertrophy of the horn.

From the position on the os pedis of the indentation made in it by the keraphyllocele (see Fig. 133) it has been argued that pressure of the toe-clip is a cause of the new growth. This, we should say, cannot be a very strong factor in the causation, for, while we admit that the continual pressure of the clip, and the heavy hammering that sometimes fits it into position, is likely to set up a chronic inflammatory condition of the sensitive laminæ in that region, we must still point out that the rarity of keraphyllocele, as compared with the fact that clips are on every shoe, does not allow of the argument carrying any great weight.

Symptoms.—Except under certain conditions this defect is difficult of detection. As a rule, lameness is not produced by it. In making that statement we are led largely by the conclusion arrived at by Professor Walley. This observer noted the fact that ingrowths of horn such as we are describing nearly always take place in false quarter, or after a sand-crack has been repaired, and that they commonly occur after the operation of grooving the wall in the manner we have just shown.

Now, we know that quite often under these circumstances the horse goes perfectly sound. Thus, while we know that in all probability keraphyllocele is in existence, we have ocular demonstration that the animal is quite unaffected by it.

In some cases, however, lameness is present. During the early stages of the growth's formation it is but slight, increasing as the keraphyllocele enlarges. Should this be the case, other symptoms present themselves. The coronet is hot, and tender to the touch, sometimes even perceptibly swollen, and percussion over the wall is met with flinching on the part of the animal. In other cases one is led to suspect the condition by the prominence of the horn of the wall of the toe. This is distinctly ridge-like from the coronet to the ground, while on either side of it the quarters appear to have sunk to less than their normal dimensions. We believe this to be an illusion, as a ridge of any size at the toe readily gives one the impression of atrophy behind it, without this latter condition being actually present.

Should this ridge-like formation and the accompanying symptoms of pain and lameness occur after repair of a sand-crack, then keraphyllocele may, with tolerable certainty, be diagnosed. When these outward signs are wanting, however, and the true nature of our case is a matter of mere conjecture, a positive diagnosis may still be made at a later stage— that is, when the abnormal growth of horn reaches the sole. In this case either there is met with when paring the sole a small portion of horn, circular in form, distinctly harder than normal, and indenting in a semicircular fashion the front of the white line at the toe, or solution of continuity between the tumour and the edge of the sole and the os pedis takes place, and the lameness resulting from the ingress of dirt and grit thus allowed draws attention to the case.

Pathological Anatomy.—With the sensitive structures removed from the hoof by maceration or other means, these growths are at once apparent. They may occur in any position, but are usually seen at the toe, and they may extend from the coronary cushion to the sole, or they may occupy only the lower or the upper half of the wall. In places the tumour (or 'horny pillar' as the Germans term it) is roughened by offshoots from it, and does not always exhibit the smooth surface depicted in Fig. 132. Commonly, the horn composing the new growth is hard and dense. Sometimes, however, it is soft to the knife, and is then found to be itself fistulous in character, a distinct cavity running up its centre, from which issues a black and offensive pus.

In a few cases the sensitive laminæ in the immediate neighbourhood are found to be enlarged, but in the majority of cases atrophy is the condition to be observed. Not only are the sensitive structures found to be shrunken and absorbed, but the atrophy and absorption extends even to the bone itself (see Fig. 133). This latter is a result of the continued pressure of the horny growth, in a well-marked case ending in a sharply-defined groove in the os pedis in which the keraphyllocele rests. The fact that the softer structures, and even the bone, thus accommodate themselves to the altered conditions is, no doubt, the reason that lameness in many of these cases is absent.

Treatment.—It is doubtful whether anything satisfactory can be recommended. When we have suspected this condition ourselves, it has been our practice to groove the hoof on either side of the toe, after the manner illustrated in Fig. 120, and, at the same time, point-firing the coronet and applying a smart cantharides blister. Certainly, after this operation, lameness has often disappeared—whether, however, as a result of the treatment adopted or by reason of the structures within accommodating themselves to the condition, we would not care to say.

FIG. 133.—OS PEDIS SHOWING THE GROOVE IN IT CAUSED BY ATROPHY AND ABSORPTION INDUCED BY PRESSURE OF A KERAPHYLLOCELE.

Other writers advocate the removal of that portion of the wall to which the tumour is attached, after the manner described on p. 182, and illustrated in Fig. 98. This, however, should be a last resource, and should be adopted only when weighty reasons, such as excessive and otherwise incurable lameness, appear to demand it.

4. KERATOMA.

In our nomenclature the terms 'Keratoma' and 'Keraphyllocele' are both used to indicate the condition we have just described. There are some, however, who reserve the term 'Keratoma' for horny tumours occurring only on the sole, and for that reason we draw special attention to the word here. Keratoma may thus be used to describe what we have called keraphyllocele directly that growth makes its appearance at the sole, and is there able to be cut with the knife. Similar hard and condensed growths may, however, make their appearance on the sole in other positions quite removed from the white line, plainly being secreted by the villous tissue of the sensitive sole, and having no connection whatever with the sensitive laminæ. They appear as circular patches, varying in size from a shilling to a two-shilling piece. Compared with the surrounding horn, they stand out white and glistening, while in structure they are dense and hard, and offer a certain amount of resistance to the knife. They are of quite minor importance, and, beyond keeping them well pared down, need no attention. Keratoma probably offers us the best analogy we have to corn of the human subject.

5. THRUSH.

Definition.—A disease of the frog characterized by a discharge from it of a black and offensive pus, and accompanied by more or less wasting of the organ.

Causes.—The primary cause of this affection is doubtless the infection of the horn, and later the sensitive structures, with matter from the ground. Those factors, therefore, leading to deterioration of the horn, and so exposing it to infection, may be considered here. Such will be changes from excessive dampness to dryness, or *vice versâ*; work upon hard and stony roads; prolonged standing in the accumulated wet and filth of insanitary stables, or long standing upon a bedding which, although dry, is of unsuitable material.

127

In this latter connection may be mentioned the harm resulting from the use of certain varieties of moss litter. This we find pointed out by J. Roalfe Cox, F.R.C.V.S.[A] Tenderness in the foot was first noticed, and, on examination, the horn of the sole and of the frog was found to be peculiarly softened. It afforded a yielding sensation to the finger, not unlike that which is imparted by indiarubber, and on cutting the altered horn it was almost as easily sliced as cheese-rind. The outer surface being in this way slightly pared off, the deeper substance of the horn was discoloured by a pinkish stain. The horn of the frog was in many instances found detaching from the vascular surface, which was very disposed to take on a diseased action, somewhat allied to canker, and became extremely difficult to treat.

[Footnote A: *Veterinary Journal*, vol. xvi., p. 243.]

Conditions such as these, although not constituting the disease itself, certainly lay the frog open to infection, especially if afterwards the animal is called upon to work in the mud of the streets of a large town, or to stand in a badly drained and damp stable.

A further cause of thrush is to be found in the condition of the frog, brought about by contraction of the heels (see p. 118). We have already seen that one of the most prominent factors in the causation of contraction is the removal of the frog from the ground by shoeing, with its consequent diminution in size and deterioration in quality of horn. This leads to fissures in the horny covering, and favours infection of the sensitive structures beneath. Thrush is, in fact, nearly always present in the later stages of contracted foot.

By some thrush is believed to be but the commencement of canker. With this, however, we do not hold. We believe both to be due to specific causes as yet undiscovered, but that the cause of thrush is not the one operating in canker. In arriving at this conclusion we are guided by clinical evidence. The two conditions are quite dissimilar, even in appearance, and, while one is readily amenable to treatment, the other is just as obstinately resistant.

Symptoms.—The symptoms of thrush are always very evident. Probably the first thing that draws one's attention to it is the stench of the puriform discharge. The foot is then picked up and the characteristic putrescent matter found to be accumulated in the median, and often in the lateral, lacunæ. The organ is wasted and fissured, the horn in the depths of the lacunæ softened and easily detachable, and portions of the sensitive frog often laid bare.

With a bad thrush lameness is present, the frog itself is tender to pressure, and often there is considerable heat and tenderness of the heels and the coronet immediately above. More especially is this noticeable after a journey.

It is, perhaps, more common in the hind-feet than in the fore, and more often met with in heavy draught animals than in nags. The hind-feet are, of course, more open to infection by reason of their being constantly called upon to stand in the animal discharges in the rear of stable standings, while it is a well-known fact that heavy animals have their stables kept far less clean, and their feet far less assiduously cared for, than do animals of a lighter type.

In a nag-horse with thrush of both fore-feet lameness becomes sometimes very great. The gait when first moved out from the stable is feeling and suggestive of corns, while progress on a road with loose stones is sometimes positively dangerous to the driver.

Treatment.—When this condition has arisen, as it often does, from want of counter-pressure of the frog with the ground, this pressure must be restored after the manner described when dealing with the treatment of contracted foot (see p. 125) either by the use of tip or bar shoes, or by suitable pads and stopping.

So far as direct treatment of the lesion itself is concerned, the first step is to carefully trim away all diseased horn and freely open up the lacunæ in which the discharge has accumulated. Good results are then often arrived at by poulticing, afterwards followed up by suitable antiseptic dressings. With us a favourite one is the Sol. Hydrarg. Perchlor. of Tuson, used without dilution. Others use a dry dressing, and dust with Calomel, with a mixture of Sulphate of Copper, Sulphate of Zinc and Alum, or with Subacetate of Copper and Tannin.

With restoration, so far as is possible, of the frog functions, and with careful dressing, a cure is nearly always obtained.

6. CANKER.

Definition.—Under this unscientific, yet expressive term, is indicated a chronic diseased condition of the keratogenous membrane, commencing always at the frog, and slowly extending to the sole and wall, characterized by a loss of normal function of the horn secreting cells, and the discharge of a serous exudate in the place of normal horn.

Causes.—The exact cause of canker has still to be discovered. Therefore, before expressing an opinion as to what the *probable* cause may be, we may state here that such opinion can only be based upon clinical observation. Such being the case, we are almost duty bound to give the views of older authors before those of more modern writers.

From the mass of material ready to hand we may select the following as serving our purpose.

The earliest opinion appears to have been that canker, as the name indicates, was of a cancerous or cancroid nature. This was also believed by Hurtrel D'Arboval, who looked upon canker as carcinoma of the recticular structure of the foot. The same theory we find enunciated in the *Veterinary Journal* so late as 1890. Although the word 'cancer' or 'carcinoma' is not there used, the author employs the terms 'Papilloma' and 'Epithelioma' with the evident intention of expressing his belief in the malignant nature of the disease.

Another early opinion was that the disease was a *spreading ulcer*, gradually extending and changing the tissues which it invaded.

A further early theory, and one which if not still believed in, has died a hard death, is the constitutional theory. This was believed in by nearly all the older writers, and is mentioned so late as 1872 by the late Professor Williams. In his 'Principles and Practice of Veterinary Surgery,' he says: 'Canker is a constitutional disease due to a cachexia or habit of body, grossness of constitution, and lymphatic temperament.' This, we believe, is credited to-day by some, and yet, quite 100 years before the date of the 1872 edition of Williams's work—in 1756, to be exact—we find a veterinary writer when talking of grease (a disease, by-the-by, very closely allied to canker) exclaiming against this habit of referring everything which we do not rightly understand to some ill-humour of the body. The wisdom his words contain justifies us in giving them mention here. 'It is a very foolish and absurd Notion,' he says, 'to imagine a Horse full of Humours when he happens to be troubled with the Grease. But such Shallow Reasoning will always abound while Peoples' Judgments are always superficial. Therefore, to convince such unthinking Folks, let them take a thick Stick and beat a Horse soundly upon his Legs so that they bruise them in several Places, after which they will swell, I dare say, and yet be in no danger of Greasing. Now, pray, what were these offending Humours doing before the Bruises given by the Stick?'

At the present day it is safe to assert that neither the ulcerative, the cancerous, nor the constitutional theory is believed in widely, and, among the mass of contrary opinions as to the cause of this disease, we may find that even quite early many of the older writers had discarded them.

Quoting from Zundel, we may say that Dupuy in 1827 considered canker as a hypertrophy of the fibres of the hoof, admitting at the same time that these fibres were softened by an altered secretion; while Mercier in 1841 stated that canker was nothing more than a chronic inflammation of the reticular tissue of the foot, characterized by diseased secretions of this apparatus.

Saving that they make no mention of a likely specific cause, these last two statements express all that we believe to-day. As early as 1851, however, the existence of a specific cause was hinted at by Blaine in his 'Veterinary Art.' We find him here describing canker as a *fungoid* excrescence, exuding a thin and offensive discharge, which *inoculates* the soft parts within its reach, particularly the sensitive frog and sole, and destroys their connections with the horny covering.

The use of the word 'fungoid,' and particularly that of 'inoculate,' is suggestive enough, and is evidence sufficient that either Blaine or his editor recognised, simply through clinical observation, the working of a special cause.

Four years later, Bouley is found holding the opinion that canker was closely allied to tetter, thus recognising for it a local specific cause. The same observer also pointed out that the secretion of the keratogenous membrane instead of being suspended was greatly increased, taking care to explain, as did Dupuy, that the products of the secretion were perverted and had lost their normal ability to become transformed into compact horn.

In 1864 this slowly growing recognition of a specific cause received further impetus from the statements of Megnier. This observer claimed to have discovered in the cankerous secretions the existence of a vegetable parasite (namely, a cryptogam, as in favus), which he termed the keraphyton, or parasitic plant of the horn.

Modern research, though failing to substitute anything more definite, has not confirmed this. The exact and exciting cause of canker is therefore still an open question, and a matter for research. We may, however, sum the matter up by briefly discussing the causes, so far as clinical observation teaches us. This we shall do under two headings—namely, *Predisposing* and *Exciting*.

Predisposing Causes.—Starting with the assumption that the disease is due to local infection, we may relate as predisposing causes anything having a prejudicial effect upon the horn, disintegrating it, and so laying the tissues beneath open to attack. The most prominent in this connection is certainly a continued dampness of the material on which the animal has to stand. Particularly is this the case when the material is also excessively foul and dirty, contaminated with the animal discharges, and presumably swarming with the lower forms of animal and plant life. We shall therefore find bad cases of canker in stables where the "sets" are irregular, or where no paving at all is attempted, where the drainage is defective, and where darkness and want of proper ventilation favours organismal growth. The fact that with modern drainage and a general hygienic improvement in stabling, canker has to a large extent died out, supports this contention.

Again, as with thrush, anything removing the counter-pressure of the frog with the ground and throwing that organ out of play, may be looked upon as a predisposing cause. The atrophy of the frog thus occurring, the deterioration in the quality of its horn and the fissures in its surface lay it specially open to infection. That one of the principal factors in the treatment of canker is a restoration of ground-pressure to the frog and the sole is sufficient proof of this.

Further, it is well to note that, although playing no part in the actual causation, certain constitutional conditions may in some measure predispose the foot to attack. Clinical observation teaches us that animals of a lymphatic nature, with thick skins and an abundance of hair, with flat feet and thick, fleshy frogs, are far more liable to attack than are animals with reverse points.

Exciting Causes. Those who give this subject careful consideration cannot fail to arrive at the conclusion that canker is most certainly due to local infection with a specific poison, and that poison a germicidal one from the ground. The symptoms arising may be due to the action of a single germ, or to two or more germs acting in conjunction. As to whether the parasitic invasion is single or multiple we cannot feel certain, but that it *is* parasitic we feel absolutely assured.

It is simply the light that bacteriological advance has made during the last two decades that enables us to make the statement with such feelings of assurance. We arrive at our conclusions by reasoning from analogy. Here we have a disease always exhibiting the same symptoms, more or less peculiar to one class of animal, always with a similar characteristic appearance and smell, always obstinately refractory to treatment, showing always a tendency to spread to the other feet of the same animal, and often to the feet of other animals *near enough to become* infected, and always cured—when cured it is—by a treatment which may be summed up in two words as 'rigid antisepsis.' Other diseases, with points in common with this, have been directly proved to be due to a specific cause. Common regard for logic compels us to admit the same for canker.

FIG. 134.—A FOOT, THE SUBJECT OF CANKER, SHOWING DESTRUCTION OF THE HORNY FROG, AND A FUNGOID-LOOKING HYPERTROPHY OF THE TISSUES BENEATH.

Symptoms and Pathological Anatomy.—The symptoms of canker are seldom noticeable at the commencement of an attack. The disease is slow in its progress; for some time confines its ravages to the sub-horny tissues unseen, and is quite unattended with pain. It is not observed, therefore, until considerable damage has been done, and the disease is far advanced. What is usually first seen is a peculiar softening and raising of the horn of the frog. The infective material has set up a chronic inflammation of the keratogenous membrane, leading to abnormal secretion, and, in place of the horny cells it should normally secrete, is thrown out an abundance of a serous fluid.

This upraised and softened horn once thrown off is not again renewed, and the whole of the sensitive frog and perhaps a portion of the sensitive sole is left uncovered. In place of the normal horn, however, is often found a hypertrophy of the elements of the keratogenous membrane leading to huge fungoid-looking growths with a papillomatous aspect, damp in appearance and offensive in smell, and readily bleeding when injured (see Fig. 131).

The horn immediately surrounding the lesion is loose and non-adherent to the sensitive structures. This indicates, of course, that the disease has spread further beneath the horny covering than is at first sight apparent. Portions of this loose horn removed reveal beneath it a caseous foetid matter, easily removed by scraping (the perverted secretion of the keratogenous membrane). When this is carefully scraped away, the sensitive structures appear to be covered with a thin, smooth membrane, gray in colour and almost transparent, while beneath it may be seen the red appearance of normal sensitive structures.

If the horn surrounding the lesion is not touched with the knife, but little is seen of the extent of the disease, for that removed by natural means is often very small in quantity. To all intents and purposes the disease appears to be confined to the frog. This appearance is misleading, especially if the disease has been in existence for some time, for it may have easily spread to the whole of the sole, and even to the greater portions of the laminæ secreting the wall.

It is, in fact, not until the pressure exerted by the normal horn is removed by its breaking away that the vascular structures of the keratogenous membrane begin to swell, and the perverted secretions to enlarge in size. Once the pressure is removed, however, this quickly comes about, and the characteristic fungoid growths rapidly make their appearance.

This tendency to spread is highly indicative of canker. The serous matter exuding from the diseased keratogenous membrane appears, in fact, to be highly infective. Once its flow is commenced, it slowly, but surely, invades the sensitive structures near it, appearing, as Elaine has put it, to 'inoculate' them. What is really the case, of course, is not that the discharge itself is infective, but that it is contaminated with infective material.

The fungoid-looking growths to which we have before referred are, in reality, nothing more than the villi of the sensitive frog and sole greatly hypertrophied and irregular in shape. At times the hypertrophy is as a huge and compact enlargement occupying the position of the frog. Sometimes, however, it occurs as numerous elongated and twisted fibrous bundles, separated from each other by deep clefts, and the clefts filled with the offensive cankerous discharge (see Fig. 134).

FIG. 135.—LOWER ASPECT OF CANKERED FOOT, SHOWING DESTRUCTION OF WALL.

At a very advanced stage canker leads to destruction of much of the horny sole and frog; or even parts of the wall may become separated from the tissues beneath, and break away from the foot (see Fig. 135). At other times the disease brings about a deformity of the whole of the foot. Its longitudinal and transverse diameters become enormously increased, and the whole foot apparently flattened from above to below (see Fig. 136). This indicates that not only has the horny sole been entirely destroyed, but that the destructive process has also extended to the greater part of the lower half of the wall, with a consequent hypertrophy of exposed soft structures, and a sinking of the bony column, similar to that which occurs in laminitis, but not so pronounced.

FIG. 136.—FOOT WITH ADVANCED CANKER.

A further aspect of the badly-cankered foot is to be found in an apparently enormous increase in the length of the wall. This we have seen protruding for quite 5 inches beyond the plane of the sole. It simply indicates that, in order to keep the animal at work, the smith has at every shoeing spared the wall, so that the diseased structures might be kept from contact with the ground.

As we have said before, pain and other symptoms of distress are quite absent. Animals affected with canker for a long time maintain their condition, feed well, and are quite capable of performing work under ordinary conditions.

Differential Diagnosis and Prognosis.—Perhaps the only disease with which canker may be confounded is thrush. They should, however, be easily distinguishable. The discharge from thrush is not so profuse, and is thicker and darker in colour, while the loosening of the horn is almost entirely absent. Furthermore, thrush shows no tendency to spread, and, even when left untreated, may remain confined to the frog for months, and even years. Canker, on the other hand, is slowly progressive, and soon shows the characteristic fungoid excrescences, which growths are in thrush never seen. A further point of difference is discovered when treatment is commenced. Canker is found to be refractory to a point that is absolutely disheartening, while thrush, with careful attention, is soon got under hand, and a permanent cure effected.

The prognosis must be guarded. By many canker has been said to be incurable. This, however, has been clearly shown to be wrong. When the animal is young, and treatment may reasonably be judged to be economical, then a favourable prognosis may be indulged in, provided the veterinary surgeon intends to put into that treatment a more than ordinary amount of individual care and attendance. Even then, however, he will have to be very largely guided by the condition of his case. He should see that it is not too far advanced, and that a great deformity of the hoof, or actual exploration, does not indicate disease of the greater part of the wall.

Treatment.—From what has gone before, it will be seen that the eradication of canker is no easy task, that it is, in fact, a most difficult matter, and one not to be lightly undertaken. At the risk of recapitulating what we have said before, we may mention here the two points which the veterinarian must bear in mind. (1) That there is no actual disease or alteration in structure of the deep layers of the keratogenous apparatus. It is only the superficial, or horn-secreting, layer that concerns us. (2) That the disease of this superficial layer is infection with a material that may reasonably be presumed to be infective.

Put thus, treatment of canker would at first sight appear to be easy. One would imagine that a simple and long-continued soaking of the entire foot in a strong enough antiseptic would be all that was needed. Clinical observation, however, shows that this is not so, and for this there must be reasons.

The reasons are these: (1) Between us and the diseased layer upon which our attention must be directed is often a layer of normal horn, effectually protecting the tissues beneath from any dressing which we might consider beneficial. (2) Anything applied with the object of destroying septic material, but strong enough, or caustic enough, to injure the membrane upon which we are working, only makes the case worse. The superficial layer of the keratogenous membrane in which we have judged the disease to exist is, after all, but a delicate structure. When attacked by the application of too potent a drug its horn-secreting layer is easily destroyed, and thus, although we may succeed in establishing asepsis, we cannot expect at the point of injury a growth of horn. In its place we are confronted with large outgrowths of inflammatory fibrous tissue. (3) Shedding of the diseased horn and removal of the pressure exerted by the hoof faces us with hypertrophy of the exposed villi.

The difficulty of meeting this with an adequate and evenly-distributed pressure is well enough known, and we find in that a further reason that the treatment of canker is superlatively difficult. (4) The material on which the animal has to stand is a distinct bar to the maintaining of a strict asepsis.

When we have said this, it is easy to understand that canker is not to be successfully met with any so-called specific—that it makes but little difference what the application may be so long as it is antiseptic, and is used by a man thoroughly conversant with the difficulties he has to contend with, and with his mind firmly set upon surmounting them.

With this point established, we will not devote more of our space to a consideration of the various dressings that have at different times been highly advocated in the treatment of the disease. It is interesting, however, to note that intensely irritating and caustic applications have been greatly in favour. Nitric acid, sulphuric acid (either alone or its action reduced by the addition of alcohol, oil, or turpentine), arsenic, butter of antimony, creasote, chromic acid, carbolic acid, arsenite of soda, and the actual cautery, have all been used.

Without dwelling further on that, we may say at once that a correct treatment consists in (1) the removal of all horn overlying infected portions of the keratogenous membrane, (2) the application of an antiseptic not too powerfully caustic in its action, (3) frequent changes of the dressings in order to insure a maintenance of antisepsis, and (4) the application of an adequate pressure to the exposed soft structures. Thus combated, canker is curable.

The man who, at the expense of much time and trouble, has demonstrated the truth of these axioms is Mr. Malcolm, of Birmingham. The determination with which he clung to his point that canker was, with correct treatment, in every case curable, was some years ago provocative of much discussion in veterinary circles. That he was successful in proving his contention is more to our point here. It is his method of treatment, therefore, that we shall give, and this we shall do by liberal extracts from Mr. Malcolm's own writings.

'On the first occasion of operating upon and dressing the cankered foot, it is usually necessary to cast the horse, and this may have to be done at intervals for a second or even third time; but in most cases once is sufficient, subsequent dressing being usually accomplished without much difficulty, frequently even without the aid of a twitch. After the horse has been secured, the drawing-knife is first employed; and if the frog alone is affected, it is unnecessary even to pare the sole, the removal of all frog horn not intimately adherent to its secreting surface being all that is required. But if both sole and frog be involved, the whole of the sound horn should be first thinned until it springs under the thumb, and then, using a sharp knife, every particle of diseased horn must be carefully removed from both sole and frog, a process much more easily, and with far greater certainty, secured by the previous thinning of the horn.

'The removal of diseased horn should always commence at the most dependent part of the foot, so that any hæmorrhage produced may be below the parts still to be operated on, a matter of considerable moment for effective treatment. But with due care there will be little hæmorrhage, as, except in the initial stage, there is no real union between the diseased horn and the diseased vascular secreting surface.

'After all apparently diseased horn has been removed by the knife, any still remaining should be at once destroyed by the actual cautery, by which it can be identified. All the diseased secreting surface should be *carefully scraped with a thin hot iron*,[A] fungoid growths excised and cauterized, and, indeed, every particle of cankered tissue should, if possible, be eradicated. In securing this more reliance can be placed on the actual cautery than on any other, whether liquid or solid: it is more under control in application, more decisive in effect, and its results can be anticipated with a far greater certainty. Moreover, its aid in diagnosis is of immense value; applied to the thinned horn or secreting surface it unmistakably demonstrates the presence or absence of canker. Healthy tissue chars black; cankered tissue, on the contrary, bubbles up white under the hot iron, and presents an appearance not unlike roasted cheese.

[Footnote A: The words in italics are alterations in the original article made by Mr. Malcolm in a private letter to the author (H.C.R.).]

'Although this test is certain for horn thinned to the quick, it is not to be relied upon with thick horn, the outside of which may be practically healthy and char black, while its underlying surface may be cankered. With this exception the test is an infallible one, as by it the demarcation between cankered and healthy tissue can be clearly traced, and as a result we can with equal confidence radically *remove*[A] all cankered tissue, and conserve all healthy. As the object of that abominably cruel and barbarous operation of stripping the sole is the exposure of all canker, and as this can be done with equal certainty with the aid of the hot iron, there can be no necessity for performing it. The pain of cauterizing cankered tissue, which is a necessary operation, is infinitesimal (canker largely destroying sensation), compared with the pain produced in the totally unnecessary process of tearing healthy horn from a highly sensitive tissue.

[Footnote A: The words in italics are alterations in the original article made by Mr. Malcolm in a private letter to the author (H.C.R.).]

'Having by means of the knife and cautery removed every known particle of disease, the next procedure is to pack the surface of the sole and frog thus exposed with a *mild dressing, such as vaseline; but if the cankered surface has not been efficiently, scraped, than there is required a more* [A] powerful astringent or caustic dressing, which may vary considerably according to the individual fancy. A great favourite of mine consists of equal parts of sulphates of copper, iron, and zinc, mixed with strong carbolic acid, a very little vaseline being added to give the mass cohesion. The dressing, covered by a pledget of tow, is held in position by a shoe with an iron or leather sole, and the dressing and tow together should be of sufficient bulk to produce slight pressure on the sole when the nails of the shoe are drawn up. This insures contact between the dressing and the exposed surface, as well as any benefit derivable from pressure.

[Footnote A: The words in italics are alterations in the original article made by Mr. Malcolm in a private letter to the author (H.C.R.).]

'The dressing of the foot and nailing of the shoe can usually be more expeditiously performed when the horse is on his feet than when prone. If only the frog, or the frog and a small part of the sole, be involved, the horse should be kept at work, but if a large part or the whole of the sole a few days' rest may be necessary; but as soon as the condition of the foot will allow, work should be resumed, and it is simply marvellous how sound a horse will walk while minus the greater part of his sole from canker.

'On the second day following the shoe should be removed, and the foot redressed. To effect this it is necessary to recast the horse. Commencing at the edge of the sound horn, at the most dependent part of the foot, all new horn, no matter what its condition, must be pared to the quick, especial care being taken to effectually remove any lingering disease. Want of success is frequently attributable to neglect of this precaution. A small particle of canker remains undetected, forms a new centre of infection, and just when success is anticipated, much to your chagrin you have to deal with a fresh outbreak of canker, instead of a rapidly-healing foot. Parenthetically, I may here remark that the amount of more or less imperfect new horn produced by a cankered surface after an effective but not too destructive cauterization is almost incredible, and one cannot fail to be struck with the very active proliferation here compared with the meagre production of new horn by the healthy surface.

'After all disease has been excised, carefully clean the foot with waste, thoroughly protect any raw surface resulting from overcauterization by some mild agent, such as a saturated calomel ointment, reapply an astringent dressing over the whole affected surface, and nail on the shoe. This method of procedure should now be thoroughly carried out daily for a time, and as it is proceeded with a successful issue soon becomes assured in nearly every case. Where, in spite of these efforts, the disease still persists, depend upon it the fault is with the operator, who has failed to eradicate some centre of infection. Under these circumstances it may be necessary to recast the patient, repare the foot, and by the aid of eye, knife, and cautery, endeavour to find the cause, and having found it, which can invariably be done, remove it. The usual treatment will then speedily become successful. As the case proceeds dressing every other day will soon be sufficient, then twice a week, and finally, once a week until sufficiently cured.

'During this healing process, and after the complete eradication of canker it may be again repeated, no agent seems to have a more beneficial effect than calomel, and for this purpose it is best used as a dry powder. Under this dressing any remaining spot of canker is readily detected by the wet condition of the calomel when the shoe is removed the next day. In dealing with such a spot, a very good plan, after all apparently diseased tissue has been excised, is to touch the cankered part with solid nitrate of silver, or a feather dipped in one of the strong mineral acids, and then reapply calomel over the surface. The result of this treatment is frequently very gratifying.

'In successful treatment the shoe must be removed each time—an adjustable plate will not do, as no man can thoroughly pare and examine a foot with the shoe on, and imperfect dressings are worse than useless. Indeed, it is better not to pare or thin the horn at all, than to imperfectly pare, since canker, if undestroyed, develops far more rapidly under thin horn than under thick.

'In conclusion, I would again urge the necessity, at the very first operation, when the horse is down, of removing *every single particle* of the diseased tissue, either by excision or effectual cauterization, but at the same time taking very great care to guard against the latter being too destructive. The cautery should be laid aside as soon as the tissue cauterized ceases to *burn white*. The moment at which the canker has thus been eradicated without destroying sound tissue is indicated by the appearance of healthy horn, by the intimate union of that with the secreting surface, and by the healthy aspect of the exuded blood when paring has been carried to the quick.

'Should subjacent healthy structures be destroyed during the process, that is shown by the production of a raw sore, or of a sore to which a "sit-fast," coextensive to the injury, is firmly attached. This seriously retards recovery. The secreting surface having been destroyed, no new horn can be produced directly from the part, and a new secreting surface and new horn have now to grow inwards from the surrounding undestroyed tissue, and that is a slow process. At the same time, on the principle of choosing the least of two evils, practical experience teaches that it is better to produce a small sore or a "sit-fast" than to leave a part of the canker undetected; but, on the other hand, it is better to leave a small part of canker undetected, which can be recognised and removed at the next examination, than to cause a large slough. The object of the skilful surgeon is, naturally, to avoid both extremes; and if trouble be taken to carry out the procedure described, there need be no fear of the result.'[A]

[Footnote A: *Journal of Comparative Pathology and Therapeutics*, vol. iv., p. 24.]

Treated in this way, the horse with cankered feet may be usually kept at work during the whole time that treatment is carried out, and a cure is obtainable in periods varying from six weeks to six or even twelve months.

The same essentials in treatment—namely, removal of diseased horn, antiseptic dressings, and pressure—are insisted on by other writers. Bermbach,[A] in 1888, treats canker as follows: The horse having been cast, the undermined hoof-horn is removed with the knife, and the hypertrophied sensitive structures, if necessary, reduced in the same manner. The chief difficulty in removing the latter is experienced in the lateral lacunæ of the frog, where it is most conveniently scraped away with a spoon or sharp curette. Professors Hoffmann and Imminger also operate in the same way, applying an Esmarch's hæmostatic bandage, and using the knife and curette freely.[B]

[Footnote A: *Ibid.*, vol. ii., p. 68.]

[Footnote B: *Veterinary Journal*, vol. xxxv., p. 433.]

Hæmorrhage is afterwards arrested, and a dressing of perchloride of mercury (a solution, 1/2 per cent., in equal parts of alcohol and water) applied. The after-dressings succeeding best are those of *slightly* caustic and astringent agents, preferably in the form of a powder, and held in position by carbol-jute pads and linen bandages applied with a certain amount of pressure.

The same author draws attention to the fact that caustic agents such as nitrate of lead, chloride of zinc, etc., act too powerfully if the bleeding has been arrested and the wound disinfected. They then form a thick crust, under which profuse suppuration takes place. The same agents are likewise contra-indicated when hæmorrhage is still present. In this latter case they combine with the blood to form metallic albuminates, which lie as an impenetrable layer on the surface of the wound, and so hinder the action of drugs on the tissue below.

During his after-treatment, Bermbach advocates removal of the dressings every second day, all cheesy material to be scraped away with the knife, and the sublimate lotion to be used again. He also insists on the animal being kept standing in a *dry stable*,—nothing but a stone pavement kept clean—and put to regular work in a plate shoe after the first or second week. Cure of advanced cases is said to be obtainable in from four to six weeks.

As illustrative of the value of pressure in the treatment of canker, we may also draw attention to a treatment advocated by Lieutenant Rose.[A] This observer holds that adequate pressure is unobtainable by packing the foot, and, to obtain it, removes the wall from heel to heel, much after the manner of preparing the foot for the Charlier shoe, so that the *whole* of the weight is taken by the sole and the frog. Tar and tow is then lightly applied, the foot placed in a boot, and the patient turned into a loose-box. The dressing is repeated at intervals of four or five days until the animal is cured.

[Footnote A: *Veterinary Record*, vol. xi., p. 435.]

Those who have followed this method of treatment have modified it by actually shoeing the animal Charlier fashion, and keeping him at work, attention, of course, being at the same time given to a proper antiseptic dressing.

Reported Cases.—1. (Malcolm's Treatment[A]). The subject was a five-year old horse belonging to a client of Mr. Giver's, of Tamworth. The case was an exceptionally bad one, for not only was the whole of the frog and sole of the near hind-foot cankered, but the disease on the outside quarter extended to within 1/2 inch of the coronet, and on the inside quarter to within 2 inches of it. As the owner, a farmer, had not proper convenience for Mr. Olver to treat the case, the latter asked me, while visiting him, if I would care to undertake the treatment, saying at the time it would be a very good test-case, as the disease was so far advanced. I readily agreed, and, after the necessary arrangements, had the horse removed to Birmingham on July 2. In this case it was found necessary to cast the animal and cauterize the foot a second time before a healthy granulating surface was secured; but after this the progress towards recovery was uninterrupted, although necessarily slow, on account of the large amount of new secreting surface which had to be formed.

[Footnote A: *Journal of Comparative Pathology and Therapeutics*, vol. v., p. 48.]

The horse was finally discharged, after inspection by Mr. Olver, absolutely cured and free from canker, on January 7.

The illustration (Fig. 135, p. 312) is from a photograph, and it gives a somewhat imperfect representation of the state of the foot two months after it came under my care.

2. (Rose's Treatment.[A]) This was a bad case of canker, which had been for two or three months treated in the ordinary manner, with but little sign of ultimate success. Commenced in June and carried on until the end of September, the ordinary treatment consisted in burning down the fungus growth with the hot iron, and dressing with copper sulphate, zinc sulphate, and boracic acid. The cauterization was repeated every five days.

[Footnote A: *Veterinary Record*, vol. xi., p. 435.]

The treatment of Lieutenant Rose was commenced at about the end of September, at which date the disease extended from the toe on one side of the foot right back to the heel, involving the sole, half of the frog, and the bulb of the heel. One week after treatment the diseased surface was drier, and granulations were more healthy. At the expiration of a fortnight the new horn had commenced to grow from the wall, and also from the frog, right round the diseased surface, the diseased part of the bulb of the heel being divided from the sole by new horn.

Three to four weeks later the diseased surface was gradually getting smaller, while in about six weeks it was quite healed up, the last place to heal being a strip outside the bar, between it and the wall, and a smaller spot on the bulb of the heel. These healed up simultaneously, and left the animal sound.

3. (Treatment by Pressure, H. Leeney [A]). I was consulted in the early part of last summer, before the dry weather had begun, as to a farm-horse with canker in three feet. Her shoes were in the 'disgruntle' condition we so often find on farms, that, to give her a level bearing until I should call another day with a farrier to help me to pack the foot up in the old-fashioned way, I had the remaining shoes pulled off. The case somehow dropped out of my list, and I neglected to call, until asked one day to see something else.

[Footnote A: *Veterinary Records*, vol. xi., p. 447]
I then found that, under a pressure of work, the animal had been used in the shafts of a farm-cart on tolerably level ground, and when the dry weather had already set in. There was a distinct improvement in all the diseased feet, and as she was badly wanted I contented myself with rasping off some broken crust, and supplied some caustic dressing for use at night. Without shoes she worked continuously on the dry and hard meadow-land for several weeks, and was practically cured in something less than three months. My astringent or caustic lotion may have had something to do with the cure of the deep-seated parts, but the bare recital of the case should be sufficient to show that it is all a question of bearing, or nearly so.

7. SPECIFIC CORONITIS.

Definition.—In describing this condition under the above heading, we are following the lead of Mr. Malcolm. We may define it as a chronic inflammatory condition of the keratogenous membrane, usually confined to that of the coronary cushion, the ergots and the chestnuts, but sometimes extending to that of the frog and the sole, characterized by a malsecretion of the affected membrane similar to that observed in canker.

Causes.—The cause which we have indicated for canker—namely, a local specific one, is in all probability the one operating here. Apparently there is a variance of opinion as to whether the condition is actually canker or not. We think, however, that the character of the secretion of the affected membranes, the appearance of the growths, the manner in which they react to the hot iron, the comparative absence of pain, and other points of similarity, point to the fact that the two conditions are actually identical. In other words, the cause is precisely the same, and the only point of difference is the alteration in the point of attack.

Symptoms.—Like canker, the disease is insidious in onset. In precisely similar manner the horn, and in this case the skin of the coronet, is underrun. Later there is the partial shedding and fissuring of the undermined horn and the exuding of the characteristic discharge—in this case not so watery as that of canker. The caseous material of canker is also present, as is a disposition to hypertrophy of the exposed sensitive structures. What horn is left becomes rough and irregularly fissured, and has been likened by some observers to deeply-wrinkled bark of an old tree. A peculiar characteristic of this condition is the state of the ergots and chestnuts. Here the keratogenous membrane participates in the diseased process, and their horn becomes dry and brittle, and readily splits into small fibrous bundles very similar to the fibroid growth described in canker. These excrescences are easily separated from the sensitive structures beneath, and the exposed surface is seen to be more or less moist, or even exhibiting a slight oozing of blood.

Again, as in canker, the deeper layers of the sensitive structures appear to be normal, the horn-secreting layers being the only ones affected. According to Malcolm, the disease is in its nature equally as inveterate as canker, but it is easier to treat, on account of its more exposed position.

Treatment.—This is exactly that as described for canker.

FIG. 137.—SPECIFIC CORONITIS OF ALL FOUR FEET.

FIG. 138.—OFF FORE-FOOT AFFECTED WITH SPECIFIC CORONITIS.

Recorded Case.—The subject of this case was a young black cart gelding. The disease is reported as having begun as thrush, and then extended to the coronet. When I saw him he had been in a similar condition to that depicted in Fig. 137 for, it was said, two or three months, the driver of the horse meanwhile endeavouring to effect a cure by some potent drug of his own. The animal was in good condition, but walked with difficulty owing to the pain. The coronary bands were swollen to two or three times their natural size, and this caused the hair immediately above to curl upwards. Just below the coronary bands there was a line of separation between them and the wall. They themselves were covered with the cheesy substance typical of canker, and they bled on friction. Down the wall of the off fore-foot some blood had trickled, which may be seen in Fig. 138. The frogs of all four feet bulged backwards, and were badly affected. The soles were covered with normal horn, but I did not resort to paring to see if they were affected. One very curious feature about the case was the fact that all the callosities (ergots and chestnuts) seemed to participate in the morbid process, and they, too, were covered with a thin layer of soft cheesy horn. The animal used to bite at his coronets and also the callosities above the knees and hocks until they bled, which they did quite easily. The owner would not go to the expense of having him treated, so he was destroyed.[A]

[Footnote A: Henry Taylor, *Veterinary Record*, vol. xvii., p. 311.]

CHAPTER X
DISEASES OF THE LATERAL CARTILAGES
A. WOUNDS OF THE CARTILAGES.

To a consideration of this we shall devote but little space. It is sufficient to say that any wound in the region of the coronet should always be given the most careful attention. More particularly should this be so when it is ascertained that the wound has involved one of the lateral cartilages. Wounds of non-vascular bodies such as these are always slow to heal, and, by reason of their slowness, invite septic infection. In many cases, in fact, it happens that they do not heal at all. Instead, the injured part becomes necrotic, is unable to cast itself off, and remains as a centre of infection in the depths of the wound, thus constituting what is known as a quittor.

Apart from this, it will be remembered that the internal face of the cartilage is in intimate contact with the pedal articulation, especially anteriorly. Wounds in this situation are, therefore, likely to penetrate the joint, giving us as a complication of the injury the conditions of synovitis and arthritis.

Immediately a wound is inflicted in this position, attempts should be made to insure thorough asepsis of the part. When possible, by far the better way of accomplishing this will be to wholly immerse the foot in a tub of cold antiseptic solution, and keep it there for an hour three times daily. During the time the foot is out of the solution the wound should be protected with a pad of carbolized tow or other suitable dressing, and wrapped in a linen bandage or clean bag. If unable to use the bath, then antiseptic solutions of more than moderate strength should be freely applied to the wound and the adjacent parts, a carbolized or other antiseptic pad placed over it, and the bandage adjusted as before. Repeated injuries to the cartilages, even if not attended with an actual wound, are apt to bring about their ossification and end in the formation of side-bones.

B. QUITTOR.

Definition.—A fistulous wound of the foot, usually opening at the coronet, and variously complicated according to the structures invaded by its contained pus. For the reason that quittor is in every-day veterinary nomenclature *usually* associated with necrosis or other abnormal condition of the lateral cartilage, we include its description in this chapter.

Classification.—It has been customary with Continental authors to classify quittor according to the extent and position of the diseased process. There were thus distinguished:

(a) The *Simple* or *Cutaneous Quittor*, in which had occurred nothing more than necrosis of a portion of the coronary skin and the structures immediately underlying it—that is, the superficial portion of the coronary cushion.

(b) The *Tendinous Quittor*, in which not only the immediately subcutaneous tissues were attacked, but also portions of tendon and ligament.

(c) The *Sub-horny Quittor*, in which the diseased process had invaded the deeper portions of the coronary cushion, and continued a downward course until the laminal tissue below the upper margin of the wall was involved, or any other case, no matter what the starting-point, in which pus existed within the horny box and was discharging itself by a fistulous opening.

(d) The *Cartilaginous Quittor*, in which a portion of the lateral cartilage had become attacked and rendered necrotic.

We believe that—in this country, at any rate—the word 'quittor' is usually held to indicate one or other of the two latter conditions, and probably the last of these; and that the two first are held of small account, or hardly of sufficient gravity to allow of the word 'quittor' being applied to them. In fact, by defining quittor as a 'fistula,' or little pipe, we have ourselves already indirectly restricted the use of the word to the two latter conditions, for in those varieties known as Simple or Cutaneous and Tendinous, the wound is generally broad and open, or, at any rate, superficial, and can scarcely be strictly described as 'fistulous.' In the two latter, however, a true fistula exists. These, however, have only one essential difference, and that consists simply in the position of the lesion and the structures it has attacked. In the main the symptoms will be the same, the disease in each case about equally serious, and in each the same essentials of treatment will have to be regarded.

In our opinion, therefore, a lengthy classification serves no useful end, and we think matters will be simplified by considering quittor under two headings only—namely, 'Simple or Cutaneous' and 'Sub-horny,' and discussing the other varieties as simply complications of either of these two.

1. SIMPLE OR CUTANEOUS QUITTOR.

Definition.—This condition is simply a sloughing of a portion of the skin of the coronet, together with a portion of the immediately underlying soft structures.

Causes.—This form of quittor has its origin more often than not in contusions, punctures, or wounds of the region severe enough to cause death of a small portion of the tissues. In this case the low vitality of the parts does not allow of the dead portion being removed piecemeal by a process of phagacytosis, as is usually the case with similar injuries elsewhere. Instead, the tissues around, aided by a process of suppuration, cast the offending portion off as a slough. It is the wound remaining after the slough which we may really regard as a quittor. In this connection may be considered as causes blows from falling shafts, self-inflicted treads, or treads from other horses, overreach, etc. On the other hand, simple or cutaneous quittor may occur without ascertainable cause. In this case we can only explain its appearance, as we did that of simple coronitis (see p. 231), by attributing it to septic infection through a wound or a blow that is able to inoculate the skin, yet which is insufficient to cause pain, or in any other way attract the attendant's notice. Meanwhile, the spot of infection thus started spreads, and the end result is an abscess in the coronary region, again accompanied with necrosis and sloughing of more or less skin and other tissue, which terminates by discharging its contents and leaving behind a wound which again constitutes a cutaneous quittor. Thus, as with simple coronitis, anything lowering the vitality of the parts, and so favouring infection of the skin, may bring about a quittor. Walking through much water in the winter months, through the dirt and mud of our streets, through melting ice and snow, or through anything in the nature of a chemical irritant, may be looked upon as a cause.

Symptoms.—Whether commencing from an ascertainable injury, or beginning at first unnoticed, cutaneous quittor is characterized sooner or later by the appearance of an inflammatory swelling, usually confined to the seat of injury. Heat and tenderness are present, and the animal is lame.

Later the inflammatory swelling becomes more profuse, the animal is fevered, and the symptoms of lameness increased. Poulticing is at this stage perhaps resorted to. By its means the process of suppuration is aided, and the swelling (at first tense and hard) either becomes gradually softened, its contents discharged, and a simple abscess cavity left behind, or the suppuration runs immediately round the necrosed structures, and casts them off bodily as a slough. This latter condition is always manifested, where the hair does not hide it, by the colour of the skin. At first this is only red in colour—the angry red of an inflamed spot. As its intention to slough away becomes evident, the red gradually gives way to a gray, or even blue-black appearance, while from around it oozes a slight discharge of pus, yellow in colour and non-offensive, or blood-stained and dark in appearance, and foetid to the smell.

Almost invariably these symptoms are added to by a more or less diffuse and oedematous swelling of the lower portion of the limb, extending in some cases to as high as the fetlock or the upper third of the cannon.

With the casting off of the slough the phenomena of inflammation to a great extent subside, the pain ceases, and the case under ordinary conditions commences to mend.

Pathological Anatomy.—In its early stages the condition of simple or cutaneous quittor is really a condition of acute coronitis (see p. 229), and consists in an inflammation of the subcutaneous tissue, and the more superficial portions of the coronary cushion. The tissues implicated are destroyed outright, become infiltrated with the inflammatory exudate and escaped blood, and act as a source of irritation to the still living tissues around. Under the irritation the latter, as we have said before, cast the necrosed portion away by a process of sloughing.

Always, however, it is found that the portion to be sloughed off, while easily separated from the tissues adjacent to its sides, is closely connected on its lowermost or deeper face with the structures below, and cannot be torn away without hæmorrhage and the causing of acute pain.

Prognosis.—With wounds about the feet our forecast should always be guarded. Even with this, the most simple form of quittor, no decided opinion should be given until the progress of the case warrants one in reasonably assuming that complications are absent. Once this point is decided, a favourable prognosis may be given.

Complications.—With cutaneous quittor various complications may arise, according to the extent of the invasion of the septic matter. Necrosis of tendon, of ligament, or of cartilage, caries of the bone, or a condition of synovitis and arthritis may be met with. As these complications are equally common to sub-horny quittor, we shall reserve their description until dealing with that condition. *Treatment (Preventive).*—Immediately after the infliction of an injury in this position, more especially if it is such as to lead one to judge that necrosis will follow to any large extent, the patient should be rested. Ill effects may then be probably warded off by having the foot immersed in a cold antiseptic solution, and afterwards bound with an antiseptic pad and bandage.

Curative.—When the condition has gone undiscovered until commencing necrosis and suppuration are plainly discernible, then the wisest course we can follow is to do all we can to hasten removal of the necrosed portion.

This is best done by promoting the suppurative process by means of warmth or stimulant applications.

To this end hot poultices, or, better still, hot baths, should be resorted to. Under their influence a greater supply of blood is directed to the still healthy tissues enabling them to actively continue the inflammatory processes necessary to the detaching of the portion necrosed, while, at the same time, the pus organisms, stimulated by the heat, are stirred into greater activity, and the readier accomplish their purpose of destroying the adhesion still existing between the necrotic portion and the surrounding living tissues.

When prolonged poulticing or bathing cannot be practised, then the swelling should be stimulated with a sharp cantharides blister, repeated, if the case demands it, at intervals of a few days.

Should the swelling show distinct signs of pointing, and an abscess is plainly the condition to be dealt with, its contents should be liberated by a free use of the knife. In this connection it is important to insist on the fact that the opening should be made large enough. One bold incision from the uppermost limit of the swelling down to the coronary margin of the wall is usually sufficient.

Even when pointing is not very evident, and suppuration is plainly more or less diffuse, benefit may still be derived from the use of the knife. In this case a deep scarification of the part is indicated. Three, four, or more vertical incisions are made in the swelling, and from them obtained a flow of blood mingled with a small quantity of pus from several different centres. By this means sloughing of the diseased portion is quickly obtained, and nothing but an ordinary open wound left for treatment. It should be mentioned, however, that when sloughing can be in any way induced to take place naturally it is better to allow this to take place. Even when the necrosed portion is freely movable, and only adherent by its base, it should not be forcibly removed, but left to the slower but more effectual action of the tissue reactions. If torn forcibly away, we in all probability leave in the bottom of the wound remnants of the dead tissue, which, being small and consequently less productive of inflammatory phenomena, are not so readily sloughed as the larger portion. These remain as centres of infection, and prolong the case.

Once a suitable slough has occurred, the after-treatment is simple. It consists in dressing the wound with reliable antiseptics, and maintaining the parts in a healthy condition until Nature completes the cure by repairing the breach. Solutions of carbolic acid, of perchloride of mercury, of zinc chloride, or of moderately strong solutions of copper sulphate, are all of them useful (see also treatment of coronitis on p. 236).

It is sometimes found that even with careful attention the wound left by the removal of the slough shows a marked disinclination to heal. The greater portion of the cavity becomes filled with granulation tissue, and the epidermis gradually closes round until all is covered except a spot of perhaps the size of half a crown or a crown piece. Here the regenerative process stops, and the wound obstinately refuses to effectually close.

In such cases we have derived excellent results with the actual cautery. The animal is cast, the foot firmly secured by fastening it upon the cannon of another limb, and the animal chloroformed. A practical point to be remembered in this connection is that all necessary fixing of the limb is easier performed if the chloroform is administered first. With the patient thus secured we first of all ascertain by means of the probe whether or no the non-healing of the wound is due to the presence of a fistula. Decided in the negative, we take an ordinary flat firing-iron, and with it cut away a portion of the skin immediately around the still open wound, carrying our incisions deep enough to 'scoop' out a large portion of the new inflammatory tissue beneath. With the loss of pressure from beneath, occasioned by the removal of so much of the cicatricial tissue, the epidermis the more readily closes over the wound. To a large extent also this new growth of epidermis is helped by the renewal of the inflammatory phenomena brought into being with the cauterization.

2. SUB-HORNY QUITTOR.

Definition.—A fistulous wound of the foot in which the lower and blind end of the fistula is situated below the level of the coronary margin of the wall.

Causes.—These, again, will be practically the same as those mentioned in the cause of cutaneous quittor—namely, bruises, punctures, wounds—in fact, any injury upon the coronet severe enough to cause death of tissue and a suppurating wound. We may thus expect sub-horny quittor to follow upon treads, overreach, accidental injuries with the stable-fork, and kicks from other animals.

Sub-horny quittor may also arise without original injury at all to the coronet. Either from a violent blow upon the hoof, or from the animal himself kicking violently against a wall, death of a portion of the sensitive structures takes place within the hoof, suppuration ensues, and the formation of quittor commences. With the escape of the pus at the coronet the quittor is fully formed.

Any other diseased condition of the foot in which suppuration is present may in like manner terminate in quittor. In complicated sand-crack, suppurating corn, or in ordinary pricked foot quittor may be a sequel. In these conditions the pus formation either goes unnoticed or is neglected, and after seriously invading the sensitive structures within the hoof, breaks out at the coronet. Again, too, as with the simpler form of quittor, and as with coronitis, we may always regard as a predisposing cause the action of excessive cold in promoting septic infection of the wound when occurring at the coronet.

Symptoms and Diagnosis.—Where the fistulous wound has had its starting-point in an injury to the coronet diagnosis is, of course, easy. The history of the case explains it. Nothing in this instance remains but to probe the opening, and ascertain its direction, depth, and extent.

An animal with the wound thus open at the coronet, and freely discharging its contents, may, if no serious complications exist, walk tolerably sound. It is only when put to the trot that symptoms of lameness are apparent.

It may so happen, however, that we first see the case when the symptoms are wholly those arising from a painful suppuration within the horny box. This occurs when the original injury has taken place at a more dependent position than the coronet. Either from violent blows upon the hoof, puncture from below, from corn or from sand-crack, or any other causes we have enumerated, suppuration is occurring deeply within the hoof, with as yet no opening upon the coronet.

Even when an opening has already occurred on the coronet, the same condition of sub-horny suppuration may be met with in cases when the opening of the fistula has by some means or other become occluded. Granulation tissue, for instance, may have temporarily closed the mouth of the fistula. The pus, instead of continuing its discharge thereat, is made to burrow in other directions.

In either of these cases pain is excessive, the animal walks on three legs, the foot is painful to percussion, and grave constitutional disturbance is noticeable. The presence of pus is immediately suspected, and, in the absence of any indication of an opening having existed at the coronet, searched for at the sole. It may or may not be found. If found it is given exit, and the case ends as one of ordinary pricked foot, of suppurating corn, or some other condition equally simple when compared with quittor. In those cases where the pus is not discovered at the sole, one adopts the expectant treatment of poulticing. This, if pus is present, is followed by a painful swelling of the coronet. At one point there forms a hot and tender enlargement, with the hairs on it standing straight up from the skin, which latter is seen below red and inflamed in appearance.

Later, the abscess—for abscess it is—discharges its contents, the opening is explored, and we find that in extent it is not confined to the coronary region, but that it is deep enough to constitute a true sub-horny quittor.

This discharge of the abscess contents may take place at a well-defined spot on the coronet, or it may ooze out at the junction of the wall with the skin. In appearance the discharged pus varies. When the softer structures only are attacked it is thick, and yellow or white in colour; when bone is involved it is ichorous; and when attacking the horn itself black or gray. It may or may not be extremely foetid, and often it is mingled with blood.

When evidence of a previous opening upon the coronet is plain, then it is not considered wise to attempt a paring of the sole. Instead, poulticing is at once resorted to, to induce the discharge of the pus through its original channel. Once this has occurred a fistulous wound remains, which is open for treatment upon one or other of the lines we shall afterwards indicate.

COMPLICATIONS—*(a) Necrosis of the Lateral Cartilage.*—This is the so-called 'cartilaginous quittor' of other writers. In all probability it is the condition generally understood when the word 'quittor' is used by one practitioner to the other. Its tendency to keep the disease existing in a chronic form renders it of grave importance, and for that reason we give it first mention among the complications.

It may occur as a sequel either of cutaneous or of sub-horny quittor, and may result either from actual wounding and infection of the cartilage, or from an attack on it of septic matter originating elsewhere.

Unless there has been discovered a fistula, which on probing is seen to lead direct to the position in which we know the cartilage to be, we know of no precise means by which the existence of this condition may be diagnosed. When free from other complications, the horse with his foot in this state may travel fairly sound. This is so when the necrosis is situate in the posterior half of the cartilage, in which case the irritation set up by the disease is confined to the comparatively non-sensitive tissues of the cartilage itself and the fibrous mass of the plantar cushion. When attacking the anterior half of the cartilage, the close contiguity of the joint renders the disease of a more serious nature. It is then that we have acute pain, and with it extreme lameness, for in this position it is more than likely that we have involved either the synovial membrane of the articulation or the tops of the sensitive laminæ. It will be remembered that here the synovial membrane protrudes as a small sac between the antero- and postero-lateral ligaments of the joint. More or less easily then it is bound to come into intimate contact with the septic matter attending the necrosis of the cartilage, and so share in the inflammatory processes, afterwards communicating them to the interior of the articulation.

With necrosis of the lateral cartilage is always swelling and thickening of the skin and subcutaneous structures of the coronet. This is the greater the longer the disease has been in existence. Upon the swelling is seen the mouth of the fistula, or it may be the mouths of several, and from them all a discharge of pus.

The mouth of each fistula is generally filled with a mulberry-like granulation tissue, standing above the level of the skin, and bleeding easily if touched. The exuding pus is thin and pale gray in appearance, gritty to the touch, and generally free from pronounced smell. At other times its colour is reddened with contained blood, and floating in it are tiny particles of a pale-green substance, which when picked up and rubbed between the fingers are seen to be small fragments of the diseased cartilage.

Should the mouth of a fistula become occluded with the granulations filling it, and the discharge prevented from escaping, it soon happens that we have close to the fistula that has closed a tender fluctuating swelling. This points and breaks, and pus is again discharged from another opening. In this manner is accounted for the multiplicity of scars and fistulas seen on the swelling of an old-standing quittor.

The continued, inflammation thus kept in existence has the effect of rendering the skin and subcutaneous tissues in the neighbourhood greatly thickened and indurated. This in time leads to a tumour-like enlargement, and causes the structures of the coronet to greatly overhang the hoof. At the same time the constant inflammation has made its stimulant effects noted in a great increase in the growth of the horn of the wall.

Although more abundant, however, the quality of the horn is deteriorated. The perioplic ring has become obliterated, and the varnish-like appearance of the healthy wall destroyed. Cracks and fissures in its surface are numerous, and sometimes deep enough to lead to exposure of the sensitive structures beneath, complicating the quittor with a sand-crack of a peculiarly objectionable type.

Pathological Anatomy of the Diseased Cartilage.—The bulk of observers appear to agree in the statement that in quittor the necrotic cartilage is pea-green in colour, and recognise it by that characteristic. In size the necrotic portion thus recognisable varies from the tiniest speck to a portion the size of a horse-bean. Commonly, however, it is about as large only as a pea. It is seen to be more or less detached from the rest of the cartilage, to which it is adherent by one of its extremities only. In general appearance we can best liken it to the split half of a green pea, whilst others have compared it with the green sprouting of a seed. The portions of cartilage nearest the necrotic piece are also slightly green in colour, thus indicating that here also the diseased process has commenced. This peculiar change of colour in the affected cartilage is of great importance to the surgeon. It enables him when operating to distinguish with some degree of certainty those portions of the cartilage which are healthy and those which are not.

(*b*) *Necrosis of Tendon and of Ligament.*—This complication of quittor is, as we have said before, treated by other writers as a distinct form of the disease, and described by them under the heading of Tendinous Quittor.

This simply means, of course, that the diseased process has extended to either of the flexor tendons, to the tendon of the extensor pedis, or, perhaps, to the ligaments of the pedal articulation.

Of the flexor tendons, the perforans is the one commonly attacked, by reason, of course, of its more superficial position. At times, however, especially when its aponeurotic expansion is diseased, the necrosis of the perforans spreads until the aponeurosis is eaten through and the phalangeal sheath penetrated. Septic materials gain entrance thereto, and commence to multiply. In this way the flexor perforatus is invaded, and comes to share in the diseased process.

The extensor pedis is usually attacked by extension of the disease from a necrotic cartilage, or results from the infliction of a severe tread in a hind-foot. In this case the diseased structure has nothing between it and the articulation, the synovial membrane in one position actually lining its inner face. The result is that a condition of synovitis is easily set up, and the case aggravated by that and by arthritis.

With the flexor tendons attacked pain is always very great, and lameness is excessive. This, however, is not sufficiently characteristic to enable us to determine the precise seat of the necrotic changes. Later, however, a tender but hard enlargement made its appearance in the hollow of the heel, which enlargement, later still, became soft and fluctuating. At this stage there is also considerable swelling along the whole course of the tendons, as high up as the knee or the hock. The foot is carried forward with all the phalangeal articulations flexed, and in many cases the limb is unable to take weight at all. Manipulated after the manner of examining the tendons for sprain, this swelling is found to be extremely painful. The animal flinches from the hand, and shows every sign of acute suffering. This condition may, in fact, be mistaken for sprain, and is only to be distinguished from it by carefully noting the history of the case—first, the appearance of the swelling in the hollow of the heel, and, secondly, the *after*-swelling of the upper portions of the tendons.

The formation of the abscess, the after-discharge of its contents, and the final establishing of a fistula, are processes greatly prolonged in this form of quittor. It will readily be understood why this should be so when one remembers the depth at which the suppurative process is going on, the thickness of the metacarpo-phalangeal sheath, and the resistant nature of the material of which this latter is made, and which must be penetrated before the condition becomes observable.

After the opening of the abscess, which usually takes place in the hollow of the heel, there is left the fistulous wound which obstinately refuses to heal. Or it may be, again, that there are several of these fistulas, each opening in the heel, and the mouth of each marked by a small, ulcer-like projection. The discharge continually oozing from these keeps the heel constantly wet with a thick purulent discharge, which is nearly always blood-stained, and very often foetid.

This constitutes what is known as tendinous quittor in its worst form, for more often than not there is associated with it inflammation of the navicular bursa, caries of the bones, or arthritis of the pedal articulation.

With the extensor pedis attacked matters are not quite so grave, in spite of the fact that the articulation is closely situated thereto, for in this case the more superficial position of the diseased structure allows both of readier exit of the discharges and of easier removal of the necrosed portion and after-treatment of the wound.

(c) Caries of the Bones.—Portions of the os pedis, more especially of its wings, and therefore usually occurring in conjunction with necrosed cartilage, become carious in quittor. In many cases it is impossible to say with certainty when this has occurred. In a few instances, however, the exuding discharge gives evidence of what has happened. It is thin, but extremely offensive, with the characteristic odour of decayed bone or tooth, and with a feel that is gritty with contained particles of broken-up bone. If, with a discharge of this nature present, the probe also conveys to the fingers the sensation that bone is reached, then diagnosis may be sure.

(d) Ossification of the Cartilage.—This may take place in part or in whole. It, of course, constitutes Side-bone, a fuller description of which will be found in a later portion of this chapter.

(e) Penetration of the Articulation.—This may occur either as a result of the suppurative changes or as an accident in excision of the diseased cartilage. Unless it is followed by a severe purulent arthritis, it is not so grave a complication as at first sight it would appear.

(f) Synovitis and Arthritis (Purulent).—Should this complication arise, the case is a most serious one. Beyond here mentioning the fact that it may occur, we shall not dwell on it. Fuller consideration is given to it in Chapter XII.

Treatment.—The various treatments adopted for the cure of sub-horny quittor offer the veterinary surgeon a large number to select from. We will describe them in the order in which they are, perhaps, most commonly practised.

Poultices and Hot Baths.—As in cutaneous quittor, and as in coronitis, when the pus formation is only suspected, and has not yet broken out at the coronet or elsewhere, then the first indication in treatment is the use of warm poultices or of hot baths. Their application is in most cases productive of pointing at the coronet.

Directly this appears it is a wise plan to thin the wall down with the rasp immediately below the swelling. To some extent it relieves the pressure of the inflammatory products within, and at the same time paves the way for operative measures which may be necessary later on.

With the breaking of the abscess and the discharging of its contents, we may in some measure ascertain the condition we have to deal with. The probe is used, and the abscess cavity explored. The size of the wound, its depth below the upper margin of the wall, the structures involved, and other information, may be thus obtained.

At first, however, the nature of the wound, and the character of the discharges, must largely guide us as to the treatment we adopt. In many cases, even where the abscess cavity is far below the upper margin of the wall, and is presumably in an unfit position to drain and heal, a a regular application of an astringent and antiseptic dressing is sufficient to bring about resolution. If, however, the discharge from the wound continues to be liquid, and the wound itself at one spot refuses to heal, it may be judged that a portion of necrotic tissue is situated under the wall, and affecting the laminæ, the cartilage, or ligament, as the case may be. If this is so, then operative measures must be determined on (see Removal of the Wall, p. 349).

Blisters.—Instead of the poultice and hot baths, the pointing of the abscess and the casting off of the slough may be brought about by the application of a sharp cantharides blister. We have, in fact, seen many cases where this treatment was adopted prior to the formation of a fistula, and also in cases where one or more fistulous openings already existed, where repeated blisters to the coronet have alone been sufficient to effect a cure.

We are bound to admit, however, that the treatments of poulticing and blistering are only expectant—we might almost say empirical. At any rate, we admit to ourselves that what we have advised and carried out is not in itself curative, but only a means of assisting Nature to satisfactorily work her own ends. Empirical or not, however, we believe that in every case of quittor it is wise in practice to at first adopt some such simple measure, for in nearly every instance where operative measures are practised, the patient must be laid aside for at least several weeks, whereas in this way he may be kept at work and a cure effected at the same time.

The Actual Cautery.—Largely of the same empirical nature, yet doing something a little more calculated to destroy necrotic tissue and bring about its sloughing is the use of the cautery, both actual and potential.

The actual cautery may be beneficially employed for the relief of sub-horny quittor in at least two ways.

In the first place, it is often used—a blunt 'point-firing' iron being the instrument—instead of the knife as a means of evacuating the contents of the coronary abscess. Those who use it for this purpose are able to say this in its favour: it brings about the opening of the abscess without the unsightly hæmorrhage attending the use of the knife, and at the same time just as effectually empties it. The opening made is not nearly so likely to close prematurely—that is, before a proper course of treatment of the wound has been carried out—and so leave necrotic tissue at its bottom. The intense tissue reaction it sets up is productive of a large slough, cast off by highly active inflammatory phenomena, which means that the remaining wound is one in which no dead tissue is left, and which is more amenable to treatment.

We have also seen the actual cautery used in sub-horny quittor, where that disease has reached a chronic fistulous stage, as a means of cauterizing the whole length of the lining of each fistulous passage.

At the present day this method is regarded as barbarous, and savouring too largely of the methods and practice of the old empirics. There is no denying the fact, however, that it is at times followed by a speedy and complete cure of what has for months been an intractable and apparently incurable quittor; and, honestly speaking, we ourselves can see nothing very greatly against the operation in certain cases save its appearance. In that it is certainly rough, and is not calculated to favourably impress the more critical of our clientele.

With the animal chloroformed, however, much of what can really be urged against it disappears, and on farms and other places where a skilled and competent dressing of an operation wound cannot be looked for, it is sometimes wise to advise this method of treatment in preference to more advanced methods of operating. So far as we can judge, the after-effects are very little worse than those following other operative measures, more especially when a suitable case has been chosen.

This method of treatment is particularly applicable to cases of chronic sub-horny quittor in the more posterior parts of the foot. Here, if one or more fistulas exist, their openings are probed and the direction of the sinuses determined. In all probability they are burrowing down along-side the wall to the sole, where, for want of outlet, they are invading the substance of the plantar cushion or the plantar aponeurosis.

Should this preliminary probing demonstrate that neither of the fistulas run dangerously near the joint, then the operation may be decided on.

The animal is cast and chloroformed, the foot firmly fixed, and the horn of the quarter rasped away quite thin. The sole of the same side is also pared with the knife until the horn of both the quarter and the sole yields easily to pressure of the thumb. All that is then needed is three or four long, round, and pointed irons (about 1/4 to 3/8 inch in diameter) heated to redness. These are inserted into the fistulas, and the false mucous coat of these passages thus destroyed. When the iron, on being directed into the fistulous opening at the coronet, is found to travel alongside the wall, and to easily reach the sole, it should be made to go further still. The sole is penetrated, and a dependent opening thus made for the escape of the discharge that afterwards accumulates.

What happens now, of course, is that an intense and acute inflammation is set up along the whole track of the fistula, in which position the inflammatory changes were heretofore chronic. The whole lining of the fistula, and with it, we hope, all necrotic tissue, is cast as a slough, leaving nothing but healthy tissue behind. This, with a suitable dressing, heals and gives no further trouble.

The after-treatment consists in the application of hot poultices. These tend to greatly ease the pain, and at the same time to facilitate the removal of the slough. The poulticing should be continued, therefore, until the sloughing comes about, which happens, as a rule, at about the fifth or seventh day.

Immediately the slough is cast off, the poultices may be discontinued and dressing of the wound carried out. This consists of injections of solutions of zinc chloride 1 in 200, perchloride of mercury 1 in 1,000, carbolic acid 1 in 20, of Villate's solution, or of such other antiseptic as the surgeon may think fit. The dependent orifice at the sole should be kept open for as long as possible, being occasionally trimmed round with the drawing-knife, and scooped out with a sharp-edged director.

Directly a healthy and pink-looking granulation is observed along the track of the iron, and the discharge therefrom takes on a thick and yellow appearance, the strength of the antiseptic solutions should be gradually diminished. This point, in fact, is of great importance in treating all wounds of the foot. There is a great temptation, on account of the known excessive liability of the parts to septic infection, to use an antiseptic solution unduly strong. What must be remembered is that used *too* strong they themselves give rise to dead tissue, or to impermeable layers consisting of compounds of the discharges with themselves, and so create substances that prove a source of irritation and subsequent trouble.

The Potential Cautery.—This is employed in the treatment of sub-horny quittor, either in the solid form (in sticks, in lumps, or in the powder), or in the liquid form, when it is injected with a quittor syringe.

In the former method such drugs as perchloride of mercury in the lump, or nitrate of silver, chloride of zinc, and caustic potash or soda in the stick, are introduced into each of the sinuses present. This is done by means of a director or a probe.

A better method, however, when the dressing lends itself to the purpose, is to use it in the form of a powder, wrapped in the form of small cubes in extremely thin paper, such, for instance, as is used for rolling cigarettes. It is then conveniently inserted into each fistula. Introduced in this more finely divided form the drug is, perhaps, a little more active in bringing about the desired result.

146

This method of 'plugging,' although practised by many, we cannot recommend in preference to the use of the hot iron or of liquid injections. Our reasons are these: the action of the drug is a protracted one. Almost immediately after its introduction into the fistula there is formed about it an almost impermeable layer of a metallic albuminate, which effectively prevents further rapid action of the caustic. In addition to thus preventing further action of the dressing, this combination of the tissue albumin with the metal of the salt, together with much necrotic tissue that it has caused, is extremely hard to remove from the healthy tissues. This we explain by pointing out that the action of the caustic, prolonged as it is, sets up a tissue reaction which partakes largely of the type of a chronic rather than an acute inflammation. With a chronic inflammation there is sooner a tendency to the production of fibrous tissue (and thus the firmer attachment of the necrosed portions) rather than an active phagocytosis and the casting-off of a slough. Again, careful though we may be with the probe, it is extremely difficult to be certain that we have discovered the whole extent of any fistula. An equal difficulty, therefore, exists in being certain that we have placed the caustic in the position in which it is most wanted—namely, at the furthermost end of the fistula where the necrotic tissue is to be found.

When a caustic is used at all, it is far better to employ it in the liquid form, when either of the drugs we have just mentioned may again be used. In the first place, the liquid is far more likely to be brought into contact with the diseased structures than is the solid salt. Also, its action may be regulated by altering the strength of the solution, and the liability to form impermeable albuminates thus diminished.

Probably the best solution for use in this way is the old-fashioned Villate's solution (see p. 199).

This liquid should be injected at least every day, and, in a bad case, even two or three times daily. Practical hints to be borne in mind when attempting to cure quittor by means of injections are these:

If the fistulas are numerous, the fluid should be injected into their various orifices.

In order to force the fluid to the bottom of each diseased track, it is necessary, when injecting one opening, to firmly close all others.

Several injections should be made at each time of injection. In other words, we must not be content with just forcing fluid in. It must be forced in, and again forced out by a further syringeful. The fistulous tracks must, in fact, be washed in the liquid.

The effect of the injection during the first eight or ten days is to render suppuration more abundant and whiter. After two weeks of the treatment sloughing of the inside of the sinuses occurs, and healing of the wound commences. Signs that this is occurring are—slight hæmorrhage at the end of each injection, and a gradually increasing difficulty in forcing in the fluid.

The Making of Counter-openings to the Fistulas.—Although Villate's solution or any other caustic used in the manner we have described often effects a cure, many practitioners insist on the fact that a counter-opening to the fistula must also be made.

The probe is used and the direction and depth of the fistula ascertained. Through the wall is then made an opening at exactly opposite the lowest point found by the probe, or through the sole if the probe should there lead us. This opening is best made with a sharp-pointed iron, and may afterwards be kept large enough by an occasional trimming with the knife. Many of the older authors, and with them writers of the present day, declare that unless this is done the ordinary injection is likely to fail in a great many instances where it would otherwise have been successful.

Where a counter-opening is thus made it is found that it very readily closes with granulation tissue, and the purpose for which it was made defeated. This may be avoided by the use of a seton. In preference to the seton, however, we ourselves would advise that the opening be kept free by the occasional use of a sharp-edged director or a fine scalpel.

An interesting modification of the practice of making a counter-opening is that related by Veterinary-Captain S.M. Smith.[A] In point of severity it runs a middle course between the making of a simple counter-opening and the removal of a wedge-shaped portion of the coronary band and the wall, a method which we shall later describe.

[Footnote A: *Veterinary Record*, vol ii., p. 157.]

To perform this operation, the animal is cast and chloroformed. The foot is fixed and the parts thoroughly cleansed. The horn of the wall is then sawed through in a direct line from the coronary margin to the solar edge, the saw-line running exactly over the seat of the sinus.

A strong scalpel is now introduced at the coronary opening, with its cutting-edge outwards, and is gradually passed down the opening made by the saw. In this way the sinus is completely destroyed, and from end to end converted into an open wound. The parts are then washed in a perchloride of mercury solution, covered with a mixture of powdered iodoform and boracic acid, over which a pledget of carbolized tow is placed, and then a bandage over the whole. This dressing should be left on three or four days, after which the injury should be treated as an ordinary wound. In conclusion, the author says: 'I can safely recommend this line of treatment to any practitioner having an obstinate case under treatment.'

Removal of the Wall and Excision of the Necrotic Tissue.—This we may term the radical operation for sub-horny quittor, for it is often productive of a successful issue when all other means have failed. No matter in what position the sinus is, whether at the extreme anterior portion of the coronet, or whether in the region of the heels, it is to be thoroughly opened up. To do this, the fistula is carefully explored with the probe and a knowledge of its exact dimensions arrived at. This is carefully noted, and the horn of the wall for some little distance around it then rasped down quite thin. Immediately over the sinus, and for a short distance on either side of it, the horn is stripped away to the sensitive structures. The cavity of the fistula is then opened up with a scalpel, and every particle of diseased tissue removed with this instrument and a pair of forceps. After-dressing consists simply in the application of suitable antiseptics.

When the Complication of Necrosed Tendon or Ligament exists.—We may take it as an axiom that wherever this exists, whether it is in the extensor pedis, in the lateral ligaments of the joint, or in portions of the flexors, all diseased structures should, where possible, be removed. This is done either with a scalpel or with a curette.

When septic matter has gained the sheath of the perforans, and the formation of pus therein is indicated by inflammatory swellings in the hollow of the heel, it is sometimes advisable to lay the sheath open for 1 to 2 inches along the course of the tendons. This, if a fistula is present, may be best done with a blunt-pointed bistoury, or with a cannulated director and a scalpel. With the pus thus given exit, and an antiseptic dressing regularly applied, the case sometimes ends in rapid resolution. More often than not, however, it is found that the pus has been liberated too late, and that it has gravitated in the sheath to the extent of affecting the plantar aponeurosis. Or it may be, of course, that it was in the plantar aponeurosis the disease commenced. Whichever may have been the case, we have in the hollow of the heel one or more fistulous openings, or an opening we have made ourselves, leading down to a necrosed portion of the terminal expansion of the perforans.

In such cases we ourselves have derived benefit from a regular flushing of the sinuses with a 1 in 2,000 solution of perchloride of mercury, introduced by means of a glass syringe, followed later by flushing in the same manner with a 1 in 40 solution of carbolic acid, the hollow of the heel meanwhile being kept clean with an antiseptic pad and bandage, or by liberal applications of an antiseptic powder.

The septic materials are in this way destroyed, and the wound heals without further complication. We must admit, however, that the cure of the lesion is generally at the expense of slight lameness, due, in all probability, to inflammatory tissue adhesions between the flexor perforans and the perforatus, and to a partial destruction of the synovial membrane of the sheath.

If, in spite of the antiseptic irrigations, the fistula persists, then nothing remains but to resort to excision of the aponeurosis, as described on p. 222.

When Necrosis of the Lateral Cartilage is present.—In this case we may at first try the ordinary treatments of poulticing; and blistering, of antiseptic caustic injections, and of plugging. In some cases a cure is effected. Should these fail, however, and we intend to see the finish of our case, then operative measures must be determined on. This means cutting down upon the diseased cartilage, and either removing the necrosed portion, or excising the cartilage in its entirety.

The latter method is seldom practised in this country. As it is the most radical of the two, however, we shall describe it here first.

Extirpation of the Lateral Cartilage.—The operation of extirpating the lateral cartilage is by no means a new one, being introduced, according to Zundel, by the senior Lafosse in 1754. It consisted in removing a portion of the wall by grooving and stripping it, and of excising the exposed cartilage by means of a sage-knife.

As to what portion of, and how much of the horn of, the quarter should first be removed, and as to what particular direction each groove should take, opinion among the older writers varied considerably. This we know now is not an important matter, and it is sufficient to say that the first preliminary is a thinning down of the horn of the quarter with the rasp over the position occupied by the cartilage. At the present time there are two or three modifications of the operation as originally introduced. In all, however, the preliminary steps are the same. We shall therefore describe them collectively, as applying correctly to either of the three methods of operating we are about to show.

Preparation of the Subject and Preliminary Steps in the Operation.—On the day previous to the operation the horn of the wall immediately over the cartilage must be so thinned with a rasp as to yield readily to pressure of the thumb in any position. It should be so thin as to only just avoid wounding the sensitive structures below.

The whole of the foot must then be thoroughly cleansed, and rendered as nearly aseptic as possible. The use of warm water, soap, and a stiff brush is the readiest means of removing the surface dirt. Afterwards the foot should be soaked for some time in a reliable antiseptic solution, a 1 in 1,000 solution of perchloride of mercury being the most suitable. When removed from the solution the foot must be packed round with wool or tow impregnated with corrosive sublimate, and then bandaged, the whole afterwards wrapped in a thick cloth, or protected with a boot.

On the following day the animal is brought out and cast, and the foot desired to be operated on firmly secured, after the manner described on p. 81. The bandages and sublimate pads are then removed, and the skin of the coronet over the seat of operation shaved of hair. An Esmarch rubber bandage is next run up the limb, and the tourniquet applied, thus rendering the operation a nearly bloodless one.

This done, the animal is chloroformed, and an antiseptic douche played over the foot.

So far, the steps in the operation are common to all methods. There are now, however, three slightly differing modes of extirpating the cartilage, which modes vary simply according to the structures severed by the knife.

First Method.—This is the oldest method of the three, and consists in making (1) a horizontal incision through the sensitive laminæ along the lower border of the cartilage, and (2) a vertical incision through the skin of the coronet, the coronary cushion, and a portion of the sensitive laminæ (see Fig. 139).

The flaps (Fig. 139, *a, a*) are now held back by tenaculæ, and the whole of the cartilage, or only the necrosed portion, carefully excised by means of right- and left-handed sage-knives. Fistulous openings in either of the flaps *a, a* must now be carefully curetted and dressed, and the flaps allowed to fall into position. They are then sutured with carbolized gut, and the wound finally dressed as to be described later (p. 357).

FIG. 139.—EXCISION OF THE LATERAL CARTILAGE (OLD METHOD).
The wall covering the lateral cartilage first thinned and stripped off; the two flaps (*a, a*) of skin and the coronary cushion made by the vertical incision turned back. *a*, The operation flaps; *b*, the exposed cartilage; *c*, the sensitive laminæ; *d*, the coronary cushion.

Second Method (after Holler and Frick[A]*).*—These operators deem it wise to leave untouched the skin of the coronet and the coronary cushion. They therefore make their first incision along the lower border of the coronary cushion (see Fig. 140), afterwards exposing the lower half of the cartilage by removing a half-moon-shaped portion of the thinned horn and underlying sensitive laminæ (see Fig. 140, *b*).

[Footnote A: Two cases of quittor successfully treated by this method are reported by R. Paine, M.R.C.V.S., in the *Journal of Comparative Pathology and Therapeutics*, vol. xv., p. 81.]

FIG. 140.—EXCISION OF THE LATERAL CARTILAGE. (AFTER MOLLER AND FRICK.) *a*, The thinned horny wall covering the coronary cushion; *b*, the lateral cartilage exposed by stripping off the thinned wall; *c*, the sensitive laminæ.

This done, the external face of the cartilage is separated from the skin of the coronet. To do this a double sage-knife is run flatwise between the coronary cushion and the cartilage, with the convex surface of the blade towards the skin. The knife is then passed backwards and forwards until the necessary separation is accomplished. During these movements of the knife a finger of the unoccupied hand should follow the knife, and guard the coronary cushion against injury.

Following this, the inner surface of the cartilage must be also separated from the structures lying beneath it. To this end a sage-knife (right- or left-handed, according as to whether the anterior or posterior portion of the cartilage is to be first removed) is again passed into the incision. With the cutting-edge of the knife forward, it is gradually reached round and under the hindermost end of the cartilage, and the posterior half of the cartilage separated from underlying structures, and at the same time excised by one clean cut forwards. Using the second sage-knife in a similar manner, the cutting-edge this time backwards, it is reached in front of the cartilage, whose anterior half is then excised by a careful cut backwards. Any small portions of cartilage remaining after this are sought for with the finger, and carefully removed by means of a scalpel and a tenaculum.

The fistulous opening or openings in the skin of the coronet should now be thoroughly curetted, and the whole of the wound dressed as to be described later.

In removing the anterior half of the cartilage it is highly important to remember the close contiguity to it of the synovial membrane of the pedal articulation. This projects as a small sac between the antero- and postero-lateral ligaments of the joint. Risks of injury to it may be diminished by having the foot secured with a line, and pulled forward by an assistant while the cut is being made.

Third Method (after Bayer).—This operator recommends that, after stripping a half-moon-shaped piece of horn from the seat of operation, instead of raising the skin of the coronet and the attached coronary cushion in two flaps (as Fig. 139, a, a), that the cartilage be exposed by raising up one flap only (Fig. 141, a), consisting of a portion of the sensitive laminæ, the coronary cushion, and the skin and underlying structures of the coronet.

With the horse cast and the preliminary steps over, the thinned horn of the quarter is incised in a semicircular fashion, and the half-moon-shaped piece thus separated from its surroundings stripped off. At about 1/4 inch from the incision in the horn, a second incision of similar shape is made through the sensitive structures, which incision is also carried up into the skin and structures of the coronet. This incision severs, from bottom to the top, (1) the sensitive laminæ covering a portion of the pedal bone and a portion of the lateral cartilage, (2) the coronary cushion, and (3) the skin of the coronet and such structures as lie between it and the cartilage.

FIG. 141.—EXCISION OF THE LATERAL CARTILAGE. (AFTER BAYER.) The horny wall is stripped off over the seat of operation. *a*, Semicircular flap of sensitive laminæ, coronary cushion, and skin; *b*, the lateral cartilage; *c*, the sensitive laminæ; *d*, the coronary cushion.

That this incision of the sensitive structures should be kept at 1/4 inch from the one in the horn has a reason. It is that when this flap is again placed into position (as later it will have to be) we have round its circumference a rim of soft structures into which to place the sutures. And in this connection it is well to advise the operator that the thinness of the keratogenous membrane (the laminal portion of it) should warn him that the portion of it to be turned up—namely, that forming the tip of the flap—should be *scraped* away quite close to the os pedis. Unless this is done, there will not be a sufficient thickness left to afterwards bring into position and suture.

The half-moon-shaped piece of tissue incised is now carefully dissected away from the external face of the cartilage, until it may be turned up as a flap (see Fig. 141, *a*), and held from off the cartilage by a tenaculum.

The exposed cartilage is now carefully removed by the aid of a sage-knife and a stout pair of forceps, the same precaution of holding the foot well forward being again taken in order to avoid wounding of the articular capsule.

At this stage in the operation considerable care is required. The operator must remember that close beneath him, and more particularly in front, is the pedal articulation. It is better, therefore, to excise the cartilage piecemeal, and to do it carefully, than to attempt, at the risk of injury to the joint, to make the operation 'showy.'

During removal of the cartilage, the terminal branches of the digital arteries are wounded, as also are the veins of the coronary plexus. Should either of these stand out with extra prominence from the others, it should be picked up with a pair of forceps, and ligatured with either carbolized gut or silk.

Attention should then be given to the flap of skin and coronary cushion. Wherever a sinus has existed in it, it is to be carefully scraped, and all dead portions of tissue removed. This done, the flap is allowed to fall into position, and is there carefully sutured, not only at the skin of the coronet, but along the whole circumference of the incision.

Dressing of the Wound and After-Treatment.—The whole secret of the success of this operation is in afterwards maintaining a strict asepsis of the wound. Unless there is reasonable room for belief that this may be done, the operation had far better not be advised, for if the wound is afterwards suffered to get into a suppurating and dirty condition, the last stage of the case may be worse than the first Synovitis and arthritis, with certain anchylosis of the joint, and a probable loss of our patient, is almost bound to follow.

We cannot, therefore, too strongly insist upon the advice that the whole of the preliminary antisepticising of the foot that we have described, and the after maintaining of asepsis that we are now about to relate, *must* be methodically and thoroughly carried out. It is of even *more* importance than little details in the operation itself.

In the first and second methods of operating, directly the actual operation is over, the surface of the wound and both surfaces of the skin-flaps should first be thoroughly douched with a 1 in 1,000 solution of perchloride of mercury. Bayer prefers a 1 in 5 solution of iodoform in ether.

Next, either iodoform or chinosol in the powder should be dusted over the whole surface, including again both inner and outer faces of the reverted skin-flaps. This done the flaps are allowed to fall into position and sutured there with carbolized silk or gut.

Another liberal application of an antiseptic dressing follows this. Iodoform, iodoform and boracic acid, or chinosol, is freely dusted over the wound and for some distance around it. Bayer, however, again prefers a dressing of the wound, and especially the moistening of the line of sutures with the 1 in 5 solution of iodoform in ether.

Over the wound is then placed a protective layer of gauze, impregnated either with boric acid, with a mercuric salt, or with iodoform.

Finally, numerous small and lightly-rolled balls of dry carbolized tow are packed regularly over the whole of the operation wound, and the foot bandaged.

Practical points to be remembered in this after-dressing are: (1) The balls[A] of tow should be numerous enough to exercise pressure upon the sutured flap when the foot is finally bandaged. (2) The bandage should be run on from the coronet downwards, in order to insure pressure being exerted in the exact position over the sutured flap. (3) Bandages should be used in abundance, commencing always from the coronet, and carefully applied so as to exert an even and uniform pressure. (4) The bandages should be of clean, unused linen.

[Footnote A: Bayer recommends that the tow be rolled into cylindrical tampons, each long enough to cross the wound. These are placed on the wound in alternate horizontal and vertical layers, so that when rolled round by a bandage they are pressed into an even and compact pad.]

Once the bandages are adjusted, the hobbles may be removed, and the tourniquet loosened. Directly the tourniquet is removed there is a steady oozing of blood through the bandages, no matter how many we have put on. This should occasion no alarm, as experience has taught that the careful attention to antiseptic measures observed throughout the operation has the effect of maintaining the lowermost dressings, those next to the wound, in a state of asepsis. The bandaged foot should now be wrapped in a piece of thick clean cloth or placed in a boot.

If our antiseptic precautions have been thorough, the dressings and bandages so adjusted may be allowed to remain without disturbance for from eight to fourteen days. In this, however, the veterinary surgeon must be largely guided by the symptoms of his patient. If, at the end of the first three or four days, the animal maintains a vigorous appetite, if he commences to place a little weight on the foot, and if the thermometer gives no indication of a rise beyond the one or two degrees of ordinary surgical fever, then the surgeon may know that things are proceeding satisfactorily. Pawing movements with the foot, inability to place weight upon it, loss of appetite, an increase in the number of respirations, and a serious rise of temperature, denote the opposite state of affairs. The wound is in all probability suppurating. The bandages and dressings should therefore be removed, and the wound either redressed and bandaged, or treated as an ordinary open wound.

Ordinarily, however, if the operation has been properly performed, healing takes place by first intention, and the wound when the bandages are removed at the end of the first or second week appears clean and *dry*.

Having assured ourselves that such is the case, we dress the foot in exactly the same manner as before, save that so many bandages are not put on. A similar dressing is repeated weekly until such time as the wound shows sufficient growth of horn—quite a thin pellicle—to act as a protective. It may then be left undressed, except for some simple hoof dressing and a bandage.

Complete healing of the wound takes from about four to eight weeks, at the end of which time the animal can be again gradually put into work. The labour, however, should be light, and quite three or four months should be allowed to elapse before any attempt is made to put him to heavy work.

Should the second method of operating have been the one adopted, then there is one slight difference in the after-dressing that needs attention calling to it. In this case we have more or less of a *hidden* cavity left to deal with rather than the broad and *open* wound left in either of the other methods. This cavity, left by the extirpation of the cartilage, must be thoroughly dressed with iodoform or chinosol, or with Bayer's iodoform in ether. The packing with carbolized tow and the bandaging may then be proceeded with as before.

In conclusion, we may say that the operation is one of some delicacy, and needs a good surgeon for its successful performance. Furthermore, no one of the antiseptic precautions we have advised can be omitted. It is, perhaps, these two considerations (and in justice to the English surgeon we should say most probably the latter of them) that have prevented this operation from being generally adopted.

That it is successful there is no gainsaying. Professor Bayer, of the Vienna School, with whose name is associated the last of the three methods of operating we have described, is enthusiastic in praise of the operation, and says: 'The favourable results that I have got by this operation have caused me wholly to abandon the medicinal treatment, and to prefer in all cases the surgical operation as being the best means to the end.'

Partial Excision of the Lateral Cartilage.—Discarding the somewhat elaborate methods we have just described, there are English operators who removed the necrosed portion only

152

of the cartilage, and do so in what appears at first sight a comparatively rough-and-ready manner.

The apparent roughness is that they do not concern themselves with conserving the coronary cushion, and hesitate but little in cutting portions of it bodily away. One would imagine that in this case the quarter of the side operated on would be always more or less bare of horn. Such, however, is not the case.

To perform this operation the animal is again cast and chloroformed. Some operators, however, use the stocks and dispense with the anæsthetic. The foot is first well cleaned with soap and water and a stiff brush, and the hair of the coronet over the seat of operation shaved. Again, too, the horn of the affected quarter is rasped until it yields easily to pressure of the thumb, and the whole of the foot washed in an antiseptic solution.

A probe is now inserted into the opening at the coronet, and the direction of the fistula noted, after which the foot is firmly secured, and an Esmarch bandage and tourniquet applied to the limb.

This done, a triangular or wedge-shaped portion of skin, coronary cushion, and thinned horn is removed with a strong sage-knife or scalpel.

The base of the wedge-shaped portion removed contains the opening of the fistula, and the apex of the wedge should reach to the bottom of the sinus (see Fig. 142).

After the horn is removed and the fistula followed up, it is sometimes found that what we at first thought was its end, it may now be continued in an altogether different direction.

It is again followed up with the probe, and the horn and sensitive structures excised until we are quite certain we have reached its furthest extent.

Attention should next be paid to the cartilage. Wherever spots of necrosis are found, as indicated by the pea-green colour of the affected parts, they must be *carefully* excised. Care should be taken in so doing to carry the line of excision some little distance around the visibly affected parts. This is done that we may be quite certain nothing at all remains calculated to give rise to further trouble.

It goes without saying that, in addition to the necrosed cartilage, all other diseased and necrotic tissues should also be removed. The os pedis is occasionally found necrotic just where the cartilage joins it, or it may be that a small portion of the sensitive laminæ, by reason of its *liver-red* or even gray coloration, gives evidence of death of the part.

The former must be well curetted, and the latter cleaned carefully with a scalpel and forceps.

FIG. 142.—PARTIAL EXCISION OF THE LATERAL CARTILAGE BY REMOVING A PORTION OF THE CORONARY CUSHION. The dotted lines show the outline of the wedge-shaped portion of structures to be removed, including skin, coronary cushion, horn, and sensitive laminæ. *a*, The opening of the fistula.

The operation finished, the foot is again douched in an antiseptic solution, the wound mopped dry with carbolized tow, dressed with either of the dressings described on page 358, and finally bandaged. The dressing should be changed every three days only, unless in the meanwhile pawing movements and other symptoms of distress indicate their removal.

The length of coronary cushion removed in this operation is from 1/4 to 1/2 inch (we ourselves, however, have seen it more), and yet its loss seems to occasion no serious after-trouble beyond a slight deformity of the parts beneath. The sensitive structures become sufficiently covered with horn, and the animal in nearly every case is returned to work, while in a great many instances he may also trot perfectly sound.

Simple though the operation may appear, and apparently rough in its method, it is nevertheless successful in effecting a cure in cases where blisters, plugging, injections, and other means have failed.

Mr. W. Dacre, M.R.C.V.S.,[A] after reading an article on the operation before the members of the Lancashire Veterinary Medical Association, says: 'My observations have not been based on a single case, and having had nine of them, and all of them successful, I felt it to be my duty to bring this subject before the Society.'

[Footnote A: *Veterinary Record*, vol. v., p. 407.]

Mr. T.W. Thompson, M.R.C.V.S.,[A] says: 'In a great number of cases I have removed a 1/2 inch of the coronary band.... I have performed the operation a great number of times, and have never seen a foot that has been damaged by it.'

[Footnote A: *Ibid.*]

Professor Macqueen[A] says: 'I do not spare the coronary band or sensitive laminæ when I find those parts diseased. I do not unnecessarily damage those structures. At the same time, I am confident that excision of a piece of the coronary band or removal of a few sensitive laminæ has not the untoward consequences so much dreaded in former days.'

[Footnote A: *Ibid.*, p. 714.]

Mr. John Davidson, M.E.C.V.S.,[A] says: 'The treatment described, if carefully carried out and details attended to, will be found a success in dealing with the majority of cases of quittor. If I may be permitted to say so, without being considered boastful, I have yet to see the first case that has resisted the treatment.'

[Footnote A: *Ibid.*, vol. xiv., p. 769.]

Should our case of quittor be complicated by caries of the bone, this must, where possible, be scraped or curetted until the whole of the diseased portion is removed, and a healthy surface is left. After-dressing must then be carried out as in other cases.

The treatment of ossified cartilage will be found under treatment of side-bones, and the methods of dealing with penetrated articulation and purulent arthritis are treated of in Chapter XII.

Surgical Shoeing in Quittor.—In the case of simple or cutaneous quittor, no alteration in the shoeing is necessary.

When the condition becomes sub-horny, however, and particularly when it is situated in the region of the quarters, ease is afforded to the diseased parts by removing the bearing of the shoe in that position.

Should there be no dependent opening at the sole, then the best shoe for the purpose is an ordinary bar shoe (Fig. 68), with the bearing eased under the affected quarter.

If, however, there is a dependent orifice, or one is expected, then it will be necessary either to leave the animal unshod or to provide him with a shoe that admits of dressing the lesion. In the latter case the most suitable shoe will be found to be either a three-quarter shoe (Fig. 102) or a three-quarter bar shoe (Fig. 103). Many operators, however, keep the animal unshod. We must say ourselves that we consider a shoe useful after either of the operations for removal of the cartilage, if only to assist in maintaining the bandages and dressings in position.

In this case a very useful shoe will be the three-quarter bar shoe. With a little manipulation the bandages are easily run under the bar portion of the shoe, and a few of their turns every now and again wrapped round the bar in order to keep the whole firmly in position.

In connection with tendinous quittor, when septic matter has gained the sheath of the flexor tendons, there is, for a long time after healing of the fistula, a marked tendency for the animal to go on his toe. To a large extent we judge this to be due to slight adhesions between the two tendons brought about by the growth of inflammatory fibrous tissue. In such cases benefit is sometimes derived from the application of a shoe with an extended toe-piece (see Figs. 84 and 108).

C. OSSIFICATION OF THE LATERAL CARTILAGES, OR SIDE-BONES.

Definition.—An abnormal condition of the lateral cartilages, in which the substance of the cartilage becomes gradually removed and bone formed in its place.

FIG. 143.—OSSIFIED LATERAL CARTILAGES (SIDE-BONES).

Symptoms and Diagnosis.—Side-bones are nearly always met with in heavy draught animals, and are rarely seen in the feet of nags. They are, moreover, nearly always confined to the fore-feet. In the ordinary way little need be said concerning their characteristics, and the way in which they may be detected. Neither need any concern be ordinarily manifested with regard to the effect they may have on the animal's gait and future usefulness. Seeing, however, that side-bone constitutes one of the recognised hereditary diseases, and that at the various agricultural and horse shows its existence or otherwise in a certain animal is a matter of great importance, some little attention must be given to these two points.

With a side-bone anywhere approaching full development, diagnosis is easy. The thumb is pressed into the coronet over the seat of the cartilage, when, in place of the elasticity we should normally meet with, we have the solid resistance offered by bone. In some instances diagnosis is even easier still. We refer to those cases in which the side-bone stands above the level of the coronet with such prominence as to be readily *seen* and recognised without manipulation, and where its growth has caused distinct enlargement and bulging of the wall of the affected quarter. It seems that in such cases the bone-forming process does not end with simply depositing bone in place of the removed cartilage, but that, after that is accomplished, the bone still continues to be produced, as in the case of an exostosis elsewhere.

Although diagnosis in cases such as these is easy, it becomes a very different matter when we are called upon to give an opinion in cases where ossification of the cartilage is only just commencing. Whether the result of our examination is to decide the sale or purchase of an animal, to determine his fitness or otherwise to enter the show-ring, or to merely advise a client as to whether or no a side-bone is in course of formation, our position is equally difficult, and in either case our examination must be searching.

Perhaps the best advice we can give is to say that the whole of the cartilage must be manipulated both with the foot *on* and *off* the ground. What the reason may be we do not pretend to say, but it is a well-known fact that in many instances the cartilage, with the foot bearing weight, is so rigid as to at once convey the impression that ossification has commenced or is even far advanced. And yet that same cartilage, with the foot removed from the ground, is as pleasantly yielding to pressure of the thumb as the most exacting of us could wish for. In any case, then, where doubt exists, the foot should be lifted to the knee, and the cartilage carefully examined with the foot in that position. If, then, at any spot above the normal contour of the os pedis we meet with hardness or rigidity, we are to look upon that foot with suspicion. Nevertheless, providing our conscience is sufficiently elastic, the animal may be passed *sound* so far as the *existence* of a side-bone is concerned. We know, however, that with commencing rigidity we may ere long expect one, and if our opinion is asked with regard to that particular, it must be admitted that with rigidity of the cartilage once commenced it is usually not long afterwards before a fully-developed side-bone makes its appearance.

As is only to be expected, the first noticeable hardening of the cartilage is to be found near the normal bone. We may thus look for it more particularly in the lower portions of the cartilage. We think we may say, too, that in the vast majority of cases the ossification of the cartilage commences in its anterior half. It is thus brought about that often we are called upon to examine and report on the condition when we have *anteriorly* a side-bone in course of formation, and *posteriorly* a perfectly normal cartilage. It is to the latter half of the cartilage that dealers and others mainly, if not wholly, devote their attention. A horse with the cartilage in this transition state will therefore pass muster, and a nice little point of ethics has again to be decided by the veterinary surgeon before giving his signature to a certificate of examination of an animal in this condition.

With regard to alteration in gait, we may say at once that side-bones in heavy animals are not often the cause of lameness. In fact, where the foot is well developed, when neither the foot as a whole nor the phalangeal bones give evidence of disease, and where the pasterns are fairly oblique and well formed, this alteration of the cartilages may be looked upon as of no serious import at all. Neither is the side-bone due to blows or other injuries likely to be productive of lameness—that is, always supposing, of course, that the foot in other respects is of good shape. If lameness is met with at all, then it is where we have a foot that is in other respects unsound, with badly contracted heels and upright 'stumpy' hoof, or where side-bones have occurred in a young animal, and have already reached a large size before the horse is put to labour. In this latter case, the added effects of concussion and the evil influences of shoeing are sufficient to turn the scale. Directly the animal, previously sound, is asked to work, lameness is the result.

It follows, therefore, that side-bone in the feet of young animals is of far more serious import than when occurring in older horses. In a nag animal they constitute a positive unsoundness, and lameness in this case is more often than not an accompanying symptom.

Causes.—To commence with, we may remark that, although met with sometimes in very early life, side-bones are seldom, if ever, congenital, and that more often than not they may be looked for in animals of three years old, or older, seldom earlier. They appear, in fact, only when the animal is shod and commences work.

This at once suggests two of the principal factors in their causation—namely, concussion and loss of normal function. Directly the horse is put to work he has for a great part of his time to travel upon roadways—either macadamized roads or town sets—where everything is calculated to bring concussion about. In addition to that he has the lateral cartilage itself thrown largely out of action by shoeing. We explained in Chapter III. (p. 66) that the chief function of the cartilage was to take concussion received by the plantar cushion and direct the greater part of it outwards and backwards. Now, with the animal shod, the plantar cushion does not itself, as normally it should, receive concussion. By the shoeing the frog is lifted from the ground, and the plantar cushion, together with the cartilage, taken largely out of active work. In other words, the normal outward and inward movements of the cartilage are enormously reduced.

It is fair, we think, to take it that the mere fact of the lateral cartilage persisting *as* cartilage is due in large measure to its constant movement. Directly, therefore, it is placed in a state of comparative idleness, then it commences to ossify, more particularly if there should at the same time be a tendency to a low type of inflammation of the parts.

Does this latter exist? We may safely say that it does. It is in this way: The secondary effect of loss of ground-pressure upon the frog and plantar cushion is to bring about contraction of the heels. With this we get compression of the parts within, with a certain amount of irritation and the exact low type of inflammatory phenomena calculated to assist in the bone-forming process.

The fact that concussion acts as a cause explains in great measure how it is that side-bones are more frequent in cart animals than in nags, and also why they should be more common in the fore-feet than in the hind. Taking, in both animals, a rough calculation as to the weight of body carried by feet of a certain size, we notice at once that the cart animal has proportionately more weight to carry than has the nag. Concussion to the foot is therefore greater. The greater part of the body-weight is borne by the fore-limbs. Concussion is therefore greater to the fore-feet than to the hind.

This, however, does not explain altogether the comparative immunity of the nag animal from this defect. He, too, must also be subject to the effects of concussion, especially when his higher and faster action is taken into account. To our minds there is only one explanation to be offered here. We point at once to the years of constant and judicious breeding of the nag. Compare that with the relatively few minutes that have been devoted to a more careful selection of the cart animal, and we at once see a possible explanation. That the explanation holds some amount of truth is borne out by the fact that, since a greater attention has been paid to the selection of our cart animals, side-bone has grown a great deal less common.

Is side-bone hereditary? We can best answer that by saying that, some several years ago, the Council of the Royal College of Veterinary Surgeons, at the request of the Royal Commission on Horse Breeding, drew up a list of those diseases 'which by heredity rendered stallions so affected unfit as breeding sires,' and that in that list was included side-bone.

Side-bones, therefore, are hereditary. We think, however, the statement needs qualifying. It is in this way: side-bones occur only at a certain, usually well-defined, time after birth, and we might say are *never* congenital. They occur only after the animal has been put to work, and are more or less plainly due to mechanical causes—namely, the ill effects of shoeing and concussion. The cause of their appearance, in short, is more plainly extrinsic than intrinsic, and side-bone in the horse is, as Professor McCall puts it, about as much due to heredity as is corn on the human foot.

Between these two opinions—that they are plainly hereditary, and that they just as plainly are not—it is well to strike a middle course. They are, we will say, hereditary in this way: So long as a cart animal is bred, to put it vulgarly, 'top-heavy' (that is, with a body out of reasonable proportion to the feet that have it to support), so long will the foot be subjected to a greater concussion, and so long will side-bones in such animals commence to make their appearance at about middle life.

In addition to the causes we have now mentioned, side-bones are often the result of other diseases of the foot. They thus occur as a sequel to sub-horny quittor, to suppurating corn, to complicated quarter sand-crack, or to the inflammation of the parts occasioned by a prick. They also arise in many instances from the effect of a prick or injury to the coronet. Among the latter we may mention treads from other animals, and treads inflicted by the animal himself with the calkin of an opposite shoe, or the repeated injury occasioned by the shafts being carelessly allowed to drop on to the foot. In severe cases of laminitis, too, the cartilages are nearly always affected. In this instance the inflammatory phenomena in the os pedis no doubt give rise to an abnormal activity of bone-forming cells. The cartilage is invaded, and the side-bone formed (see Fig. 118).

Treatment.—In the ordinary way the 'treatment' of side-bone is a thing but rarely mentioned. The explanation lies, of course, in the fact that side-bones are so rarely the cause of lameness. When lameness does occur with a side-bone, and we have reason to believe that the said side-bone is the cause of the lameness, it is well before talking of treatment to question ourselves thus: 'In what way does the side-bone cause lameness?' The now generally-accepted answer to that query is the explanation put forward several years ago by Colonel Fred Smith—namely, that the pain, and therefore the lameness, was due to the compression of the sensitive laminæ between the ossified and enlarged cartilage and the non-yielding and often contracted wall of the quarters. That, in fact, constitutes the basis upon which Smith's operation for side-bone (that of grooving the wall of the quarters) is founded.

Before describing the operation, however, we may say that we are now able to understand that older operators who claimed success for other methods of treatment, were to a very great extent justified in so doing.

For instance, take the combined treatments of firing and blistering, and the use of a bar shoe. Here the beneficial action of the cautery and the blister may be largely problematical. The bar shoe, however, would be almost certain to give good results. Frog-pressure with the ground would be again restored, and the contraction of the heels removed. Pinching of the sensitive structures would be diminished, and the lameness cured.

Take, again, the treatment of 'unsoling.' It was barbarous, we know barbarous, because unnecessary and easily avoidable. It was practised, however, certainly very little more than two decades ago, and practised by men of standing in the profession. Without dragging the case to light again by mentioning the names of those concerned, we may mention that not many years ago a highly respected member of the profession was, at the instigation of the Royal Society for the Prevention of Cruelty to Animals, prosecuted for practising unsoling for the relief of side-bone. Practically only one other member of the profession was able to come forward and defend the operation on the score of its utility. We see now, however, that—as does Smith's operation—unsoling does permit of the greater expansion of the heels. The contraction is done away with, the pressure on the sensitive laminæ again diminished, and the lameness relieved.

Not that we are attempting to defend the operation—far from it. We simply mention it as interesting, and quote this and the use of the bar shoe (with both of which methods older operators have claimed success) merely as evidence that the operation of Smith is based on a logical foundation.

When treatment is decided on, therefore, we may first advise blistering and the use of a bar shoe. After that, should the lameness continue, and should we still judge the side-bone to be the cause of it, the operation may be advised.

As we have said before, the operation consists in so grooving the wall as to allow of the quarters widening sufficiently to relieve pressure on the parts within. In one or two previous portions of this work we have considered operations involving this procedure. Before detailing the operation here, therefore, we will first describe the instruments necessary, and the most satisfactory methods of incising the horn.

To begin with, it must be remembered that all methods of hoof section have for their object the after-expansion of the horny box, and that this can only be brought about by making each groove complete from coronary margin to solar edge of the wall, and carrying it, throughout its length, *deep enough to reach the commencement of the sensitive structures.*

To this end, therefore, the operator must bear in mind the comparative thickness of the various parts of the wall, and must, in particular, remember the relative thinness of that portion of horn forming the outer boundary of the cutigeral groove, and accommodating the coronary cushion.

For the making of the incisions there is the special saw devised for this operation by Colonel F. Smith, A.V.D., and which we illustrate in Fig. 144. With this the wall is sawn through *until the depth arrived at is equal to what is indicated by a previous examination of the thickness of the crust as viewed from the solar surface.* Here Colonel Smith says: 'I strongly advise everyone to use a metal gauge (a thin piece of material) to introduce into the incision made by the saw, and run it up and down to ascertain whether the wall is properly divided throughout. The depth to which this should be done we know from the previous measurements of our gauge on the crust.'

FIG. 144.—SMITH'S SIDE-BONE SAW (EARLY PATTERN).

Should the saw be of a pattern in which the set of its teeth makes only a narrow incision,[A] it should, while operating, be kept well oiled, and should be withdrawn every few seconds in order that the horn-dust lying in its teeth may be examined. If this is getting slightly blood-stained, we know, of course, that the sensitive structures are reached, and the incision has been carried far enough. In so judging the depth of the incision, however, care must be taken to see that the top of the coronary cushion is not injured with the saw, for if this is done the blood trickling into the depth of the incision will tinge the horn-dust, and give the false impression that the incision is sufficiently deep.

[Footnote A: That is Smith's older pattern. The newer pattern (Fig. 145) has the teeth so set as to make an incision wide enough to be looked into. In this case the depth arrived at is to be judged by the appearance of the bottom of the incision.]

If the operator has had no previous experience of the use of the saw in this operation, he must also be careful to avoid placing too great a pressure on the teeth of its lower third. This is done by keeping the hand too greatly depressed. Again, this leads to wounding of the sensitive structures (this time at the lower end of the incision), and again the operator is confused by the blood thus allowed to run into the groove.

The only portion of horn difficult to operate on is that immediately under the coronet. This is best severed with a succession of downward movements, and is easier performed with Smith's later pattern of side-bone saw (Fig. 145) in which the set of the foremost teeth is reversed.

FIG. 145.—SMITH'S SIDE-BONE SAW (IMPROVED PATTERN).

In making these grooves we must say that we think the use of the special saw may be dispensed with, and the incisions just as easily, or, at any rate, just as successfully, made with the knife. Those who select to use this instrument should choose a narrow-topped and sharp searcher, or a modern shaped drawing-knife of suitable size, such as those depicted in Fig. 46, *a* and *b*, and they will find their work much easier if they will make the first steps in the incisions with an ordinary flat firing-iron. By the use of the latter instrument the grooves are made conveniently open along their tops, and room left for nicely finishing the more delicate manner of removing with the knife the softer horn near the sensitive structures.

Those whose leaning is towards the use of special instruments, but who, at the same time, do not care to use the saw, will find their wants supplied in the hoof plane (Smith's), Fig. 146, or the hoof chisel (Hodder's), Fig. 147. With the hoof plane the groove in the wall is made by a succession of downward scraping movements, while with the chisel the cut in the wall is made either from below upwards, or from above downwards, according as the foot is held forward or backward—whichever, in fact, comes most convenient.

FIG. 146.—HOOF PLANE (SMITH'S).
When using the knife or the hoof plane it is not often that the sensitive structures are injured. In all cases, however, no matter what the instrument used, the metal gauge should be employed when the sensitive structures have been touched, and the operation obscured by blood.

FIG. 147.—HOOF CHISEL (HODDER'S).
Our instruments at hand, the operation may be proceeded with. The first step is to ascertain the extent of the side-bone, and to determine the position of the incisions. To do this the coronet is felt with the thumb, and the anterior extremity of the side-bone noted. This is marked on the horn with a piece of chalk, and a vertical line dropped from this position to the inferior margin of the wall (Fig. 148,1). The line crosses the horn fibres obliquely, and is purposely made in that direction in order that its inferior end may be far enough back to avoid the last nail-hole. Should the side-bone reach very far forwards, it may be wise to cause this line to slant from before backwards (see dotted line *a*, Fig. 148). Unless this is done, it is found that in some feet so much of the wall is isolated at the bottom that insufficient is left to nail the shoe to.

The next line to be made is the rear one. Its correct position is ascertained by first noting the junction off the wall with the bar (see groove 2, Fig. 149); and its inferior end must be just anterior to the inflexion of the wall. This is done that we may avoid cutting the bar. The position of the lower end of the rear line thus ascertained, it is run upwards with the chalk in the direction of the horn fibres.

FIG. 148.—DIAGRAM ILLUSTRATING THE POSITION OF THE GROOVES IN THE WALL IN COLONEL SMITH'S OPERATION FOR SIDE-BONE. 1,2, and 3, mark the grooves in the order in which they are made; the dotted line *a* marks the position taken by the anterior line when the side-bone, is one reaching far forward, while the dotted lines *b* and *c* mark the position of the additional grooves to be made if thought necessary.

The third line is made in such a position as to divide into two equal portions the wall between lines 1 and 2. Here, however, some operators prefer to make two, or even three, lines, adding those as at *b* and *c*, Fig. 148; and Smith himself says that a multiplicity of lines is an advantage rather than not.

In any case, having once determined the position of the lines, they should be plainly marked out with chalk, and then viewed from a distance with the foot on the ground, in order to judge of their regularity. If we are satisfied with them, we then lightly mark them with the saw, with the hot iron, or with the knife, whichever instrument we may be intending to use.

Unless the details are methodically carried out as here described, it is probable that more of the foot will be isolated than is necessary, and that as a consequence very little is left to which to nail the shoe.

FIG. 149.—DIAGRAM ILLUSTRATING THE POSITION OF THE GROOVES MADE IN THE HOOF IN COLONEL SMITH'S OPERATION FOR SIDE-BONES. 1, 2, and 3, show the grooves in the wall in the order in which they are made; 4 shows the groove made at the junction of the sole with the wall.

The incisions are then made with the saw or the knife, with the foot held in a convenient position by an assistant. That usually found most comfortable for the first incision is with the foot held forwards and placed on an assistant's thigh in the position adopted for 'clenching up' when shoeing, while that for the rear incision is with the animal's knee flexed, and the foot held well up to the elbow. In this, however, each operator will suit himself.

Should the preliminary steps in making the incisions be performed with the iron, it will be easiest done with the foot on the ground.

When the incisions through the wall are complete, our attention must be given to the sole. A drawing-knife is here used, and a further incision made over the white line so as to destroy the union of the sole with the wall between incisions 1 and 2, and so completely isolate the portions of wall included within the four grooves (see groove 4, Fig. 149). When this is done it should be found that the portions of the isolated wall spring readily to pressure of the thumb.

The inferior or wearing margin of the isolated wall must now be so trimmed that it takes no bearing on the ground when the opposite limb is held up by an assistant and full weight placed upon the foot.

For a day or two after the operation lameness is intense. This is to be treated with hot poultices or hot baths, and and soon disappears. Three to four days later a bar shoe is nailed on (taking care that the bearing of the quarters is still eased), and the hot poultices still continued. Four days later still walking exercise may be commenced, to be followed shortly afterwards by trotting. At about the twelfth day some animals may conveniently be put to work, while in other cases a fortnight, or even a month, must elapse before this can be done. When put to work early, it is wise to fill in the fissures made in the wall with hard soap, with wax, or with a suitable hoof dressing, in order that irritation of the sensitive structures with outside matter may be prevented.

This operation is soon followed by remarkable changes in the shape of the foot. At about the third week the coronet shows signs of bulging, and the upper part of the wall operated on is often so protruding as to render the foot wider here than at the ground surface. This is a sign that the case is doing well.

Should no improvement be noticed at the end of three weeks or a month, or should the grooves become filled from the bottom (which they do remarkably fast), then the incisions must be deepened, the exercise reduced, and the fomentations or poulticing repeated. So treated, many cases of side-bone lameness will be relieved, if not entirely cured, and, should the worst happen, and no alteration in the lameness is noticeable, no harm will have been done to the foot. In this connection, the originator of the treatment says: 'I may assure those induced to doubt either their diagnosis or the value of hoof section that no harm is done to the foot, even should the operation be of no value. It may do much good; it cannot do harm. The operation will never succeed until the inherent timidity of sawing or cutting into the wall is overcome. The *incisions must be deep, and of the same depth from the coronet to the ground.*'[A]

[Footnote A: *Journal of Comparative Pathology and Therapeutics*, vol. iii., p. 313.]

It is well to remark here that the operation of hoof section cannot be expected to succeed in every case. The last man in the world to claim that for it would be its originator. Failure to relieve the lameness may be accounted for in a variety of ways. First, of course, will come errors in diagnosis. No one of us is infallible, and the lameness we have judged as resulting from side-bone may arise from another cause. There are, too, complications to be reckoned with, the existence or absence of which cannot always be definitely ascertained. Such are: Ringbone, especially that form of ringbone known as 'low'; bony deposits on the pedal bone, either on its laminal or plantar surface, or even changes in the navicular bursa.

CHAPTER XI
DISEASES OF THE BONES
A. PERIOSTITIS AND OSTITIS.

We head this section, Periostitis *and* Ostitis, for the reason that in actual practice it is rare for one of these affections to occur without the other. The periosteum and the bone are so intimately connected that it is difficult to conceive of disease of the one failing to communicate itself in some degree to the other. Pathologically, however, and for purposes of description, it is more convenient to describe separately the abnormal changes occurring in these two tissues.

With the main phenomena of inflammation occurring elsewhere we presume our readers are aware. Briefly we may put it, that under the action of an irritant, either actual injury, chemical action, or septic infection, the healthy tissues around react in order to effect repair of the parts destroyed. Also that this reaction involves the distribution of a greater blood-supply to the part, with an abundant migration of leucocytes, and the outpouring of an inflammatory exudate, together with symptoms of heat, pain, redness, and swelling of the affected area. And that in chronic inflammations, owing to persistence of the cause, the process of repair thus instituted does not stop at mere restoration of lost tissue, but continues to the extent of forming an abnormal quantity of such tissue as normally exists in the parts implicated.

The process of inflammation in bone is essentially the same. It takes place along the course of the bloodvessels, and is only modified in its attendant phenomena by the structure of the parts involved. Swelling, for instance, cannot take place in the centre of compact bone tissue. Otherwise, other changes occur exactly as in inflammations of other structures.

When the causal irritant has been excessively severe and the migration of leucocytes abundant, actual formation of pus may occur, the bony tissue being broken down and mingled with it, and an abscess cavity formed. In milder cases, affected and necrotic tissue is removed by a process of phagocytosis, and new tissue (this time osseous) formed in its place.

In the periosteum we may take it roughly that inflammation runs a course similar to that occurring in soft tissues elsewhere. There is but one exception, and that, as we shall mention shortly, is connected with its deeper layer.

As we know, the periosteum consists of two layers, an outer fibrous and an inner yellow elastic, and is extremely vascular. Numerous bloodvessels ramify in it, and, with their attendant nerves, break up to enter the numberless canals of the Haversian system. This extreme vascularity, of course, favours abundant exudation. The exudate, however, is, as it were, shut in by the dense fibrous layer of the membrane, and the result is that in periostitis it collects between the membrane and the bone, causing swelling and raising of the membrane, and giving rise to excruciating pain from pressure upon the nerves.

Should the periostitis be complicated by the formation of pus, then the vessels entering and supplying the bone are, in the suppurative area, destroyed. With their destruction it may happen that we get also death of a portion of the osseous tissue. This, however, when the suppuration is abundant, cannot commonly occur, as the bloodvessels within the bone—those of the medulla—commence to supply blood to the affected part. In cases of trouble with the bones of the foot, these last few remarks have a special significance. Here we have three bones whose medullary cavity is extremely small—almost nil, in fact—which explains in some measure how easy it is when suppuration exists to get necrosis and exfoliation of, say, portions of the os pedis. Necrosis and sloughing of the periosteum itself may also happen, but as the extreme vascularity of the membrane is a fairly strong safeguard against that it is of only rare occurrence.

In connection with the deep layer of the periosteum, and forming part of it, are found numerous bone-forming cells (*osteoblasts*). These, under ordinary conditions, are relatively quiescent. Under the slightest irritation or stimulation, however, their bone-forming functions are stirred into abnormal activity, thus explaining how easy it is (especially with bones so open to receive slight injuries as are those of the foot) to get ossific deposits, the starting-point of which we are quite unable to account for.

With this brief introduction we will now describe such pathological changes as occur in the separate structures, and which we are likely to encounter in the various diseases of the foot. While so doing, we shall draw attention to such diseases as we have previously described in which the pathological conditions we are considering may be met with.

1. PERIOSTITIS.

This we shall consider under *(a)* Simple Acute Periostitis, *(b)* Suppurative Periostitis, *(c)* Osteoplastic Periostitis.

(a) Simple Acute Periostitis.—This is the periostitis that follows on the infliction of a slight injury to the membrane—an injury without an actual wound and free from infective material. It is one, therefore, which we always judge as existing in those cases where we have distinct evidence or history of injury, but in which the injury has not been severe enough to lead to fracture or to the infliction of an actual wound.

Such cases may be those of lamenesses persisting after violent blows upon the foot—cases where the animal has been kicking against the stable fittings, or where the foot has been partially passed over by the wheel of a waggon. It may be, too, that in a case of 'nail-bound' a great deal of the pain and lameness is due to a simple periostitis caused by pressure of the bulged inner-layer of horn upon the sensitive structures.

Simple acute periostitis may also occur in cases where an actual wound is in existence, but where such wound, fortunately, remains aseptic. We may thus have this condition accompanying ordinary cases of pricked foot, of treads in the anterior region of the coronet, and of accidental injuries of other kinds.

In simple acute periostitis the membrane is thicker and redder than normal, and is easily stripped from the bone. As it is pulled off it is noticed that there are numerous fibril-like processes hanging to its inner surface, and which draw out from the substance of the bone. These are simply the vessels (bloodvessels and nerves) which, loosened by the inflammatory exudate, are readily detached and drawn from the Haversian canals into which they normally run. In addition to its increased redness, the membrane has a swollen and gelatinous appearance owing to its infiltration with the inflammatory discharges. Simple acute periostitis may and often does end in resolution. On the other hand, it may end in suppuration or may become chronic. If the latter, then the osteoblasts of the innermost layer become active, and abnormal deposits of bone are the result.

(b) Suppurative Periostitis.—This condition simply indicates that the inflammation is complicated by the presence of pus organisms. It is, therefore, a common termination of the simple acute form attending the infliction of a wound. The wound becomes contaminated, and the case of simple periostitis is soon changed into the suppurative form. Once having gained entrance to the wound, the pus increases in quantity, and slowly runs between the

membrane and the bone. This, however, it does not do to any large extent, showing rather a tendency to penetrate the outer fibrous layer and gain the outside of the membrane.

Suppurative periostitis is met with in foot cases, commonly in connection with punctured foot. It occurs, too, as a complication in suppurating corn, in severe tread, in complicated sand-crack, as a result of the spread of suppurative matter in acute coronitis, and in sub-horny quittor.

In ordinary cases of suppurative periostitis the pus formed is yellow in colour, creamy thick, and free from pronounced odour—the so-called 'laudable' pus of the older writers. It so happens in many cases of foot trouble, however, that putrefactive organisms gain entrance side by side with those of pus. In this case the characters of the discharge are very different. It is distinctly more fluid, is of a pink or even light chocolate colour, and extremely offensive. In these instances the pus shows a marked tendency to spread, strips the periosteum from the bone, perforates the outer layer of the membrane, and finally infiltrates the surrounding tissues.

This forms a near approach to what is known in human surgery as an *infective* periostitis, and in our subjects is nearly always met with in cases of severe prick. Its rapidly spreading character makes it always a dangerous condition, and a punctured foot exuding a discharge of this nature should always be regarded as serious. The close contiguity of the joint (it can never be *far* distant in foot cases), the spreading character of the disease, and the rapidity with which the horse succumbs to arthritis, are all factors to be taken into consideration, and to lead to a warning-note being struck when attending a case of such kind.

A further instance of infective periostitis is that met with in acute laminitis. The discharge obtained from the sole in these cases very often bears the character we have just described, and when one considers the thinness of the keratogenous membrane, one is bound to admit that changes so grave occurring in it cannot fail to spread and infect the periosteum.

(*c*) *Osteoplastic Periostitis.*—This is more particularly a chronic process, and is, as the suffix '*plastic*' indicates, associated with bone-forming changes in the membrane. It may occur as a consequence of slight but continued irritation, often without ascertainable origin (see Case 2, p. 392), or it may be the sequel of acute disease.

In this form of periostitis the membrane is again swollen and more vascular than in health, and is also easily separable from the bone. The exposed bone is generally rough, in some cases even spicular, and the inner layer of the removed membrane is rough and gritty to the touch—characters imparted to it by numerous minute fragments of bone that have been torn away with it from the more compact osseous tissue beneath.

The results of an osteoplastic periostitis are frequently met with in the bones of the foot, and are described by veterinary writers under such headings as 'Pedal Exostoses,' 'Ossifying Ostitis,' and 'Pedal Ossification' (see Figs. 152, 153, 154, and 155). In many of these cases the disease is purely chronic, and the original cause nearly always wanting. When the foot has been subjected to laminitis of some weeks' duration, the same condition is also met with, being at the same time associated with rarefactive osteoplastic ostitis, conditions which we shall shortly describe. Cases we have examined have undoubtedly shown this condition of osteoplastic periostitis, the rarefactive and osteoplastic changes in the bone itself, met with in older cases, occurring no doubt as a result of non-expansion of the horny box. So far as we are able to ascertain, there is every reason to believe that in chronic laminitis the accompanying periostitis leads to the formation of bone, and would, if it were possible, lead to increase in the size of the os pedis. If proof were wanted of this, it is only necessary to point out the increased growth at points where resistance is nil—namely, along the upper margin of the bone (see Fig. 118). However, increase in size elsewhere is prevented by the resistance of the hoof, so that, as the bone-forming process progresses, as it inevitably*must* under the inflammatory changes going on, it is, as it were, compensated for by rarefaction or bone-absorption changes occurring simultaneously with it.

2. OSTITIS.

163

We shall next deal with the inflammatory changes occurring in the bones themselves, and shall consider them under (*a*): Rarefying or Rarefactive Ostitis, (*b*): Osteoplastic Ostitis, and (*c*): Caries and Necrosis.

Inflammatory changes occurring in the medulla we may pass without consideration, for in the bones of the foot the medullary cavity is so small, and the changes taking place in it of such minor importance, that we may do this without in any way seriously prejudicing our work.

(*a*) *Rarefying or Rarefactive Ostitis.*—By this term is indicated an inflammation of the bone attended by its absorption, the absorption being due to the action of certain cells, termed *osteoclasts*. This condition may be due to the pressure of tumours, may occur as the result of injury when a piece of bone is stripped of periosteum, or may be the result of an inflammation occurring in the periosteum elsewhere.

A piece of bone undergoing rarefactive ostitis is redder than normal, and the openings of the Haversian canals are distinctly increased in size. As a result a greater number of them become visible. Their increase in size is due to the inflammatory absorption of the bony tissue forming them, and in the larger of them may be seen inflammatory granulation tissue surrounding the bloodvessels. This enlargement of the Haversian canals is well seen when the bone is macerated, the whole then giving the appearance of a piece of very rough pumice-stone.

This process of rarefaction or absorption of bone tissue may be confined to quite a small portion, or it may be spread over the whole of the bone, rendering it more porous than is normal, but stopping short of complete destruction of the bone tissue (a condition which is sometimes known as inflammatory osteoporosis (see Fig. 118)). In this latter case the condition is a chronic one, and the bone tissue remaining often appears to be strengthened by a compensatory process of condensation. For an example of rarefactive ostitis as met with in cases of disease of the feet, we refer the reader to laminitis (see Fig. 118). The osteoplastic or condensing process that appears to exist simultaneously with it explains, no doubt, how it is that bones so affected do not more commonly fracture.

A further example of this process is illustrated in Fig. 133. The pressure of a tumour (in this case a keraphyllocele) has led to rarefactive changes in the bone, forming a neat indentation in the normal contour of the bone which serves to accommodate the tumour.

(*b*) *Osteoplastic Ostitis, Osteosclerosis, or Condensation of Bone.*—This, too, is essentially a chronic process. It may occur as a result of, or, as we have just shown, exist simultaneously with the condition of, diffuse rarefactive ostitis. In this case there is a formation of new bone in the connective tissue surrounding the vessels in the Haversian canals. As a consequence the bone affected is greatly increased in density, and many of the Haversian canals by this means obliterated. The end result is an increase in size of the bones in such positions as the horny box admits of it, and a peculiar ivory-like change in their consistence.

For an example of this, we again refer the reader to the changes occurring in chronic laminitis.

(*c*) *Caries and Necrosis.*—*Caries* is a word which appears to be used with a considerable amount of looseness. In addition to the meaning implied by necrosis (namely, 'death' of the part), caries is generally used to indicate that there is also a condition of rottenness, decay, and stench. It is particularly applied, in fact, when the death of the bone is slowly progressive, and is due to the inroads made upon it by putrefactive or septic matter.

Necrosis of bone may be the result of any injury, such as severe blows, or pricks and stabs. In such cases it would appear that it is loss of a portion of periosteum that is the starting-point. With death of a portion of this membrane the vascular supply to a portion of the bone is cut off, and necrosis ensues. It may also result from the extension of inflammatory affections of the structures adjoining it, as, for instance, the spread of the infective material in severe tread, or the encroaches made by pus in cases of quittor, suppurating corn, or complicated sand-crack.

When the necrosed portion of bone is small, and is free from infective properties, it is quite possible that it may, as is the case with small spots of necrosis in softer tissues, be removed by a process of absorption. It must be remembered, however, that where the necrosis has occurred as a result of septic invasion this cannot be looked for, for in every case such reparative changes are worked solely by healthy tissue. If the tissues around the necrosis are engaged in dealing with organismal invasion and the poisonous products thus poured into their working area, their state of health is so weakened that they are unable to successfully combat with the two conditions simultaneously. As a consequence, the necrotic piece of bone persists, and acts as a permanent source of irritation.

It must be remembered, too, that if the dead portion of bone—even though it be free from septic matter—is very large, that it may itself act as a continual irritant, in which case it again persists, and cannot by natural means be removed.

In our cases necrosis of bone may be met with in punctured foot, in severe cases of tread, in cases of complicated crack, and in suppurating corn. It is met with, too, in navicular disease, in the extension of irritating discharges in cases of quittor, and in cases of chronic laminitis where the solar margin of the os pedis has penetrated the sole. In this latter case the protruding portion of bone is quickly denuded of its periosteum. Its blood-supply is destroyed, and necrosis follows.

Treatment.—In simple cases of periostitis, those caused by a blow but free from an actual wound, the most beneficial treatment is the continued application of cold by means of a hose-pipe or by swabs. If by these means we are successful in holding the inflammatory phenomena in check, any large formation of new bone is prevented, and the case does well.

When the case is complicated by a wound, then antiseptic measures, such as those described in the treatment of punctured foot, will at the same time have to be practised.

It must be admitted, however, that in all but the most simple cases ordinary treatment such as this is of very little use; for with only a slight exostosis in almost any position in the foot, excessive lameness presents itself and remains. In such cases nothing is left to us but the operation of neurectomy.

When the periostitis and ostitis is the result of a wound, and is complicated by caries or necrosis of the bone, the diseased portion of bone must in every case be laid bare and removed. It so happens that the majority of cases of this kind occur in positions where the diseased bone is easily got at. The lower margin of the os pedis or portions of the wings are commonly the seat of such changes. We meet with the former in cases of pricked foot, and with the latter in severe cases of tread, or as a complication in suppurating corn or in quittor. In such cases the animal must be cast and the foot secured. The wound is then followed up, the horn if necessary removed, and the bone curetted with a Volkmann's spoon; or, if showing itself as a sequestrum, removed with a scalpel and a strong pair of forceps. Care must be taken that every particle of the diseased bone is removed, and that no part of it is left to act as an after-source of irritation. With removal of the diseased portion and a strict attention to antisepsis healing soon takes place.

Reported Cases of Periostitis and Ostitis.—1. 'Figs. 150 and 151 represent the phalangeal bones of the off fore-leg of a thoroughbred horse named Osman, who was well known as a hunt steeplechaser of considerable merit in the Midland counties some twenty years ago. I may say that this horse was under my observation pretty regularly during the whole of his career, and up to the time of his death, from ruptured aorta, when eight years old. My attention was called to him as a yearling by his owner, who told me that he sometimes fancied the colt was lame. I went over to see him, and found that he was unmistakably lame on the off fore-leg. Careful examination showed no heat or enlargement anywhere. I advised rest and the colt became pretty sound, though not quite so—in fact, he never did become quite sound, and sometimes he was very lame indeed.

FIG. 150.—EFFECTS OF PERIOSTITIS ON THE PEDAL AND NAVICULAR BONES.

'Every imaginable sort of treatment was tried short of neurectomy, without avail. The curious part of the case was that there never was much heat or any apparent change of structure, nor was "pointing" a very noticeable feature. The foot always remained a good-looking one. As the horse won a good number of races he was of some value, and was seen by a good many members of the profession, who were by no means unanimous as to the cause of lameness. The favourite theory was that it was a sequence of "split pastern." A post-mortem examination showed that there was no fracture. There was no adherence of the tendon to the navicular bone nor any ulceration. The morbid changes consisted entirely of osseous deposit as shown in the photographs. The under surface of the navicular bone was much enlarged and roughened by this bony deposit, which extended on to the os pedis, causing complete anchylosis at each extremity of the navicular. The lateral cartilages were healthy. The interesting points in connection with the case are the insidious commencement of osseous disease, its extensive development, and the entire absence of any external manifestation, through its being confined entirely within the limits of the hoof.

FIG. 151.—EFFECTS OF PERIOSTITIS ON THE PEDAL AND NAVICULAR BONES.

'It should also be noted that the animal was able to undergo a severe course of training for some years, and to gallop successfully over some of the most trying courses in England. During the whole of this time he walked and galloped apparently sound, but trotted always lame, and generally dead lame.'[A]

[Footnote A: W. E Litt, M.R.C.V.S., *Veterinary Record*, vol. viii., p. 527.]

FIG. 152.—EFFECTS OF PERIOSTITIS ON THE OS PEDIS.

2. 'I herewith send you photographs of three cases of the above disease, occurring in the internal surfaces of the wings of the os pedis. The photos were kindly done for me by Dr. A. Lingard, Imperial Bacteriologist to Government of India. It is a cause of many cases of obscure foot lameness in India, and frequently accounts for the numerous entries on veterinary medical history sheets under the heading "Contused Foot."

'The course of the disease is as follows: The disease makes its appearance very soon after arrival in India, the animal being admitted to hospital suffering with undoubted foot lameness, generally slight. One is soon led to suspect this disease by negative symptoms of other disease being in existence. No coronary enlargement or flinching on pressure to the coronet, no shrinkage or wiring in of the heels, neither is the characteristic pointing of navicular present. In the early stages one has false hopes of recovery by finding gradual improvement for a time by fomentation and poultices, followed by irrigation and stimulants to the coronet, and perhaps the animal is discharged from hospital, to be returned after a few days worse than ever. The disease then becomes insidious and more pronounced, the nodding of the head, even at a walk, more exaggerated, and, in fact, the animal seems afraid to put his foot to the ground, and much resembles a horse with an abscess in his foot, either from prick or picked up nail. He absolutely nurses his foot. There is a certain amount of heat always present. The disease being now well developed, pressure is caused by the ends of the navicular bone, and they become involved at their points by bony deposits. The causes of this disease I attribute, firstly, to hereditary predisposition; and, secondly the exciting cause, standing confined on board ship, where no doubt pedal congestion takes place. And perhaps some subjects start it in their marches in mobs down country in Australia. Concussion may be the cause among older horses, but the specimens photographed were taken from remounts, that had either done no work or only very gentle work, in a deeply littered riding school.

166

FIG. 153.—EFFECTS OF PERIOSTITIS ON THE OS PEDIS.

Treatment.—It is obvious from the position of this disease that treatment will be of no avail in producing a cure. As already stated, the disease is insidious and progressive, and it is hopeless to expect to arrest the growths once they are started. Unnerving would no doubt remove the symptom (lameness) of the disease, but an unnerved horse is not of much good for army purposes. I therefore consider that once the disease becomes firmly established it is an unfortunate and incurable one.

F   F

IG. 154   IG. 155

FIG. 154, 155—EFFECTS OF PERIOSTITIS ON THE OS PEDIS.

'Post-mortem reveals the small nodular growths on the inner surfaces of the wings of the pedal bone, and if long established the ends of the navicular bone are also involved. Exudation and gradual growth of false material around the nodules takes place, which also serves to increase pressure.'[A]

[Footnote A: Captain L.M.Smith, A.V.D., *Veterinary Record*, vol. xi., p. 229.]

3. 'This case was brought for my opinion. The horse was lame, and walked similar to one that had had laminitis, putting the heel down first upon the ground. I ordered the patient to be destroyed. You will note the ossification of the flexor pedis at its attachment to the pedal bone. I enclose photos of the ground, also of the articular, surfaces of the bone.'[A]

[Footnote A: F.B.Jones, M.R.C.V.S., *Veterinary Record*, vol. xi., p. 230.]

B. PYRAMIDAL DISEASE, BUTTRESS FOOT, OR LOW RINGBONE.

Definition.—A condition of periostitis and ostitis in the region of the pyramidal process of the os pedis, usually preceded, but sometimes followed, by fracture of the process, and characterized by deformity of the hoof and an alteration in the normal angle of the joint.

Causes.—In the majority of cases buttress foot is brought about by fracture of the pyramidal process. Thus, although distinct evidence of such is nearly always wanting, we may assume that the original cause is violent injury to the part in question. Properly, therefore, one would say that this condition should be described under Fractures of the Os Pedis. It appears, however, that other cases of the kind arise in which fracture is altogether absent, or in which it is plainly seen to be subsequent to the diseased processes in the bone. For that reason, and also for the reason that the condition has come to be known by the name we have given, we give it special mention.

Symptoms and Diagnosis.—Even when the condition arises as the result of fracture, the ordinary manifestations of such a lesion are absent. By reason of the situation of the parts within the hoof we are unable to detect crepitation, and the resulting lameness is perhaps— in fact, nearly always is—neglected until such time as any heat or swelling caused by the injury has disappeared, in which case we are denied what evidence we might have obtained from that. All that is presented is lameness, and lameness that is at times excessive. But with the lameness there is nothing distinctive. The foot is tender on percussion, and the gait suggestive of foot lameness, that is all. We are unable, therefore, to make an exact diagnosis, and the condition goes for some time undetected.

Later, however, changes in the form of the hoof and the coronet begin to appear. The skin of the coronet, especially in the region of the toe, becomes more or less thickened and indurated, and the same remark applies to the subcutaneous tissues. The most marked change, however, is the alteration in the shape of the hoof. The wall protrudes at the toe in a manner that has been termed 'buttress-like,' and has given to the condition one of its names. This, of course, entirely alters the contour of the horny box. From being more or less U-

167

shaped, it approaches nearer the formation of the letter V, the point of the V being at the toe.

In the later stages the coronary enlargement is plainly seen to be due to an extensive formation of bone. It is, in fact, a reparative callus, and the reason it reaches so large a size is probably to be accounted for by the pull of the extensor pedis upon the detached pyramidal process. As might be expected, this displacement of the fractured portion, with its effect of giving greater length to the extensor pedis, leads to a backward displacement of the os coronæ upon the pedal bone. As a result there is a marked depression at the coronet, the depression being heightened in effect by the exostosis in front. Pyramidal disease is, as a rule, met with in the hind-feet, but occurs also in the fore.

Pathological Anatomy.—When occurring without fracture, the first observable change is a thinning of the articular cartilage of the pyramidal process, through which the bone beneath appears abnormally white. Later the thinning of the cartilage progresses until at last it becomes entirely obliterated. This destruction of the cartilage commences first at the highest point of the articular surface of the pyramid, and gradually reaches further backward into the joint. While this is taking place the new bone is being formed on the front of the os pedis, below and around the process, until, as we have already seen, an exostosis is formed, large enough to be noticeable at the coronet. This, of course, partly implicates the joint and the points of the insertion of the extensor tendon.

Finally, fracture may, or may not, take place. When it does, the exostosis is larger, and the general deformity of the hoof greater.

Treatment.—Ordinary treatment, such as point or line firing, repeated blisters, or hoof section, each of which we have tried, appears to be utterly useless. So far as we have been able to gather from the writings of other practitioners, however, neurectomy returns the animal for a time to usefulness. If the fore-limb is the seat of trouble, either plantar or median neurectomy may be practised; if the hind, then the best results are obtained by section of the posterior tibial.

Reported Cases.—1. This animal, a mare, had been rested for lameness behind for two or three weeks, and then sent out to work, going sound. This was repeated several times, and each time the coachman reported, "Goes very lame behind after she has been at work about fifteen to twenty minutes." She always pulled out sound when I saw her in a halter on the following day, so I had her ridden, and after about seven or eight minutes she began to go lame in a hind-limb. Her lameness got rapidly worse as she was being ridden, and within a quarter of mile of her first showing lameness, she dropped and carried the lame foot in a way that suggested a badly fractured pastern. There was no recognisable disease in the limb to account for this lameness.

'I divided the posterior tibial nerve, and she went back to work moving sound, and continued to work sound up to her death from one of the regularly fatal bowel lesions twist or rupture.

'She worked nearly two years after unnerving, and developed the usual thickening at the coronet.'[A]

[Footnote A: W. Willis, M.K.C.V.S., *Journal of Comparative Pathology and Therapeutics*, vol. xv., p. 366.]

2. 'The subject of this note was a chestnut mare, nine years old, and used for omnibus work.

'*History.*—For about two months the mare was lame on the off fore-leg, and in spite of treatment the condition became steadily worse. The off fore-foot was rather long and narrow, and the fetlock-joint was inclined to be bowed outwards, but the degree of lameness was out of proportion to these defects, and the diagnosis was obscure.

'Median neurectomy was performed on May 10, 1902, and reduced the lameness to about half of what it was before. On June 5 ulnar neurectomy was performed, with the result that the mare became sound, and went to work three weeks later. She continued to work soundly and well, being inspected from time to time.

'During February of 1903 the coronet began to enlarge in front and slightly to the outer side, and gradually a ridge of bone grew down from the coronet to the toe. The case, in fact, became a typical one of so-called "buttress foot," which my friend Mr. Willis has described as diagnostic of disease of the pyramidal process of the pedal bone. Meanwhile the swelling of the coronet, which appeared to be mainly composed of fibrous tissue, increased in size, until the whole of the front and sides became involved, assuming the appearance shown in Fig. 156.

'In spite of the coronary enlargement the mare worked well, and remained free from lameness till June 8, 1903, on which day the limb became swollen up to the site of the median operation. The appearance of the limb closely simulated an attack of lymphangitis. The mare was kept under observation till the 13th of the same month, during which time the swelling increased, as did also the lameness to a slight degree. During progression she brought the heel to the ground and "rocked the toe," as in a case of rupture of the perforans tendon. The mare was killed on June 13.

FIG. 156.—A CASE OF BUTTRESS FOOT.

FIG. 157.—FRACTURE OF THE PYRAMIDAL PROCESS IN BUTTRESS FOOT.

'*Post-mortem.*—In trying to pull away the hoof from the sensitive structures with a pair of farrier's pincers, the tendons and ligaments of the corono-pedal articulation gave way, leaving the pedal bone *in situ*. The flexor perforans tendon showed inflammatory softening, and was very nearly ruptured through at the level of the navicular bone. There was slight evidence of navicular disease. The articular cartilage of the corono-pedal joint had been almost completely removed, and there was sclerosis of the opposed bony surfaces, which by unequal wear had brought about deformity of the os coronæ and os pedis.

There was very old-standing fracture of the pyramidal process (see Fig. 157), with the formation of a false joint between the process and the pedal bone. There was also a recent fracture of the part of the pedal bone which carries the articulation for the navicular bone, and this and the tendon lesions probably accounted for the final symptoms of 'break-down.'

Neurectomy enabled us to get a year's useful work out of what would otherwise have been a hopeless cripple.[A]

[Footnote A: A.R. Routledge, M.R.C.V.S., *Journal of Comparative Pathology and Therapeutics*, vol. xvi., p. 371.]

C. FRACTURES OF THE BONES.

More or less by reason of the protection afforded them by the hoof fractures of the bones of the foot are rare. When occurring they are more often than not the result of direct injury, as, for example, violent blows, the trapping of the foot in railway points, the running over of the foot with a heavily-laden waggon, or violent kicking against a gate or a wall. They occur also as a result of an uneven step upon a loose stone when going at a fast pace, and as a result of sudden slips and turns, in which latter case they are met with when animals have been galloping unrestrained in a field, or when an animal, ridden or driven at a fast pace, is suddenly pulled up, or just as suddenly turned.

At other times fractures in this region take place without ascertainable cause, and cases are on record where animals turned overnight into a loose box in their usual sound condition have been found in the morning excessively lame, and fracture afterwards diagnosed.

1. FRACTURES OF THE OS CORONÆ.

Fractures of the os coronæ result from such causes as we have just enumerated, and are nearly always seen in conjunction with fractured os suffraginis. When this latter bone is also fractured diagnosis is comparatively easy, a certain amount of crepitus, even when the suffraginis is only split, being obtainable. When the os corona alone is fractured then diagnosis is extremely difficult, the smallness of the bone and the comparative rigidity of the parts rendering manipulation almost useless, and effectually preventing the obtaining of crepitus. It is, in fact, only when the bone is broken into many pieces that crepitus may be detected, and even then it is slight.

Reported Cases.—1. 'The subject was a four-year old hunter. While at exercise in the morning of August 10 he bolted, got rid of his rider, and ran about in a mad fashion, came into contact with a wheelbarrow in a narrow passage, and finally came into violent contact with a wall, which had the effect of throwing him down. The rider stated that the animal suddenly put down his head and managed to get off the bridle; he then bolted, and the only chance for the rider was to throw himself off.

'On examination I found the horse unable to place any weight on the off fore-leg, the pastern was swollen and painful, the hollow of the heel was also swollen, and there was marked constitutional disturbance.

'After a short time he would place the heel on the ground and elevate the toe to a slight degree. On manipulating the pastern slight crepitation could be discovered, and there was abnormal mobility in the corono-pedal articulation. On the near fore-leg there were extensive wounds in the region of the knee, and great laceration of the tissues. The animal was destroyed.

'On examining the leg I found the subcutaneous tissues infiltrated from below the knee to the foot, large masses of gelatinous blood-stained material being present along the flexor tendons and in the hollow of the heel. The inferior articular surface of the os suffraginis was denuded of cartilage anteriorly; the os coronæ was fractured into eight moderate sized, irregular fragments, and ten minute pieces. The surface of the perforans tendon as it glides over the smooth surface at the back of the os coronæ was lacerated, and minute portions of the bone were found embedded therein.'[A]

[Footnote A: E. Wallis Hoare, F.R.C.V.S., *Veterinary Record*, vol. xiv., p. 133.]

2. 'Here, again, fracture was the result of the animal bolting with his rider. Trying to avoid collision with a conveyance coming towards him, the animal slipped on a wooden pavement, sliding along until his near fore-leg came in contact with the wheel of a standing cab. There was considerable swelling from the knee downwards, great pain, and evidence of fracture in the region of the pastern.

'Post-mortem revealed the os suffraginis broken into about thirty pieces, and the os coronæ with a piece broken off the inside of its proximal end.[A]

[Footnote A: A.F. Appleton, M.R.C.V.S., *Veterinary Journal*, vol. xiii., p. 411.]

3. 'The patient was a brown mare used for heavy van work in London. About January 10 she was lame, and as she had a cracked heel, was treated by poulticing for a day, and then by antiseptic lotions. In a week she was sent to work, but the following day lameness returned, and continued till about February 15. No special symptom was detected which indicated the exact position of any cause of lameness. Then the lameness increased in severity, and some swelling around the coronet began to show itself.

'In consultation with another veterinary surgeon, two possible causes of this intense lameness were discussed: one, that we had septic infection of the coronet, and that probably the swelling of this part would soften, and sloughs occur; the other, that a fracture of the os pedis or os coronæ existed. The enlargement of the coronet was hard and firm, not particularly sensitive. It was decided to do nothing for a few days. In a week the pain abated, and the mare would put her foot on the ground, and ceased to "nurse" the limb as she had done. When moved over in the box she put a little weight on the foot, but limped very decidedly.

'Another week passed, and the pain and lameness further abated, but the swelling around the coronet continued. Perhaps it was a little less in front, but it had not decreased on the inside. It remained firm, and was not painful on pressure. It showed no soft places, and the upper part of the leg remained free from oedema.

FIG. 158.—FRACTURE IN SITU (OS CORONÆ).

The diagnosis was now that a fracture existed, and it was proposed to send the mare to grass for a few months. The consulting veterinary surgeon suggested that before doing so a blister might be applied to the coronet. This was done. The mare was found next day again on three legs. She had apparently been down during the night. In a few days the coronet increased again in size, and within a week "broke out" in two places.

The opinion now formed was that, with a fracture and this additional cause of inflammation around the joint, it would be most economical for the owner to have her killed. This was done, and a post-mortem examination was made by Mr. Hunting and Mr. Willis.

FIG. 159.—WITH BROKEN PORTION REMOVED.

'*Post-mortem.*—The foot, cut off at the fetlock-joint, showed extensive swelling all round the coronet. There were two wounds on the skin—one on the front of the coronet, the other on the inner side. From both pus and blood had escaped. They both communicated under the skin with a large abscess cavity. The abscess did not communicate with the joint. The pastern bone was sound. On separating the pastern from the coronet bone the articular surfaces were of a healthy colour, but the soft tissues immediately surrounding them were inflamed. On the centre of the articular surface of the coronary bone a thin red ring was noticed, and the portion of cartilage within it seemed raised. With the point of a scalpel this portion was lifted, and was found to be not only cartilage, but a layer of bone completely detached from the os coronæ. On removing the bones from the hoof the rest of the bone was quite normal, as was the pedal bone.

'Fig. 158 shows the articular surface of the coronet with the fracture *in situ*, and Fig. 159 the surface from which the broken portion is removed and laid to the side of the foot.

'Some interesting questions arise. How was the fracture caused? When did it occur? Between the broken portion and the main bone there was a layer of granulation tissue, so that it is certain the injury existed before the blister was applied, and it may possibly have existed from the commencement of the lameness.'[A]

[Footnote A: R. Crawford, M.R.C.V.S., *Veterinary Record*, vol. viii., p. 478.]

2. FRACTURES OF THE OS PEDIS.

These also are a result of the causes we have before given. The os pedis is also liable to fractures from pricks, from treads in the region of the wings, and from the malnutrition and careless use of the foot sometimes following neurectomy.

It is interesting to note that, with fracture of this bone, lameness is nearly always excessive, but that at times it may be entirely absent. Crepitus is, of course, denied us, and in nearly every instance the case is only diagnosed when the lameness persists and pus commences to form, or when grave changes in the normal shape of the foot compel our attention to the parts. When it is the continued formation of pus that draws our notice to something more than ordinarily grave, it is in giving exit to the pus that the fracture is nearly always discovered.

Reported Cases.—Two interesting cases of fractured os pedis are reported by Mr. Gladstone Mayall, M.R.C.V.S., in the *Veterinary Record*, vol. xiv., p. 54:

1. 'The horse was brought in markedly lame on the off hind-foot, knuckling at the fetlock, and taking a long stride with the injured limb. There was a punctured wound at the toe. The horn was pared, and antiseptic poultices applied. Notwithstanding the antiseptic treatment pus continued to form. At the end of a week sufficient horn was removed to ascertain the cause of the constant suppuration. A movable object was found at the bottom of the wound, and a piece of bone as large as a sixpence finally removed. Recovery was uneventful.'

FIG. 160.—FRACTURED OS PEDIS.

2. 'A filly was attended for a discharging fistula at the coronet. Externally it had all the appearances of a quittor. At first no history was given. The filly went scarcely lame at all, and had never been shod. Treatment with poultices and caustic injections was useless. Finally the filly was cast and the foot examined. A piece of bone, apparently part of the wing of the os pedis, was removed, and the case made a good recovery. Subsequent inquiries elicited the fact that the animal had kicked at and hit a gate-post, and it was judged that then the injury had occurred.'

3. 'The subject was a bay horse, nine years old, used for railway shunting. On August 7 he was found to be intensely lame of the near hind-limb, and, after inquiries, there was no evidence bearing on the cause, as is often the case, and at times this comes to light when least expected.

'I was called in consultation on September 2, and found him suffering acute pain, with great swelling around the coronet. The foot was examined thoroughly, and the diagnosis was fracture of the pedal bone, and immediate slaughter was recommended. However, that was not carried out, and he died on September 22.

'The post-mortem inspection revealed a complete fracture of nearly the whole of the articulating surface and the left wing of the pedal bone (as shown in Fig. 160).'[A]

[Footnote A: J. Freeman, M.R.C.V.S., *Veterinary Journal*, vol. xxxi., p. 324.]

4. A further interesting case is reported by Mr. William Hurrell.[A] Here the cause was presumably galloping in the field, for the subject, a cart mare running out at grass with her foal, was suddenly found to be lame.

[Footnote A: *Ibid.*, vol. v., p. 408.]

As the lameness continued to increase in severity, Mr. Hurrell was called in on August 1, and diagnosed the case as one of foot lameness. On this date the foot was pared out, and a large accumulation of pus discovered, Poulticing and antiseptic dressings were continued until August 16, when a movable piece of the os pedis was found at the toe.

On August 25 this detached portion of the bone was removed, and turned out to be the whole of the anterior margin of the os pedis, measuring 3-1/2 inches long, and varying in width from 1/2 inch to 1-1/2 inches. On September 20 the mare was working without lameness.

3. FRACTURES OF THE NAVICULAR BONE.

Hidden within the wings of the os pedis, and protected as it is by its tendinous covering and the yielding substance of the plantar cushion, the navicular bone is even less liable to fracture than either of the other bones of the foot.

The most common cause of fracture of the navicular is that of stabs or deep pricks in the region of the point of the frog (see p. 216). Following that, the next most common cause is violent injury. We thus find the navicular bone fractured, together with one or both of the other bones of the foot, when the foot is run over by a heavy vehicle. One such case is reported by Mr. J.H. Carter, F.R.C.V.S., where the horse's foot was run over by a tram-engine, in which the os pedis and the navicular were fractured in several places.[A] A further case is on record where a sharp blow on the front of the hoof was the cause. In this case the os pedis and other structures were uninjured, but the navicular bone was fractured into three large, and about half a dozen small, pieces.[B]

[Footnote A: *Veterinary Journal*, vol. xxxi., p. 246.]

[Footnote B: *Veterinarian* for 1857, p. 73.]

Fractures of the navicular may occur, however, in which history of a prick or of a violent injury is absent. See reported case below.

As with fractures of the os pedis and the os coronæ, so with this exact diagnosis is difficult—we may say almost impossible. With a history of violent injury, however, some little regard may be paid to a continued heat and tenderness of the foot, and a distinct inclination on the part of the animal to go on the toe. Even when the fracture is the result of a prick, and the bone is plainly felt with the probe, we still cannot be positive as to fracture.

Reported Case.—'The animal was a Hungarian, a troop-horse in the 3rd Hussars (G. 15). On November 22, 1881, on the march from Norwich to Aldershot, the horse suddenly made a violent stumble, very nearly coming on to his knees. The rider declared that he put his foot on a stone. The accident caused great lameness in the near fore-leg, and the horse had to be led the remainder of that day's march. On the following day he was also led; but, after going some sixteen or eighteen miles, he was so lame that he was left at the nearest billet (in Edmonton). He was here attended by Mr. Stanley, M.R.C.V.S., of Edmonton, who pronounced it a case of navicular disease. I first saw the animal on December 1, 1881, and quite agreed with Mr. Stanley that it was a case of foot lameness, though, from the horse's former history, I could not think it a case of ordinary navicular disease. I diagnosed it a case of fracture, without displacement, either of the os coronæ or the navicular bone, but was more inclined to the former than the latter. This was after a full hour's examination. I failed to find any heat in, or any flinching by manipulation of, any part of the limb; but, in walking, the horse was excessively lame, going on the toe, and, indeed, trying if possible to keep the foot entirely off the ground.

'On December 6 the horse was sent on to Aldershot by rail. He was then walking better, though still very lame. My only treatment for a short time was to apply cold water constantly to the coronet and foot. For two hours daily this was done by a hose, the remainder of the time by a cold swab. On December 14 I applied a strong blister over the coronet, reaching up to the fetlock. This was washed off about the end of December. The horse was then not nearly so lame. I then resumed the cold-water treatment, and he got gradually better, and was sent to light duty on February 18, 1882. He, however, only attended one field-day, and was taken into the Horse Infirmary again on March 8, very lame. Again, there was an entire absence of heat or pain on pressure, but the same action, viz., going on the toe. I forgot to remark that he always pointed the toe of the affected leg when standing in the stable, and this symptom continued. I put him under the cold-water treatment for a short time, and about the middle of March again applied a strong blister over the coronet up to the fetlock. This was washed off about the end of the month, and was succeeded by the cold water again. Towards the end of April there was no improvement at all, and I applied for permission to destroy the horse. This was carried out on April 27, at the recommendation of Mr. Gudgin, I.V.S., Aldershot, and a Board of veterinary surgeons.

'On making the post-mortem examination I first thought the bone was only partly fractured or cracked, but on manipulating it, after its being in hot water a short time, I saw the fracture was complete.'[A]

[Footnote A: S.W. Wilson, M.R.C.V.S., A.V.D., *Veterinary Journal*, vol. xv., p. 12.]

Treatment of Fractures of the Bones of the Foot.—It will be seen at once that in most cases anything in the way of bandaging is well-nigh useless. When the os coronæ is fractured, however, a little more may be added to the natural rigidity of the parts by enclosing the region of the pastern and the foot in a plaster-of-Paris bandage. The main treatment, however, in every case, will be a continual use of the slings for at least seven to eight weeks, by that means compelling the animal to give to the injured parts the necessary amount of rest.

With fracture of the os pedis, when such is caused by pricks and complicated by a flow of pus, then attention must be given to removal of the displaced piece of bone. The pus track is to be followed up with the searcher, sufficient horn removed with the knife, and the broken piece of bone removed with a scalpel and a pair of strong forceps, the operation to be afterwards followed up by antiseptic dressings to the opening. Until this is done the wound refuses to heal.

Fracture of the navicular bone, if in any way diagnosed with certainty, offers us an almost hopeless case, for it appears to be a commonly reported fact that attempts at reunion are rare. This, in all probability, is due to the pressure put upon it every now and again, when the animal's weight presses the bone between the os coronæ and the os pedis above and the perforans tendon below. Even should reunion take place, the resulting callus, interfering as it does with the movements of the perforans, leaves us a case of incurable lameness. When the

173

fracture is complicated by the formation of pus, as in the case of prick, then the case, with the attendant purulent synovitis and arthritis, is even more hopeless still.

Diagnosis of fracture of either of the bones of the foot is, as we have said before, extremely difficult. It so happens, therefore, in those cases caused by violent blows, that anything approaching an accurate opinion cannot be given until some months after the injury. After some time we are met with unmistakable changes in the form of the foot, and are able to assume that the persisting lameness is due to pressure of a reparative callus within the hoof. In such cases the only treatment of any use is that of neurectomy.

CHAPTER XII
DISEASES OF THE JOINTS[A]

[Footnote A: Properly speaking, we have in the foot of the horse but *one* joint— namely, the corono-pedal articulation.

Although not a joint in the strict sense of the word, we, nevertheless, intend here to consider the navicular bursa as such. In this apparatus, although we have no articular cartilage proper, and no apposition of bone to bone, we still have a large synovial cavity, and in close proximity to it bone. We may, in fact, and do get in it exactly similar changes to those termed 'synovitis' and 'arthritis' elsewhere. Therefore, we include the changes occurring in it in this chapter, and hence the plural use of the word to which this note refers.]

A. SYNOVITIS.

Definition.—By the term 'synovitis' is indicated an inflammation of the synovial membrane. It may be either (*a*) *Simple* or *Acute*, or it may be (*b*) *Purulent* or *Suppurative*.

In the simple form there is little or no tendency for the affection to implicate the other structures of the joint, whereas in the suppurative form the joint capsule, the ligaments, and the bones soon come to participate in the diseased processes, giving us a condition which we shall afterwards describe as acute arthritis.

(*a*) SIMPLE SYNOVITIS.

1. *Acute—(Causes).*—Simple or acute synovitis is nearly always brought about by injury to the joint—by blows or bruises, or by sprains of the ligaments. At other times it occurs without ascertainable cause, and is then put down to the influence of cold, or to poisonous materials (as, for example, that of rheumatism) circulating in the blood-stream.

Pathology.—Uncomplicated acute synovitis never causes death. The pathological changes in connection with it have therefore been studied in cases purposely induced, and the animal afterwards slaughtered. It is then found that, as in inflammation elsewhere, the synovial membrane is showing the usual inflammatory phenomena—that it is thick and swollen as a result of the inflammatory hyperæmia and commencing exudation. Later, the synovial fluid becomes increased in quantity, is thin and serous, and after a time is seen to be mixed with the inflammatory exudation poured into it. We then find that it has lost its clear appearance, has become thick and muddy, and has floating in it flakes of fibrin.

If the case progresses favourably these materials are soon absorbed and resolution occurs. In rarer cases the thickening and congestion of the membrane increases, and the articular capsule becomes so distended with the increased synovia and accumulated inflammatory discharges that a kind of chemosis occurs. In other words, there oozes through, without actual rupture of the membrane, a thin, blood-stained, and purulent-looking discharge.

It is an important point to note that in cases of synovitis the fringes of the synovial membrane become swollen and blood-injected, forming noticeable red elevations at the margins of the cartilages. It is then that the diseased condition soon spreads and runs into arthritis.

Further, it is important, especially with regard to the question of the degree of pain and lameness likely to be caused, to note that often granulations are thrown out upon the looser folds of the membrane. As these increase in size they come to form fringed and villous membranous projections inserting themselves between the bones forming the articulation. In such cases there is no doubt that the intense pain sometimes observed in these cases is due to pinching of these prolongations of the synovial membrane by the opposing bones of the joint.

Symptoms and Diagnosis.—Acute synovitis of a joint leads to heat of the parts, pain, distension of the capsule, and, where the joint may be easily felt, fluctuation. In the articulation with which we are dealing, however, these last two symptoms are not easily detected, for the surrounding structures—namely, the lateral and other ligaments of the joint, the extensor pedis tendon in front, and the perforans behind, together with the dense and comparatively unyielding nature of the skin of the parts—are such as to prevent distension and fluctuation becoming marked to a visible extent. We are able to diagnose the case as one of foot lameness, and, with a history of a severe blow or other injury, are able to assume that this condition, perhaps attended with periostitis, is in existence.

When other symptoms present themselves diagnosis may be more certain. The animal becomes slightly fevered, throbbing pains in the joint manifest themselves by irregular pawing movements on the part of the patient. The animal comes out from the stable stiff, even dead-lame, and the limb is carried with the lower joints semiflexed. The breathing is hurried and the pulse firm and frequent, while in a bad case patchy perspiration breaks out at intervals on various parts of the body. If with this we get a puffy and tender swelling in the hollow of the heel, our diagnosis may be certain at any rate as to the existence of joint trouble, although, from reasons we have given, we may not be able to mark its exact nature.

2. *Chronic.*—Simple synovitis may in many instances become chronic. In this case we have simply a pouring into the synovial capsule of serous fluid, and with it an increased quantity of synovia—this time with an absence of the usual inflammatory phenomena. Beyond the swelling of the capsule there is little to be noticed. The joint becomes perhaps a little weaker, but pain or tenderness and heat are entirely absent. Such a condition, by reason of the natural rigidity of the parts, is not to be observed in the foot, although at times it must most certainly occur. Examples of such a condition are to be found in bog-spavin, in hygroma of the stifle, and sometimes in the fetlock. From a study of these, we know that they may be induced by frequent attacks of acute synovitis, from repeated slight injuries or bruises, or from strains to the ligaments of the joint; or that they may be chronic from the outset. We know, too, that in such cases the synovial membrane becomes thickened, and that in places it may have extended somewhat over the edges of the articular cartilages. It is only fair to suppose that such changes occur also in the pedal articulation. In that case we may take it for certain that the natural rigidity of the surrounding structures has the effect of pushing the thickened membrane further between the bones of the joint than occurs in a like condition elsewhere, leading, of course, to a lameness that is marked in degree but occult as to cause.

In our minds there is no doubt that many of the occult and chronic forms of foot-lameness we meet with in practice are in this way to be accounted for. We may, in fact, explain them by suggesting either a chronic synovitis alone, or a synovitis complicated with periostitis.

Treatment of Synovitis.—If a joint has been injured, as we have suggested, by slight blows or other causes—in other words, if the injury is subcutaneous, and no wound is in existence—then there is no treatment which offers better results than does the continued application of cold.

At the same time, the animal should be slung, or, if non-excitable and inclined to rest, allowed at intervals to lie on a thick and comfortable straw bed, the cold fomentations during such intervals being discontinued. When the case is a marked one and the animal valuable, benefit will be derived from the application of crushed ice.

The animal's condition must be watched, and the case helped as far as is possible by the administration of a mild dose of physic, by saline drinks, and, when necessary, by the giving of small but repeated doses of Fleming's tincture of Aconite in order to relieve the pain. In a chronic case the repeated application of a blister is indicated.

(b) PURULENT OR SUPPURATIVE SYNOVITIS.

In this condition we have synovitis complicated by the presence of pus. Unlike the simple form, it shows a marked disposition to spread, and quickly involves the surrounding structures. Very soon the ligaments of the joint, the periosteum, the articular cartilages, and the bones are implicated. This, of course, constitutes a condition of acute purulent arthritis. Under that heading, therefore, the condition will be later discussed.

B. ARTHRITIS.

(a) SIMPLE OR SEROUS ARTHRITIS.

With an attack of simple synovitis it may be always assumed that the changes commenced in the synovial membrane, communicate themselves more or less readily to the surrounding tissues, and are not confined to the synovial membrane alone. We may thus have the inflammatory phenomena asserting themselves in the surrounding ligaments, in the periosteum, in the bone, and in the articular cartilages. It depends, in fact, upon the severity of our case whether we call it synovitis or arthritis. The two conditions merge so the one into the other that no hard-and-fast rule may be laid down whereby they may with certainty be differentiated. Such symptoms, therefore, as we have given for synovitis may be also read as indicating a condition of simple arthritis. The course of the case will be very similar, and the treatment to be followed identical with that just given.

(b) ACUTE ARTHRITIS.

Causes.—An attack of acute arthritis may commence with the affection of the synovial membrane, and spread from that to the other structures. In other cases the disease of the synovial membrane, and after it the disease of the joint, may be secondary to diseases commencing in the structures around the joint. This affection may therefore follow on a case of acute coronitis, a case of suppurating corn, a case of quittor, a severe case of tread, or may attend a case of laminitis.

Symptoms.—In our cases we get very little beyond a magnification of such symptoms as we have described under acute synovitis. The heat and the pain is perhaps greater, and the lameness more marked. It is rather to the constitutional disturbance we must look, however, for a confirmation of our opinion that arthritis is in existence. This is always severe, and of an acute febrile nature. The pulse is fast, thin, and thready, the respirations enormously increased, and the temperature high. The appetite is in abeyance, the animal quickly becomes what is termed 'tucked-up,' or greyhound-like, in the body, and patchy perspirations break out about him. The limb is held with the joints all semiflexed, and severe and intense throbbing pains are indicated by the frequent pawing movements the animal makes in the air. Manipulation of the foot is resented, and the agonizing intensity of the pain so caused is shown by the drawn and haggard appearance of the eyes.

In a favourable case the symptoms from now onwards may gradually subside. The appetite returns, the breathing and other signs of disturbance show a return to the normal, weight is placed on the limb, and resolution slowly but surely takes place. In many of these, our favourable cases, however, resolution is incomplete, and recovery only takes place at the expense of anchylosis of the joint, a condition we shall refer to later.

In unfavourable cases, and these unfortunately are only too common, the condition terminates in suppuration.

(c) PURULENT OR SUPPURATIVE ARTHRITIS.

Definition.—By this term we indicate an arthritis complicated by the formation of pus within the joint.

Causes.—The organisms of pus may infect the joint by extension of a suppurating process from without. For example, in the case of a suppurating corn, in quittor, in tread, or in the case of a suppurating wound caused by a prick, the pus formed may in many instances be very near the capsular ligament of the articulation. Under such circumstances, unless there is a free and unhindered flow of the pus from an outside opening, inroads will be made by it upon the thin capsule. The latter is quickly penetrated, and pus is admitted to the interior of the joint.

In other cases infection of the joint may proceed from within, from a poisoned state of the blood-stream. The condition occurs, for instance, in bad attacks of laminitis. We ourselves, too, have seen two cases where suppuration of the pedal articulation occurred in the septic pyæmia of foals, a disease known commonly as 'joint-ill,' and characterized by an

176

infected state of the circulation. Cases have also come under our notice where this condition has resulted from slight injuries in the region of the insertion of the extensor pedis inflicted by the animal himself when galloping away.

Perhaps, however, the most common cause of suppurative arthritis in the foot is direct penetration of the articulation in the case of pricks. The penetrating object is nearly always dirty—bacterially dirty, at any rate—and suppuration only too readily commences. Even should such a wound be inflicted by an aseptic body, infection would quickly ensue as a result of the wound gathering dirt from the ground, or even from admission to the joint of impure and bacilli-laden air.

Symptoms and Diagnosis.—This is one of the most serious conditions we are called upon to face when dealing with diseases of the foot, for in many cases it quickly ends in exhaustion and death of the patient, while in even the most favourable cases nothing better than a condition of complete and bony anchylosis is to be expected. The owner, therefore, should be warned accordingly.

As in the other joint affections, so here, we get all the symptoms of acute febrile constitutional disturbance. The pulse, the temperature, the respirations, and the general haggard, 'tucked-up,' and distressed appearances of the animal all tell too plain a tale. Our patient is in constant pain, and the seat of the trouble is clearly enough shown by the constant pawing movements of the affected foot. If he has room to get up and down in comfort the animal adopts for long periods at a stretch the recumbent position, and is not upon his legs long enough to take the necessary amount of food to keep him going. Even when down, it is plain to see that the animal is not at rest. The pawing movement is still maintained with the foot, and every now and again the eyes are opened and the headed lifted to give a troubled look round. The appetite, too, is capricious, and in many cases almost entirely lost.

In some slight degree the condition is less to be feared in a fore than in a hind foot— that is, so far as absolutely fatal results are concerned. With the condition confined to one fore-foot, the animal is able to get up and down with a moderate degree of comfort. At intervals, therefore, he rises to take nourishment, and as soon as his wants are satisfied again lies down.

With the disease in a hind-foot matters are not taken so comfortably. The patient finds that with each day's increasing weakness the difficulty that at first he had to raise himself with only one sound hind-foot becomes enormously increased. The consequence is that he fears to go down, and the standing position is maintained until sheer weakness overcomes him, and he goes down, not to rise again without assistance.

If judiciously attended he is, of course, put in slings before this stage is reached; but there are instances, as in the case of a cart-mare heavy with foal, where the use of slings is most decidedly contra-indicated.

If doubt before existed as to the nature of the case, it is at a later stage dispelled by the appearance, generally in the hollow of the heel, of a hot and painful swelling. This at first is hard, but later fluctuates. Finally it breaks at one or more spots, and there exudes from the opening or openings a purulent and oftentimes sanious discharge, which coagulates about each fistula after the manner of ordinary synovia.

With the discharge of the abscess contents there is some slight improvement in the symptoms. Here, with a suitable treatment, and with a patient of a particularly robust constitution, the case appears to turn, and slowly but surely progresses towards the only end we can hope for—namely, a more or less painless anchylosis of the articulation.

In less favourable cases the purulent discharge continues, and (always a bad sign) becomes more or less chocolate-like in colour, distinctly thin, and stinking. The diseased process spreads until the ligaments of the joint, both by reason of their infiltration with the inflammatory discharges, and also on account of the ravages made on them by the invading pus, either greatly stretch or altogether rupture.

The joint, after its ligaments have been destroyed in this manner, is loosened, and the bones are now freely movable. Their manipulation gives to the touch a sickening, grating sound—in other words, we have crepitus. This, of course, indicates that the articular cartilages have become greatly eroded by the inflammatory process, and so left what we may term 'raw' surfaces of bone to rub together. When the animal is put to the walk the toe of the foot is elevated, and the extreme mobility of the foot gives one the idea of fracture. With every step there is a peculiar sucking noise, comparable to that of a foot moving in a boot of water, and putrescent matter is squeezed from every opening each time the foot is put to the ground. Although we have seen cases even advanced thus far recover, it is questionable whether it is now wise to attempt to prolong life. Slaughter is far more humane, and, in our opinion, except with a valuable brood animal, more economical.

If the animal is allowed to linger, other symptoms will nearly always present themselves before death occurs. Whether in slings or not, a careful watch should be kept upon the sound limb. For some time the patient stands upon it incessantly, but sooner or later it happens that a farther visit show us the animal standing with full weight on the diseased foot, and making painful pawing movements with what before was the sound. We immediately jump to the conclusion 'laminitis.' And so it is, but it is a laminitis brought about by pyæmia. This is indicated by the swollen and oedematous nature of the lymphatics of the limb. Plainly enough they indicate the road by which the poison has travelled. It is in this way: Pus and putrefactive organisms have gained entrance to the lymphatics of the original diseased limb. From these they have rapidly gained the blood-stream and set up infection elsewhere. In this particular instance it is demonstrated by the laminitis and lymphangitis of the previously sound limb. With the poison thus circulating in the blood-stream, we often also get spots of infection commenced in one or other of the more vital organs—notably the lungs or the kidneys. The end of our case is then either a gangrenous pneumonia or complications induced by a condition of widespread pyæmia.

With the animal in slings there are one or two other symptoms that call for attention. In many cases, especially with animals of a lymphatic and indolent nature, the use made of them is inordinate. The patient rests so continually in them that alarming swellings commence to make their appearance about the rectum, or in the case of a mare about the vulva. The animal must then be let down at regular intervals and again raised when rest is obtained.

A more alarming symptom still is when the animal, instead of resting in the slings by his buttocks, casts his weight bodily into the belly-rest and hangs with a heavy head into the head-stall. This indicates complete exhaustion and a wish for death. Matters should therefore be explained to the owner, and his consent obtained for immediate destruction.

Pathology.—The pathological changes occurring in suppurative arthritis we shall pass over briefly. It is almost sufficient, in fact, to say that the whole of the joint becomes completely disorganized.

The synovial membrane becomes so tremendously thickened and injected as to be scarcely recognisable as such, the thickening in the later stages being due to large growths of granulation tissue which entirely alter the appearance of the membrane as we know it normally. In the early stages the contents of the joint are composed of thin pus and synovia. Later, as destruction of the synovial membrane proceeds, the flow of synovia is stopped, while the pus formation goes on until finally nothing but pus and dead tissue products fill the cavity.

If the suppurative process has commenced from within, the pus that is formed is, as a rule, thick and creamy, comparatively unstained, and free from marked odour. If, on the other hand, air has gained access to the joint, or the suppurative process has started from the materials introduced by a foreign body, the joint contents are thin, blood-stained, and stinking.

The inflammatory changes in the joint soon spread to the ligaments, and to the soft structures in contact with them. This means that the ligaments become infiltrated with inflammatory exudate, that the fibrous bundles composing them become separated, and that the ligaments are weakened and easily stretched. As a consequence, a certain amount of displacement or dislocation of the bones is allowed.

In like manner the inflammatory changes keep spreading until we have the periosteum next the ends of the bones affected. The periostitis thus set up invariably takes the osteoplastic form, and as a result of this we have growths of new bone in the near neighbourhood of the joint. It is in the later stages of the disease—that is, when the pus has been evacuated and reparative changes commenced—that this osteoplastic periostitis is most marked, and it plays a large part in bringing about the condition of anchylosis, which we shall afterwards describe.

Grave changes also occur in the articular cartilages. They quickly lose their peculiar glistening polish, their semitransparency is lost, and the natural tint of a pearl-like blue gives way to a dirty yellow. Later this is followed by erosion of the cartilages at such points as they happen to be in greatest contact. The ends of the bones are thus exposed, and their medullary cavities exposed to infection. As a result we get in them the changes we have already described under Ostitis.

Treatment—(a) Preventive.—Seeing that many of these cases have their starting-point in stabs or penetrating wounds of the sole, we shall be concerned first with a consideration of the correct treatment to be adopted when we know the wound to have reached the articulation.

Only too frequently the treatment practised is that of poulticing. In other portions of this work we have pointed out the advantages that a continued antiseptic bathing has over the application of a poultice, the greater readiness with which the solution comes into contact with the deeper parts of the wound, and the far greater chance there is of maintaining water in an antiseptic condition than there is of keeping a poultice in the same state. There is no doubt, that in this case also, the cold or warm antiseptic bath is to be preferred to the poultice. It is questionable, however, whether even the bath is sufficient for our purpose here. We have in this case a deep punctured wound, and a wound that in every probability is infected with the organisms of pus or of putrefaction. It is a wound, moreover, which is likely to impede the thorough access to it of the solution in which the foot is fomented, on account of the flakes of coagulated fibrin which fill it.

The most rational treatment, therefore, if we get to the case early enough, is to irrigate the wound freely with a solution of carbolic acid in water (1 in 20), or with a solution of perchloride of mercury (1 in 1,000), injected by means of a glass syringe, or the pattern of syringe devised for quittor. This injecting should be done thoroughly, and by that we mean that several syringefuls of the solution should be injected, the joint after each injection being manipulated so as to distribute the solution as far as possible over it. When this is done the opening in the sole may be plugged with a little perchloride of mercury, or, better still, with a little piece of tow saturated with a concentrated solution of perchloride of mercury or a solution of iodoform in alcohol and an antiseptic pad of tow or lint placed over all. The foot should then be bandaged and encased in a boot or sacking protective. The bandage should be removed daily and the antiseptic pad changed. At each visit the animal's condition must be carefully noted. So long as constitutional disturbance is slight, the foot appears comfortable, is free from marked heat and tenderness, and pawing movements are absent, and so long as the discharge on the pad appears non-purulent, free from marked odour, and small in quantity, then this dressing may be persisted in.

This treatment of open joint, preventive as it is of arthritis, is also indicated in the case of open navicular bursa. In several instances we have practised this treatment for the dressing of wounds implicating the bursæ of tendons and the capsules of joints. It is also spoken of favourably by Mr. C.H. Flynn in the *American Veterinary Review* for June, 1888, whose treatment is as follows: 'Place the patient in a clean, well-ventilated, and drained stable. Have all the litter removed, and insist on the stall being kept clean. Either place the animal in slings, or tie the head so as to prevent lying down. Clip the hair and cleanse the parts well. He prefers the corrosive sublimate solution (1 in 1,000). Should the wound be of two or more days' standing, inject the joint with the corrosive sublimate solution. Now dry the parts with a clean towel and sprinkle the wound with iodoform. Over this place a thick layer of absorbent cotton-wool, filled with iodoform, bandage securely, and keep the patient on a moderate diet, preserving the utmost quietude possible. Should the bandage remain in position and the animal free from pain, leave the bandage and dressing in place from five days to a week. Then change it, and should the discharge be little, do not disturb it, but renew the iodoform and cotton dressing, leaving it on for another week.'

Other treatments for the same condition are practised, in which the wound is dusted with powdered iodoform, with potassium permanganate, or with corrosive sublimate, or

179

where the wound, instead of being dusted, has the corrosive sublimate applied in the form of a plug. In each case the preliminary irrigation with the corrosive sublimate solution is dispensed with. This, however, should on no account be omitted. In our opinion it constitutes the very essence of the rationality of the treatment.

(b) Curative.—It may happen, however, and often does, that this first injection of an antiseptic is unsuccessful in preventing organismal infection of the wound. In this case grave constitutional disturbance and other untoward symptoms such as we have already described quickly make their appearance.

The animal should now be placed in slings and preparations made for actively treating the wound with antiseptics. Whether we fail or not, we have the satisfaction of knowing that we have given to the patient the best and the only chance of recovery.

It should be remembered, however, and should be pointed out to the owner, that with purulent arthritis fully developed, with the grave constitutional changes it occasions, and with the ever-present danger of a general septic invasion of the blood-stream, that the human surgeon under such circumstances offers to his patient the alternatives of amputation or probable death. With us no such alternative is possible. It is either return the joint to some semblance of its former usefulness, or destroy the patient.

In this case we advise the injection of the original wound, and also such fistulous openings as may have formed, with the 1 in 1,000 sublimate solution. Also, in order to avoid the sometimes abortive attempts of the antiseptic pad, to maintain a condition of asepsis around the wound, we advise the continual soaking of the whole foot in a cold antiseptic bath. This may be either carbolic acid 1 in 20, or—what is less volatile, perhaps more effectual, and certainly more economical—perchloride of mercury 1 in 1,000.

It has been our good fortune, even when we have seen the foot almost detached from the limb by the devastating inroads of the pus, to see the suppurative process by this means gradually overcome, a reparative anchylosis set in, and the animal restored to good health and usefulness, if not to soundness.

Once the suppurative process is checked and anchylosis commences, it is good treatment to smartly blister the whole of the region of the coronet, the pastern, and the wound itself with a mixed blister of cantharides and biniodide of mercury, repeated at intervals of a fortnight. This prevents to some extent further infection of the wound, and assists also in promoting the changes that tend to anchylosis.

(d) ANCHYLOSIS.

The word anchylosis signifies the stiffening of a joint. When one has read the serious changes occurring within the joint in the more serious forms of arthritis, it is easy to understand how it comes about. In suppurative arthritis, for instance, we have the synovial membrane destroyed, the articular cartilages partly or wholly obliterated, and the former boundaries of the joint entirely lost. If the animal lives, nature is bound to make repair of a sort. The synovial membrane and the articular cartilages utterly destroyed, as we have described, cannot again be replaced. Nature can only build again from such materials as are left to her. In this case the material is bone.

It must be remembered, however, that often the bone has been so diseased that spots of necrosis or caries within it are bound to remain unless moved by operative interference. Such diseased portions, when dealing with the foot, are beyond reach of the surgeon's knife, and we have no alternative but to allow them to remain. We get, therefore, in many cases, a condition of rarefactive ostitis occurring side by side with a slowly progressive caries within the bone, while outside is occurring an osteoplastic periostitis. The concurrence of these conditions leads in time to great increase in size of the parts, together with increasing anchylosis and deformity.

C. NAVICULAR DISEASE.

Definition.—Chronic inflammatory changes occurring in connection with the navicular bursa, affecting variously the bursa itself, the perforans tendon, or the navicular bone, and characterized by changes in the form of the hoof and persisting lameness. The disease is commonly noticed in thoroughbreds or in horses of the lighter breeds, and is but seldom observed in heavy cart animals. Usually it is met with in one or both fore-feet. Although of extremely rare occurrence, it has been noticed in the hind.

180

History.—To English veterinarians appears to belong the credit of discovering navicular disease. As early as 1752 we find one, Jeremiah Bridges, in 'No Foot, No Horse,' drawing attention to 'coffin-joint lameness,' and advocating for its treatment setoning of the frog. It appears, too, that Moorcroft, prior to his departure for India in 1808, was acquainted with what was then known as coffin-joint[A] lameness, having drawn attention to it in 1804 in a letter to Sir Edward Codrington.[B] In 1819 Moorcroft made it even plainer still that he was fully acquainted with what we now know as navicular disease. This we learn from a letter written by him to Sewell, in which he laid claim to being the originator of neurectomy. In this letter he says:

[Footnote A: The coffin-joint at this time included the navicular bursa.]

[Footnote B: Percival's 'Hippopathology,' vol. iv., p. 132.]

'On dissecting feet affected with these lamenesses, the flexor tendon was now and then observed to have been broken, partially or entirely, but more commonly to have been bruised and inflamed in its course under the navicular or shuttle bone, or at its insertion into the bone of the foot. Sometimes, although seldom, the navicular bone itself has been found to have been fractured; at others its surface has been deprived of its usual coating, and studded with projecting points or ridges of new growth, or exhibiting superficial excavations more or less extensive.'[A]

[Footnote A: *Ibid.*]

Pathology and Point of Commencement of the Disease.—The exact position in which the diseased process starts has for a long time been a subject of discussion, and even now it is doubtful whether the point has been definitely settled. To mention but a few among many: We find Mr. Broad, of Bath, strenuously insisting on the fact that the disease commences in the interior of the navicular bone. Just as strenuously we find the editor of the journal in which the matter is being discussed, the late Mr. Fleming, asserting that the disease commences in the bursa.[A] Others, too, hold that the disease commences primarily in the tendon. Wedded to this view was the discoverer, Mr. Turner, of Croydon; while Percival commits himself to the statement that it is either the central ridge or the postero-inferior surface of the navicular bone, or the opposed concavity in the perforans tendon, that shows the earliest signs of the disease. The observations made by Dr. Brauell, the first Continental writer to fully describe the disease, led him to the statement that neither the bone nor the bursa was the *invariable* starting-point of the trouble, but that usually it commenced in inflammation of the bursa itself.

[Footnote A: Percival's 'Hippopathology,' vol. iv., p. 132.]

Without, therefore, committing ourselves to an expression of opinion as to the precise starting-point of the affection, we shall describe the pathological changes occurring in navicular disease as noted in (1) the bursa, (2) the cartilage, (3) the tendon, and (4) the bone.

1. *Changes in the Bursa.*—Upon the internal surface of the bursal membrane is first noticed a slight inflammatory hyperæmia, accompanied by more or less swelling and tumefaction, owing to its infiltration with inflammatory exudate. The portion covering the hyaline cartilage of the navicular bone has lost its peculiar pearl-blue shimmer, and become a dirty yellow.

Remembering that the bursal membrane is a synovia-secreting one, and bearing in mind what happens in ordinary synovitis and arthritis (with which, of course, this may be very closely compared), we shall first expect changes in the bursal contents. It is highly probable, though difficult of proof, that in the very early stages the chronic inflammatory stimulus has the effect of increasing the flow of synovia. In every case, however, where it can with any certainty be said that navicular disease exists, it is too late to meet with this condition. The disease has then progressed until destruction of the secreting layer of the bursal membrane has been seriously interfered with, and in this case we find a distinct deficiency in the quantity of synovia in the bursa. In advanced cases it is even found that the bursa is *absolutely dry*.

2. *Changes in the Cartilage.*—Directly that portion of the bursal membrane covering the cartilage is the subject of inflammatory change, the cartilage itself, by reason of its low vitality, soon suffers.

Under a process, which we may term 'dry ulcerative,' the cartilage covering the ridge on the lower surface of the bone commences to become eroded, and in appearance has been likened, both by English and Continental writers, to a piece of wood that has been worm-eaten (see Fig. 161).

FIG. 161.—NAVICULAR BONE (POSTERO-INFERIOR SURFACE) SHOWING THE 'WORM-EATEN' APPEARANCE CAUSED BY EROSION OF THE HYALINE CARTILAGE, AND COMMENCING RAREFACTIVE ARTHRITIS.

'At this stage, or much earlier'—we are quoting Colonel Smith, A.V.D.—'may be found calcareous deposits in the fibro-cartilage and the bone. They are scattered like fine sand here and there, generally across the inferior half of the face of the bone; they are sometimes numerous, frequently scanty, occasionally entirely absent. The amount of calcareous degeneration depends upon the lesions present. If much destruction of bone exists, there will be but few calcareous deposits; whilst if there are many calcareous deposits, there may be but slight ulceration of bone tissue, and perhaps none at all. In fact, I have held the opinion, and see no reason to modify it, that calcareous deposits are safeguards against caries.'[A]

[Footnote A: *Journal of Comparative Pathology and Therapeutics*, vol. vi., p. 195.]

3. *Changes in the Tendon.*—The effect of these calcareous deposits on the under surface of the bone is to produce a certain amount of roughness. Seeing that with every movement of the foot the perforans tendon is called upon to glide over this surface, it is clear that a secondary effect must be that of inducing erosion and destruction of the tendon. The point at which this usually commences is at the bottom of the depression that accommodates the ridge on the bone. With erosion of the cartilage and of the tendon at points exactly opposite each other, we have two surfaces come together that are prone to readily unite, and fibrous tissue adhesions often take place between the bone and the tendon. In some measure this accounts for the torn and ragged appearance of the tendon. Adhesions take place, and, under some small strain, are broken down. This may happen more than once or twice, and with each breaking of the adhesion between the bone and tendon, fibres from the latter are lacerated and torn from their place (see Fig. 162).

4. *Changes in the Bone.*—The changes occurring in the bone are essentially those of a rarefactive ostitis. These changes are described by many writers, and, whether originating primarily in the bone or not, it seems certain that extensive changes may have occurred within the bone, with but little or nothing to be noted on its outer surface. It would seem that the first change is one of congestion of the vessels of the bone's cancellous tissue. With the cause, whatever it may be, in constant operation, the congestion persists until a low type of inflammation is set up, interfering, not only with the flow of synovia in the adjoining bursa, but with the nutrition of the bone itself. As the disease progresses, there is softening and enlarging of the cancelled tissue towards the centre of the bone. The cells break up, and absorption takes place. This goes on until a large portion of the interior of the bone is in a state of dry necrosis, with, in many cases, but slight signs of mischief on the exterior of the bone.

In other cases, however, the changes in the interior of the bone are accompanied by well-marked lesions on its gliding or postero-inferior surface, and by evidences of an osteoplastic periostitis along its edges.

That an osteoplastic periostitis has been in existence is witnessed by the appearance along the edges of the bone of numerous outgrowths of bone, termed osteophytes (see Fig. 163).

FIG. 162.—A FOOT WITH THE SEAT OF NAVICULAR DISEASE EXPOSED. On the anterior surface of the perforans fibres of the tendon are seen to be torn away from their abnormal adhesion with the navicular bone, while others are seen to be still attached thereto. The surface of the navicular bone itself exhibits small defects in the bony substance, which have been brought about by a rarefactive ostitis. *a*, The perforans tendon cut through and reflected; *b*, the sole.

The interosseous and postero-lateral ligaments of the articulation often participate in the inflammatory changes, and in many cases become completely ossified. The true articulatory surface of the bone, that articulating with the os pedis and with the os coronæ, is never affected.

Causes.—In enumerating the causes of navicular disease, we shall follow the example of Colonel Smith and classify them under certain headings—namely, (1) *Hereditary Predisposition*; (2) *Compression*; (3) *Concussion*; (4) *A Weak Navicular Bone*; (5) *A Defective or Irregular Blood-supply to the Bone*; and (6) *Senile Decay.*

FIG. 163.—THE NAVICULAR BONE FROM A CASE OF LONG-STANDING NAVICULAR DISEASE. The erosion of the cartilage on its central ridge is most marked, and the porous appearance of the bone thus uncovered points to the existence within it of a rarefactive ostitis. Along its edges large osteophytic outgrowths speak of the effects of an osteoplastic periostitis.

1. *Hereditary Predisposition.*—That navicular disease is hereditary is a fact that has for a long time been insisted on, and has come to be so generally admitted that we do not intend to dwell on it here. As we have said before, it is found in the lighter breeds of horses (and, according to Zundel, especially in the English breeds), and is there seen to be frequently transmitted from parent to offspring.

2. *Compression.*—By this is meant the compression of the navicular bone between the os pedis and the os coronæ in front, and the perforans tendon behind.

In order to appreciate this explanation of the causation of navicular disease at its true value, it will be well to consider briefly the physiology of the parts in question.

The navicular bone is what we may term a complement of the os pedis. It exists, in fact, simply in order that the os coronæ may have a sufficiently large articulatory surface to play upon. One wonders at first that Nature did not arrive at this by originally placing a larger bone below. Colonel Smith explains this by suggesting that this would in all probability have meant its fracture. In progression the hind part of the foot comes to the ground first, and upon the hinder portion of the articulation would fall the first effects of concussion, together with the greater part of the body-weight. A yielding joint was in this position necessary, and that formed by the navicular bone fills all requirements.

In this connection one next considers the part played by the front limbs during progression. As Zundel expresses it, they are columns of support rather than of impulsion, and, as the body-weight is thrown forward by the hind-limbs, it is the duty of the fore-limbs to receive it. The shock or concussion of the body-weight thus thrown forwards is first received by the muscles uniting the limb to the trunk, and a great part of it there minimized by their sling-like attachment. It is further absorbed by the shoulder-joint, and from there passed on to the almost vertical bony column represented by the radius and ulna, the knee, and the metacarpus. On reaching the first phalanx, a portion of the remaining force is passed on to the front of the phalanges and loses itself in front of the hoof, while the other portion is transmitted to the flexor tendons, finally to the perforans, and to the posterior parts of the foot. During progression, therefore, the navicular bone is constantly pushed downwards and backwards by the bony column, and is just as constantly pushed forwards and upwards by the resistance of the perforans tendon. This means, of course, that the navicular bone is more or less constantly subject to compression, and constant pressure, as we know full well, is a pretty sure factor in bringing about malnutrition of the parts, with atrophy or chronic inflammatory changes as an end result.

Even with the limb at rest the pressure on both sides of the navicular bone is still constant. The only circumstances under which we can conceive of it being entirely absent, in fact, are when the tension on the tendon is relaxed, and the body-weight altogether removed by the animal adopting the recumbent position.

The compression theory as to the causation of navicular disease was, we believe, first originated by Colonel Smith. He, at any rate, has laid much stress on it in his writings. If we accept it, and we see every reason that we should, then we must, with the author, admit the possibility of navicular disease arising from long standing in one position.

3. *Concussion.*—This we are bound to admit as a cause, and in so doing partly explain the comparative, almost total, immunity of the hind-feet from the disease. The fore-limbs, as we have already pointed out, are little more than props of support, and the force of the propelled body-weight is transmitted largely down their almost vertical lines, to end largely in concussion in the foot. With the hind-limbs matters are different. 'These,' as Percival explains it, 'have their bones obliquely placed, so as to constitute, one with the other, so many obtuse angles, to the end, that by forming powerful levers, and affording every advantage for action to the muscles attached to them, they may be fitted for the purpose of propulsion of the body onward.'

The effect of these several obtuse-angled joints in the limb is to absorb the greater part of the force exerted by the body-weight before it reaches the foot. When with this we take the facts that the fore-limbs have to carry the head and neck, and that they have to bear this added weight, plus a propelling force from behind, we see why it is that they should be so subject to the disease, and the hind-limbs so exempt.

As pointing out the part that concussion plays in its causation, we may mention that navicular disease is a disease of the middle-aged and the worked animal. It is interesting to note, too, that it occurs in animals with well developed frogs—in feet in which frog-pressure with the ground is most marked. This at first sight appears to flatly contradict what we have said with regard to frog-pressure in other portions of this work. With this, however, must be reckoned other predisposing causes. In this case it is not to frog-pressure alone we must look, but to the condition of the frog itself, and that of the neighbouring parts. It is when we have a frog which, though well developed and apparently satisfying all demands as to size and build, is at the same time composed of a hard, dry, and non-yielding horn that we must look for trouble.

The foot predisposed to navicular disease is the strong, round, short-toed or clubby foot, open at the heels, with a sound frog jutting prominently out between them. Here is a frog exposed to all the pressure that might be desired for it, bounded at its sides by heels thick and strong, and indisposed to yield, and itself liable, from its very exposure, to become, in the warm stable, hard and dry, and incompressible' (Percival).

Here, instead of acting, as normally it should, as a resilient body, and an aid to the absorption of concussion, it seems rather to play the part of a foreign body, and to bring concussion about. Seeing, then, that the navicular bursa is in very near contact with it, it is conceivable that this joint-like apparatus should suffer, and the pedal articulation be left unaffected, the more so when we take into consideration the compression theory just described.

4. *A Weak Navicular Bone.*—When the disease commences first in the bone—and there is no denying the fact that sometimes, although not invariably, it does—it may be explained by attributing to the structure of the bone an abnormal weakness in build.

The navicular bone consists normally of compact and cancellated tissue arranged in certain proportions, the compact tissue without, and the cancellated within. These proportions can only be judged of by the examinations of sections of the bone, and when it is found in any case that the cancellated tissue bulks more largely in the formation of the bone than normally it should, we have what we may term a weak navicular bone. In this connection Colonel Smith says: 'Though it is far from present in every case of the disease, still I consider it a factor of great importance.'

5. *A Defective or Irregular Blood-supply to the Bone.*—This, Colonel Smith considers, is brought about by excessive and irregular work, and by the opposite condition—rest. The author points out that the bloodvessels passing to and from the navicular bone run in the substance of the interosseous ligaments, or in such proximity to them that it is conceivable that under certain circumstances mechanical interference may occur to the navicular circulation. He further points out a fact that is, of course, well known to every veterinarian, that in periods of work the circulation of the foot is hurried, and that in rest there is always a tendency to congestion; and he says in conclusion: 'I cannot help thinking that irregularities in the blood-supply in a naturally weak bone must be a factor of some importance, especially when the kind of work the horse is performing is a series of vigorous efforts followed by rest.'

6. *Senile Decay.*—With approaching age the various tissues lose their vigour, and are prone to disease. The navicular bone and surrounding structures are not exempt. With the other and more active causes we have described acting at the same time it is not surprising that navicular disease is seen as a result.

In conclusion, it is well, perhaps, to say that, no matter to which particular theory of causation we may lean, we should make up our minds to consider them as a whole. While one cause may be exciting, the other may be predisposing, and the two must act together before evil results are noticed. It may be that even more than two are concerned in bringing on the disease, and to each the careful veterinarian will give due consideration.

Symptoms and Diagnosis.—In the early stages of navicular disease the symptoms are obscure. Pointing of the affected limb is the first evidence the animal gives. This, however, more often than not, goes unnoticed, and the first symptom usually observed by the owner or attendant is the lameness. Even this is such as to at first occasion no alarm, being intermittent and slight, and only very gradually becoming marked. In a few cases, however, lameness will come on suddenly, and is excessive from the commencement. It is the lameness, slow in its onset, intermittent in its character, and gradual in its progress, however, that is ordinarily characteristic of navicular disease.

The animal is taken out from the stable sound, with just a vague suspicion, perhaps, that he moved a bit stiffly. While out he is thought by his driver or rider to be going feelingly with one foot or with both. Even this is not marked, and the driver has some difficulty in assuring himself whether or no he really observed it, or whether it was but imagination.

On the return home the limb is examined, and nothing abnormal is to be found. The leg is of its normal appearance, and neither heat nor tenderness is to be observed in it or in the foot. On the following day the animal again is sound, and the lameness of the previous day is put down to a slight strain or something equally simple. The patient is then, perhaps, rested for a day or two. When next he is worked he again moves out from the stable sound, but again during the going gives the driver the unpleasant impression that something is amiss; and so the case goes on. One day the owner fears the animal is becoming seriously enough affected to warrant him in calling in his veterinary surgeon; the next he is confidently assuring himself that nothing is wrong.

Perhaps the animal is now rested for a week or two, or even for a month or two, hoping that this will put him sound. Immediately on commencing work, however, the same symptoms as before assert themselves, and the veterinary surgeon is called in.

With a history such as we have given the veterinarian's suspicions are aroused. He has the animal trotted, and may notice at this stage that there is an inclination to go on the toes, that the lame limb or limbs are not put forward freely, and that progression is stilty and uncertain; it is such, in fact, as to at once suggest the possibility of corns being present.

In some cases there is just the suspicion of a limp with one limb, and this only at intervals during the trot. At one moment the veterinarian is positive that he sees the animal going lame; at another he is just as confident he sees him coming towards him sound.

Nothing is found in the limb—neither heat, tenderness, nor swelling. There is nothing in the gait (either a limited movement of the radius, or a circular sweep with the leg) to indicate shoulder or other lameness, and the veterinary surgeon, by eliminative evidence, is bound to conclude that the trouble is in the foot.

The foot is then examined—pared, percussed, pinched, and in other ways manipulated—but nothing further is forthcoming. In such a case the veterinary surgeon is wise to declare the abortive result of his examination, to hint darkly of his suspicions, and to suggest a second examination at some future date. It may be that two, three, four, or even more, such examinations are necessary before he can justly pronounce a positive verdict.

Later he is enabled to do this by an increase in the severity of the symptoms, and by the changes that take place in the form of the foot. The lameness is now more marked, and the 'pointing' in the stable more frequent. With regard to the latter symptom, it has been seriously discussed whether the horse with navicular disease points with the heel elevated or with it pressed to the ground. In either case, of course, the limb is advanced; but while some hold that the phalangeal articulations are flexed and the heel slightly raised, in order to relieve the pressure of the perforans tendon on the affected area, and so obtain ease, there are others who hold that the heel is pressed firmly to the ground in order to deaden the pain. It may be, and most probably is, that both are right; but, in our opinion, there is no doubt whatever that pointing with the heel elevated is by far the most common.

The lameness is now excessive, and is especially noticeable when the animal is put to work on a rough or on a hard ground. Even now, however, heat of the foot or tenderness is so slight as to be out of all proportion to the alteration in gait.

With the case thus far advanced, evidence of pain may be obtained by pressing with the thumb in the hollow of the heel. Evidence of pain may also be obtained by using the farrier's pincers on the frog. These methods, however, are never wholly satisfactory, as a horse with the soundest of feet will sometimes flinch under these manipulations.

Extreme and forcible flexion of the corono-pedal articulation also sometimes gives evidence of tenderness. In this case the foot is held up, the animal's metacarpus resting on the operator's knee, and the toe of the hoof pushed downwards with some degree of force.

The same movement of the joint is given by causing the animal to put full weight upon the diseased limb, a small wedge of wood being first placed under the toe. In this manner the pressure of the perforans tendon upon the bursa is greatly increased, and the animal is caused to show symptoms of distress.

The lameness may also be increased, and diagnosis helped, by paring the heels, so as to leave the frog prominent and take the whole of the body-weight. The same end is also obtained by applying a bar shoe. This was originally pointed out by Brauell, and is quoted by Zundel and by Möller.

The changes in the form of the hoof may now be noticed. These are largely dependent on the fact that more or less constantly the patient saves the heel. The horn of the walls in this region, and the horn of the frog, is thereby put out of action and induced to atrophy. The hoof gradually assumes a more upright shape, and the heels contract. We thus get a hoof which is visibly narrowed from side to side, with a frog that is atrophied and often thrushy, and with a sole that is abnormally concave, hard, and affected with corns.

When occurring in the hind-feet—a condition that is rare, but which has been noticed by Loiset, and quoted by Zundel—the animal is stiff behind, walks on his toes, and gives one the impression that he is suffering from some affection in the region of the loins.

One such case is reported by an English veterinary surgeon, and we quote it here:

'A gray gelding, and a capital hunter, the property of a gentleman in this neighbourhood, became lame in the near fore-foot after the hunting season of 1859. The lameness was believed to be due to navicular disease. The operation of neurectomy was ultimately had recourse to. The horse subsequently did his work as well as ever, and was ridden to hounds regularly till the end of the year 1861, when he went lame of the off fore-foot. From this date he also showed very peculiar action behind, and was at times lame of both hind-limbs without any apparent cause.

'In the year 1862, from the groom's indiscreet use of physic, super-purgation was brought on which caused the animal's death. On a post-mortem examination being made, the horse was found to have *navicular disease of all four feet*. It is worthy of note that this horse had always "extravagant" action behind, but was a remarkably quick and good jumper.'[A]

[Footnote A: F. Blakeway, M.R.C.V.S., *Veterinarian*, vol. ii., p. 21.]

Differential Diagnosis.—Navicular disease may be mistaken for ordinary contracted foot. It will be remembered, however, that in the early stages of navicular disease contraction is absent, and that it is only when the disease in the bursa is of long standing that contraction comes on. With ordinary contracted foot, too, careful paring and suitable shoeing soon sees a diminution in the degree of lameness, and a return to the normal in shape (see Treatment of Contracted Foot, p. 125). With navicular disease, however, such shoeing as is beneficial in the treatment of contracted foot (notably the various methods of giving to the frog counter-pressure with ground) soon brings on an aggravation of the lameness.

It is, perhaps, even more likely to be confounded with contraction when we have with the contraction a state of atrophy and thrush of the frog. With a frog in this condition pressure will give rise to pain, and navicular disease be erroneously judged to be present. In such a case we must rely wholly upon either extreme flexion or extreme extension of the joint to guide us, when, if contraction *only* is the offending condition, no symptom of pain will be shown.

Navicular disease may also be confused with rheumatic affections, with sprain of the posterior ligaments of the first interphalangeal articulation, and with sesamoid lameness. Mistakes are sometimes made, too, especially with a hasty observer, in confounding it with shoulder lameness.

In rheumatism the constant changing of the seat of pain, the sometimes elevated temperature, and the appearance of symptoms of heat, tenderness, and swelling in the affected area should guide one to a right conclusion.

In sprain of the posterior ligaments of the coronet and in sesamoid lameness, nothing but a careful examination and manipulation of the parts will ward off error, for in each of these cases there is 'pointing' and resting of the limb, and considerable disinclination to put weight firmly upon it. If at the same time manipulation gives distinct evidence of pain, all doubt may be set at rest.

Roughly speaking, sesamoid lameness is a condition of the gliding surface of the sesamoids, and the face of the tendon playing over them, similar to that found in navicular disease. All symptoms of pointing, the constant maintaining of the limb in a state of flexion, and a feeling manner of progression are again all present. It is plain from this that in all cases where an animal with a gait at all suggestive of navicular disease is brought for our examination, the manipulation of the limb should be thorough. The character of the lameness is almost sure to deceive us; and it is not until we are able to obtain local symptoms pointing to the one or the other of the conditions we have enumerated that a decisive opinion may be given. In sesamoid lameness the local symptoms are those of heat and pain in the fetlock on palpation, and a swelling of the affected parts, such swelling being at first slight, yielding, and barely distinguishable, and afterwards larger, bony and hard, and more marked. Later still there is distinct evidence of 'knuckling' over at the fetlock and inability to fully flex it.

In cases of shoulder lameness the gait alone should be sufficient to render liability of error small, for with nearly every case there is a manifest inability to 'get the limb forward', and this is best seen at a side view when the animal is trotting past the observer. When trotting towards one, there is a further and unmistakable symptom common to most shoulder lamenesses that serves to distinguish it at once, and that is the peculiar 'sweeping' outwards with the affected limb.

Lastly, with either of the conditions we have just mentioned, it is the exception to get contracted foot follow on. With navicular disease it sooner or later makes its appearance.

Prognosis.—The prognosis of navicular disease (once diagnosed with certainty) must almost of necessity be unfavourable. The facts that the disease has made serious progress before it is really noticeable, that the situation of the parts prohibits operative interference, and that the disease is one of a chronic and slowly progressive type, all point to an unfavourable termination.

Treatment.—We have seen from the pathology of this disease that it may commence either as a rarefactive ostitis, or as a synovitis and tenositis in connection with the bursa. With the former condition in existence, or when this and the synovitis has led to erosion of the cartilage, treatment is probably of no avail, on account of the more chronic nature of these two conditions. When, however, the condition is simply that of synovitis or tenositis, a more or less acute condition, we may assume that suitable treatment and a long rest will bring about resolution.

The first indications in treatment are those of what we may term 'nursing' the foot. It should have sufficient rest, should be placed so as to minimize as far as possible compression of the parts, and should have its posterior half treated so as to render it softer and less liable to concussion.

The period of rest required cannot be satisfactorily advised, and the practitioner is wise who makes it a long one. Best should be advised, in fact, long after symptoms of lameness have disappeared and recovery is judged to have taken place.

Compression of the parts may be somewhat minimized, if the animal be kept in the stable, by allowing the floor upon which the front-feet are to stand to be slightly sloping from behind forwards. The same effect, though not so marked, is obtained by removing the shoes, and considerably lowering the wall at the toe, while allowing that of the heels to remain. It may here be remarked that it is a good practice to allow the shoes to remain on, and this even when the animal is at grass. They should, however, be frequently removed, and the foot trimmed as we have directed.

With the foot thus trimmed so as to most suitably adjust the angles of the articulations, it should next be thoroughly pared and rasped in its posterior half, so as to render the horn of the sole and the frog and the horn of the quarters as thin as possible. The heels, however, should not be excessively lowered, *if at all*. We now have the foot in a soft condition, and easily expanded. It should, if possible, be kept so; and this may be done either by the use of poultices, by tepid baths, or by standing the animal upon a bedding that may easily be kept constantly damp. Such materials as tan, peat moss, or sawdust, are either of them suitable.

All this, of course, calls for keeping the animal in the stable. It is far better, however, more especially if a piece of marshy land is at hand, to turn him out in that. A moderate amount of exercise is beneficial rather than not, and the feet are thus constantly kept damp without trouble to the attendants.

The second indication in the treatment is that of applying a counter-irritant as near to the diseased parts as possible. Regarding its efficacy we must confess to being somewhat sceptical. The treatment has been constantly practised and advised, however, and we feel bound to give it mention here. A smart blister may, therefore, be applied to the whole of the coronet, and need not be prevented from running into the hollow of the heel.

Instead of blistering the coronet (or in conjunction with that treatment), the counter-irritant may be applied by passing a seton through the plantar cushion or fibro-fatty frog. Setoning the frog appears to have been introduced by Sewell. In many cases great benefit is claimed to have been derived from it, especially by English veterinarians of Sewell's time, and by others on the Continent. Percival, however, was not an advocate for it, and, at the present day, it is a practice which appears to have dropped out of use altogether.

FIG. 164.—FROG SETON NEEDLE.

To perform this operation a seton needle of a curved pattern is needed (see Fig. 164). This is threaded with a piece of stout tape dressed with a cantharides, hellebore, or other blistering ointment, and then passed in at the hollow of the heel, emerging at the point of the frog. The course the needle should take will be understood from a reference to Fig. 165.

The seton may be passed with the horse in the standing position. Previously the point of the frog should be thinned, and the animal should be twitched. After-treatment consists simply in moving the seton daily, and dressing it occasionally with any stimulating ointment, or with turpentine.

If, in spite of these treatments, the disease persists, then nothing remains but neurectomy.

D. DISLOCATIONS.

The firm and rigid manner in which the bones of the pedal articulation are held together renders dislocation of this joint an exceedingly rare occurrence, and then it is only liable to happen under the operation of great force. In the literature to our hand we have only been successful in discovering one reported instance, and, strange to say, in this, a well-marked case, the cause was altogether obscure. We quote the case at the end of this section.

FIG. 165.—DIAGRAM SHOWING THE COURSE TAKEN BY THE NEEDLE WHEN SETONING THE FROG. This is shown by the dotted curved line *a, b*. 1, The navicular bone; 2, the plantar cushion; 3, the os pedis; 4, the perforans tendon.

A partial dislocation of this articulation is the condition met with in 'Buttress Foot.' In this case the fracture of the pyramidal process, and the consequent lengthening of the tendon of the extensor pedis, allows the os coronæ to occupy upon the articulatory surface of the os pedis a more backward position than normally it should.

It is quite probable, too, that slight lesions of the other restraining ligaments and tendons of the articulation may bring about a similar though less marked condition. We may be quite sure of this—that whenever such lesions (as, for example, sprain and partial rupture of the lateral ligaments) do occur, and the normal position of the opposing bones is changed, if only slightly, that great pain and excessive lameness must be the result, and this with but little to show in the foot. Many of our cases of obscure foot lameness might, if capable of demonstration, turn out to be cases of sprain and partial dislocation of the pedal articulation.

Recorded Case.—'The animal, a trooper of the 8th Hussars, was found on the morning of April 17 unable to bear any weight on the limb (the near hind). Cause not known—the heel-rope I thought at first; but on investigation I found the heel-rope had been on the other leg.

Diagnosis.—Dislocation of the left os coronæ from the articulating surface of the os pedis in a backward direction.

'Every devisable means were unsuccessful in reducing the limb to its natural position. The horse was thrown, and a strong rope, with four men pulling at it, was fastened round the hoof, whilst I put my knee to the back of the pastern, using all possible force, with one hand to the foot and the other to the fetlock, but all to no purpose. Next day other means were tried. First by throwing the horse and placing him on his belly, with the fore-legs stretched out forwards, and the hind-legs backwards. This I did so as to get the injured limb placed as nearly flat on the ground as possible, with its anterior aspect downwards. Then a very heavy man, with his boots off, was made to jump on the back of the pastern, where the prominence showed most; and afterwards, when these means failed, a strong piece of wood, well covered with leather, was placed (where the hollow of the heel ought to have been) on the most prominent part, and hit several times with a heavy hammer; but all efforts were futile.

'*Prognosis.*—Unfavourable. During the latter operations I had a very strong pressure applied to the hoof, and the horse firmly fastened in every way, and it appeared as though no amount of force would ever reduce the dislocation.

'*Tautological.*—The case was destroyed on April 30, being of no further use to the service.

'*Post-mortem.*—The os coronæ was found to have slipped out of the articulating cavity of the os pedis, backwards and past the lateral ligaments. These last-named structures prevented the bone being forced forward into its proper position, being firmly locked over the lateral prominences. The capsular ligament was considerably lacerated and inflamed, causing slight effusion and swelling about the region of the coronet.'[A]

[Footnote A: T. Flintoff, A.V.D., *Veterinary Journal*, vol. xix., p. 74.]

Treatment.—After the forcible means of reduction related by Mr. Flintoff, we may add that when they are successful, they should be followed by suitable bandaging of the parts, and rest. The first is effected by applying plaster of Paris and linen, and the second by having the animal put in slings.

www.ingramcontent.com/pod-product-compliance
Lightning Source LLC
Chambersburg PA
CBHW071715170526
45165CB00005B/2023